T0177681

No More to Spend

No More to Spend

Neglect and the Construction of Scarcity in Malawi's History of Health Care

LUKE MESSAC

Foreword by

PAUL FARMER

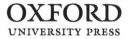

OXFORD

UNIVERSITY PRESS

OXFORD
UNIVERSITY PRESS

Oxford University Press is a department of the University of Oxford. It furthers
the University's objective of excellence in research, scholarship, and education
by publishing worldwide. Oxford is a registered trade mark of Oxford University
Press in the UK and certain other countries.

Published in the United States of America by Oxford University Press
198 Madison Avenue, New York, NY 10016, United States of America.

Library of Congress Control Number: 2020932230
ISBN 978–0–19–006619–2

1 3 5 7 9 8 6 4 2

Printed by Integrated Books International, United States of America

To my wife, Jamie

Contents

Foreword

Paul Farmer, M.D.

This is a brilliant book, and for several reasons.

The first is the topic. *No More to Spend* asks how medical impoverishment—as good a term as any to describe Malawi's long predicament as both a British colony and an independent state—comes to have what physician-historian Luke Messac terms "the ring of the tragic yet inescapable." How often do we contemplate what it might be like to face down both poverty and disease and, after the briefest reflection, and if we are spared such challenges, simply shrug? Hoping that some experts, somewhere, are on the case? This study reveals that there were experts on the case, but that their expertise—about everything from epidemic disease to health systems—was often wanting. As often as not, these and other deficiencies were attributed to want itself: by relying on the correspondence and reports of British health authorities, Messac shows that "in every era of Malawian history, scarcity was one of the most common ideas in official correspondence and public proclamations" (introduction).

Another reason this book is brilliant is that its author takes a universal concern—who among us does not hope for expert mercy when ill or injured?—and subjects it to sustained interrogation by lived experience from a single patch of real estate over a long sweep of time. The temporal continuities that lead from precolonial polities to the British protectorate of Nyasaland and on to Malawi are too rarely studied, in part because social histories like this one rely primarily on examining archives from a previous era, whereas deep understanding of present predicaments requires doing ethnographic research, or something like it. Messac has done both, having lived in rural Malawi and learned its most commonly spoken language, Chichewa.

One person who makes repeated appearances is a forty-eight-year-old farmer named Francis, with whom Messac lived in 2015. He and his wife, their children, their grandchildren, and their in-laws are not as poor as some of his neighbors, but Francis too must face down illness and injury whenever they afflict members of his extended family. As a historian, Messac complements brief interludes about Francis's travails with a chronology drawing on diverse sources: the vast and numbing colonial archive; memoirs and correspondence from the staff of the medical service; statements from political figures from Britain and what would become Malawi; commentary from the staff of its postindependence health ministry, including World Bank and other aid officials; and whenever possible, the rural farmers, porters, and traders who make up the vast majority of Malawians. Messac also quotes patients and health-care providers, but there were and still are too few of those.

A third reason *No More to Spend* is brilliant is more difficult to lay out in the clear language of Messac's concise and affecting study, since much of it treats what some schools of historiography call "mentalities." How do people come to think the way they do? In this study, Messac's subjects are sometimes people he knows, like Francis, but more often than not he cites the medical officers whose letters, complaints, and reports express frustration with medical scarcity while seeming unable to make it seem other than inescapable. The book's emotional terrain is that of conflict and discord, which can't be smoothed over during or soon after colonial rule because colonial rule is the source of the problem.

Malawi was integrated into the world's greatest empire at the height of British sway. Formal colonial rule there began more or less when it did elsewhere across the continent: At the close of the nineteenth century, when Europe's colonial powers divided up Africa like a cake. The slice that became Nyasaland was carved with the help of Cecil Rhodes. His British South Africa Company financed the administration of the protectorate in its early years, squashing African resistance to British encroachment and aiding private European estates. These required seasonal labor to grow and harvest cash crops like cotton and tobacco but did little to alleviate the deprivation of conquered Africans.

Luke Messac's study of privation and the social construction of scarcity—and of acquiescence or resistance to both—is thus a twentieth-century story. The broad arc of *No More to Spend* is tied to the contingent and specific history of Nyasaland, but the experiences of its subjects were not dissimilar to those of other British subjects in Africa. This similarity undermines the common refrain that British iterations of indirect rule led to enormous variation in policies across its vast empire. Messac's book details what will be for historians of other British colonies a series of familiar events and processes: the armed violence of conquest and pacification, which dispersed camp epidemics and ecological disruption across vast areas; the adoption of martial public health strategies focused on disease control rather than caregiving; the proliferation of rules and ordinances (many of them internally contradictory and most of them punitive); and—casting its pale beam over all—the inescapable logic of scarcity for the natives and the concomitant rise of new strains of white supremacy across southern Africa and beyond.

Equally familiar and yet rendered in fresh detail are the ways in which two world wars marked Africa's colonies; the stuttering and violent collapse of colonial rule; and after independence, a series of often-hampered efforts to build a care-delivery system. But there's not a lot to read about caregiving itself. Then again, while the British claimed control of Nyasaland in 1891, Malawi's first medical school was not opened until 1991. During the first half of that century, the delivery of clinical services was little more than an afterthought. "Curative medicine was not," as Messac wryly puts it, "a meaningful part of the experience of being governed" (chapter 1).

This is a book, in other words, about "the practice of medicine without medicines." Yet these were precisely the years when European and North American medicine and its allied sciences began to develop revolutionary new tools to prevent and cure disease. If the world was a dangerous place for humans prior to vaccines, surgery, antibiotics, insulin, antihypertensives, and the like, for some people it became less dangerous after their development. As effective preventative measures and therapies were conceived, those without access remained stuck in the Dark Ages of medicine. But many practitioners and would-be patients stuck there were well aware that a therapeutic Enlightenment was under way. The practice of medicine without medicines became increasingly frustrating as the number of effective therapies available in the global economy spiked during the prime period of colonial rule in Africa, where they remained largely unavailable.

The opposite of scarcity is abundance, and Malawi has known little of that. The synergy promised by effective preventatives (like vaccines) and therapeutics (like antibiotics) could not occur anywhere prior to World War II. That synergy could, in principle, be introduced anywhere after it. But where did the notion of scarcity come to exert its greatest hold? In the far reaches of the empire, the places from which the British and other colonial powers extracted their surplus, as well as raw commodities and raw labor. Some of the facts may be newly brought to light, but most of them won't surprise historians of colonial medicine any more than they would surprise the battered subjects of Britain's other African colonies: the tiny health budgets and the complaints about them, the racist justifications for martial disease-control efforts and the inevitable critiques of those, the parlous conditions of the porters who moved everything from point A to point B, and the fact that during these long years the British never got around to building a robust care delivery system or founding a medical school.

It comes as no surprise that the colonial subjects in question resisted this status quo. What is more interesting is that many of the personnel of the colonial medical service, even those who never questioned the utility or legitimacy of colonial rule, were among those raising their voices against the presumption of scarcity. How does a travesty become an accident? To have the ring of the tragic yet inescapable? Messac answers with "the presumption of scarcity" but is quick to remind us that not all colonial officials accepted the claim that scarcity was inevitable. There were, it transpires, experts on the case, and he shows both the reach and the limitations of the "reformist elites" who sought to improve the colonial medical service from within.

When the details of this story depict a world of vanished colonies and its long-gone medical officers, Messac turns back to the struggles of the Malawians he got to know while living there. The dilemmas of Francis-as-Everyman underline, as do his words, that stories like his—of tardily or improperly attended illness and injury—are a dime a dozen along the shores of Lake Malawi and in the rural district of Neno, two of the settings in which Messac worked.

More important, this physician-historian has a firm understanding of the varying effectiveness of varied medical interventions. Across Nyasaland and during much of its history, the natives (as they were termed) also sought to learn about the effectiveness of colonial medicine's offerings. What, they asked, about the practice of medicine *with* medicines? Surely therapies could not be blocked in customs forever? Although Messac would be sure to note that this particular experiment is ongoing, since modern-day Malawi, like Nyasaland, has yet to develop a proper health system, there are empirical data points pointing to some preliminary answers. When antibiotics were shown to cure yaws, gonorrhea, pneumonia, and malaria, the people of Nyasaland lined up for them.

Archival and ethnographic research is complemented by Messac's clinical acumen, which allows him to underline the sturdy empiricism of the Malawians. It wasn't, you build it, they will come; rather, it was, if it works, they will avail themselves of it. The utilization of the public care delivery system dwarfed attendance at mission hospitals once they were better stocked, which gave the lie to cognitivist and culturalist claims, such as those insisting that native superstition, not an absence of caregiving, is what once kept government health posts empty. As reported by anthropologists, enlightened missionaries, and ministry officials, Africans voted with their feet. They showed up, Messac writes, not because of a sudden "love of all things European," but because of that sturdy empiricism. This development does much to undermine tales about superstitious, refractory, rebellious, unreasonable natives who didn't know what was good for them. These cultural showdowns were the subject of much colonial commentary, much of it hidden in obscure reports and correspondence that come to life in Messac's study.

Since there wasn't much clinical care going on, cultural showdowns between rulers and ruled often emerged in the wake of epidemics and colonial authorities' responses to them. Take, for example, the parasitic infection trypanosomiasis, which sickens cattle and other beasts of cloven hoof. In West Africa, where it was first described, trypanosomiasis was primarily a disease of humans, in whom it causes a slow neurological decline leading, in terminal cases, to obtundation and coma. In 1803, a century before its etiologic agent and life cycle were identified, it had been described as "African sleeping sickness" by the Briton Thomas Winterbottom, Sierra Leone's first medical officer:

> The Africans are very subject to a species of lethargy, which they are much afraid of, as it proves fatal in every instance. . . . This disease is very frequent in the Foola country, and it is said to be much more common in the interior parts of the country than upon the sea coast. Children are very rarely, or never, affected with this complaint, nor is it more common among slaves than among free people, though it is asserted that the slaves from Benin are very subject to it. . . . Small glandular tumors are sometimes observed in the neck a little before the commencement of this complaint, though probably depending rather upon accidental circumstances than upon the disease itself. Slave traders, however, appear to consider these tumors as a symptom indicating a disposition to lethargy, and they either never buy such slaves, or get quit of them as soon as they observe any such appearances. The disposition to sleep is so strong, as scarcely to leave a sufficient respite for the taking of food; even the repeated application of a whip, a remedy which has been frequently used, is hardly sufficient to keep the poor wretch awake.[1]

One hundred years later, the world's most powerful empire hadn't whipped African sleeping sickness or the tsetse fly into submission. There was little reason to doubt that the winged vector—thanks to the massive dislocations of formal colonial rule—would move the parasite east, north, and south. And that, Messac shows, is what came to pass. The stakes had been elevated during the closing years of the nineteenth century, when Europeans pursued their conquest and pacification campaigns. Belgium's King Leopold called in the tropical medicine gurus from Liverpool to map the trypanosomiasis-affected areas of his vast holdings. A proxy war between Arab slave traders from Zanzibar and groups of Congolese under Leopold's boot moved the blood-hungry flies across the continent; movement of carriers, troops, and labor, to say nothing of cattle and game, meant that the first decade of the twentieth century was marked by cataclysmic trypanosomiasis outbreaks, including one that brought British East Africa to its knees. Between 1901 and 1905, colonial authorities estimated that 200,000 Ugandans perished along with their all-important cattle. Throughout that British colony, author-ities responded by setting up "isolation camps" and testing and moving thousands from the forested waterside villages preferred by the tsetse fly into these camps, which were short on supplies, including food and medicines. The therapy that most sufferers received was called atoxyl, an arsenic de-rivative, sometimes supplemented by strychnine. Alone or in combination, atoxyl didn't seem to cure many natives with sleeping sickness. The author of one major investigation of trypanosomiasis, a British military officer, noted that after years of coordinating these resettlements he had yet to see a single case of sleeping sickness cured with atoxyl, but he had seen many of those treated go blind as a consequence of therapy.[2] Many patients de-voted their waning energies to escaping these lazarets or isolation centers, which colonial authorities—British, French, Belgian, and German—tried to rebrand as "treatment centers." It was much the same story in Nyasaland. Since typanosomiasis moves between humans and game, with the tsetse fly the intermediary, epidemics of what had been previously considered an in-dolent infection exploded across the protectorate and Northern Rhodesia (present-day Zambia). This led not only to many deaths among man and beast, including the abundant game denied to the people of Nyasaland, but also to arguments about when trypanosomiasis reached Nyasaland, and how. One prominent British authority felt sure that trypanosomiasis did not exist in Nyasaland prior to 1907 or so, noting that the first medical officer to investigate rumors of mounting cases was himself bitten by tsetse flies and soon died of the disease.[3] Across the protectorate, thousands were reassured that atoxyl was a miracle drug, even as its failure became evident. The director of one lazaret in the northeast put it this way: "Strictly speaking, it was a permanent prison and should bear the inscription, 'Abandon all hope, ye who enter here.' "[4]

This is a history with profound implications for the present, as anyone working to contain and treat Ebola knows well. As Messac notes throughout this study, the shrugs over deplorable health conditions continue in discussions of and within the postcolony. "Refined over decades," he writes, "such rationalizations continue to pervade debates over health care spending in the present" (introduction). Although spending on health care for the natives "was always paltry," Messac explains, "officials were able to sustain the state of neglect."

That is, it's easy to sustain when those on its receiving end are poor and black. Messac does not elevate some mythically abundant time prior to formal colonial rule, nor does the postcolony receive much praise. But here again, the former colonial power, having shed Nyasaland, sent only two X-ray machines in response to nearly a decade of urgent requests. The book's emotional terrain, the reader realizes by its end, is sadness and shame. This is not achieved through ethnographic interludes, though they too are mostly tales of woe. It comes through just as much in the plaintive and often contradictory testimonies of elite reformists. It's hard to end on a positive note, and so Messac chides us: "We need not condemn ourselves to perpetually impoverished ambitions, not while there is still so much to do, or so much ground to make up."

No More to Spend is a beautifully rendered social history, but it is also a superb and humane ethnography. Like a good historian, Messac advances while looking backward. Like a good anthropologist and a superb doctor, he casts his eyes, and his thoughts, on people like Francis, trudging forward against long odds not of his own making.

Acknowledgments

In writing a book about neglect, I am grateful that all of my experiences with it were secondhand.

The team at Abwenzi Pa Za Umoyo, the sister organization of the non-profit Partners In Health, introduced me to rural Malawi, and continues to show that decent medical care and social protection are possible in one of the world's poorest regions. Historians and anthropologists of Malawi, including Wapumuluka Mulwafu, Joey Power, Owen Kalinga, John Lwanda, Gift Kayira, Colin Baker, John McCracken, Zoë Groves, Anna West, and Geoff Traugh, provided great advice. Two anonymous reviewers at Oxford University Press provided insightful critiques and suggestions. In Mangochi and Neno Districts, people welcomed me into their homes and histories. They gave generously of their time and trusted me with the intimate details of their lives. They allowed me to accompany them on doctor visits. A few even invited me to live with them while I conducted my fieldwork. That fieldwork would not have been possible without George Banda, who helped translate interviews, introduced me to members of his community, and gave me a much deeper understanding of the people and places I wrote about.

Librarians and archivists around the world helped me track down the papers and books that form the substrate of this work. The archivists at the Malawi National Archives in Zomba do heroic work with far too few resources. Innocent Mankhwala was particularly generous with his time. I am also grateful to the librarians and archivists at Oxford University; the University of Edinburgh; Indiana University in Bloomington; the World Bank Group Archives in Washington, DC; the Society of Malawi Archives in Blantyre; the UK National Archives at Kew; the British Library; the London School of Economics; the London School of Hygiene and Tropical Medicine; and the interlibrary loan librarians at the University of Pennsylvania.

My academic advisers at Penn opened up new worlds to me. Over the past half century Steven Feierman's work has forged a field that writes of Africans as peoples with deep histories and complex intellectual lives, with stories that are neither derivative nor stunted nor simple. Robert Aronowitz is a trailblazing historian, but thankfully he will never shake his earlier life as a clinician. He brings to every study an eye for skepticism and nuance, yet never forgets the urgent concerns and pain that the experience of illness holds. Megan Vaughan's careful, creative scholarship has long been an inspiration. Ramah McKay's advice on writing has been invaluable. The editors at the Journal of Southern African Studies graciously allowed me to reproduce material from a journal article in Chapter 6.

My copy editor, Mary Lederer, saved me from many infelicitous phrases and long-winded explanations. At Oxford University Press, editor Alexandra Dauler expressed interest in my manuscript and guided me through the review process. My second editor, Sarah Humphreville, kindly took on the project in its later stages and saw it through to publication.

Other mentors, including Philippe Bourgois, Projit Mukharji, John Tresch, David Barnes, Jeremy Greene, and Seth Holmes, have patiently answered my endless questions about academic theory and academic life. Skip Brass created a productive environment for MD/PhD students at the University of Pennsylvania. Monda Mwaya was an able teacher of Chichewa and has become a close friend. I leaned heavily on other preternaturally patient administrators at Penn, especially Maggie Krall, Helene Weinberg, Pat Johnson, and Courtney Brennan. My fellow graduate and medical students at Penn were an essential source of emotional support and intellectual stimulation. It is perilous to single people out, but I must give special thanks to Jason Chernesky, Douglas Farquhar, Allegra Giovine, Roland Li, Marissa Mika, Maxwell Rogoski, and Utpal Sandesara. More recently, my mentors and fellow trainees at Brown University's Department of Emergency Medicine have supported me as I completed this book while learning how to practice medicine with skill and compassion.

Paul Farmer introduced me to the fight for global health equity, first in a seminar during my freshman year of college and then over many years in Rwanda and Boston. His dedication to patients and students has been an inspiration to so many, including me. His advice to write about health and illness in a way that is, as he puts it, "historically deep and geographically broad" spurred me to pursue a PhD in history alongside a medical degree. The students, faculty, and staff at the University of Global Health Equity in Rwanda made me feel a welcome colleague as we explored the history and interrogated the assumptions of global health together.

I knew when I first met Matthew Basilico during our freshman year in college that his passion for justice would change the course of my life. I hope he knows how much our conversations shaped this work.

My parents, my first teachers, showed me (through their teachings and their example) the centrality of care to any meaningful life. They taught me not to be satisfied with the world as it is and to narrow the distance between my stated ideals and my everyday actions. My brothers, Owen and Patrick, have always kept me honest, made me laugh, supported my work, and traveled to visit me during my fieldwork.

I was lucky to join a great family when I married my wife, Jamie. Her parents, James and Cathy, have been unfailingly supportive since the minute I met them in a cab, where they told me to buckle my seat belt. Their entire family, including Samantha, Melanie, Nada, Nina, and Josie, have brought warmth and so many new ideas into my life.

Finally, I am grateful to Jamie. She loves with an abandon that I have never seen before and did not think possible before I met her. Her care for patients, friends, and family gives me faith that the world can become a much better place.

Abbreviations

BL	British Library, London
BLOU	Bodleian Library, Oxford University
BMJ	*British Medical Journal*
MNA	Malawi National Archives, Zomba
SoMA	Society of Malawi Archives, Blantyre
UoELA	University of Edinburgh Library Archives
UKNA	United Kingdom National Archives, Kew
UMMC	University of Malawi Malawiana Collection, Zomba
WBGA	World Bank Group Archives, Washington, DC

Introduction

The Construction of Scarcity

It was not a clean space. Cockroaches scuttled about the floor and on bedframes in the men's ward of the Mangochi District Hospital. Minutes after the floors were washed each morning, the roaches were back. The nightstands next to the beds were cluttered with half-empty bottles of the orange soda hawked by vendors outside the hospital gates.

Nor was the ward a space where anyone could seek privacy. In the large, open room, everyone's words were audible, their actions visible. That morning in early February 2015, patients occupied all thirty-six beds—that is, until an attendant and a nurse wheeled away the covered body of a just-deceased patient. A dozen family and friends followed the stretcher in silence on its way to the mortuary. An elderly man with a distended abdomen sat upright, talking to a family member who had just fetched his hospital-provided lunch of *nsima* (maize porridge) and beans. On a nearby bed, a cachectic man with blank, glassy eyes stared at the roof.

Neither the cockroaches nor his wardmates were of much concern to a fifteen-year-old patient, "Innocent." He had another problem: his right leg was rotting. Innocent had been shot in the leg a week earlier when, while walking his sister home from school, they came upon a demonstration, and he was struck by a stray bullet fired by a policeman. The bullet had torn straight through his knee, injuring the popliteal artery, which carries much of the blood supply to the lower leg and foot. Friends had taken Innocent to the nearby district hospital, where he was transferred by ambulance to a larger district hospital an hour away. Upon arriving there he underwent emergency surgery to ligate (tie off) the popliteal artery. The wound had been wrapped in gauze. He was put into a bed for observation.

This surgery helped prevent Innocent from bleeding to death. But what he really needed in those crucial hours was a vascular surgeon. Though hemorrhaging blood from the torn artery could have become life-threatening without ligation, Innocent was almost certainly doomed to lose his limb if

No More to Spend. Paul Farmer, Oxford University Press (2020). © Oxford University Press.
DOI: 10.1093/oso/9780190066192.001.0001

blood flow to the lower leg was not restored. Popliteal artery trauma is "the most limb-threatening of peripheral vascular injuries," but in the United States gunshot victims with this injury can have their limbs salvaged—and blood flow restored—with prompt surgical repair involving a vein graft. Outcomes are particularly good if surgery is performed within seven hours of injury.[1] Vein graft has been the standard of care for American soldiers with popliteal artery injuries since the early 1950s. A 2002 review of twenty-four published series of 678 penetrating popliteal artery injuries found a mean amputation rate of 11 percent, with lower rates in the more recent series.[2] But this review drew from patients treated mostly in the United States and Europe. On the day Innocent was shot, there was no vascular surgeon in the whole of Malawi, a country of fifteen million people.[3] There were vascular surgeons in South Africa, but emergency air evacuations were reserved for expatriate aid workers and government officials, not the children of subsistence farmers. Instead of receiving surgery that could have saved his leg, Innocent was left lying in a bed to rot.

Innocent's right leg steadily decayed. First he lost feeling below the knee. Then the skin began to blacken. The toes shriveled, and the toenails turned a ghostly silver hue. Ten days after the shooting, Innocent's attending physician (who made rounds three times per week) warned that he would likely have to have the leg amputated soon, to prevent gangrene from ascending from the necrotic tissue to the rest of his body. Four days later doctors wheeled Innocent into the surgical suite and amputated his right leg, just above the knee.

After the amputation Innocent was taciturn. Whenever I posed a question, he deferred to his mother. I asked if he planned to get a prosthetic leg. The look on Innocent's face was forlorn. "We would like one," his mother explained, "but it is too much money." A wheelchair would be of little use on the uneven, sandy paths near his home. The doctors had advised Innocent that he would have to let his stump heal for a few months, then he could travel to the referral hospital in Blantyre to be fitted for a prosthetic limb. He would have to pay for it himself. The cheapest leg available would cost £150. To Innocent's mother, who cultivated a small plot barely large enough to feed her children, the idea that she could ever find so much money was absurd. Innocent faced a bleak future.

To many public health experts, such stories have the ring of the tragic yet inescapable. Had Innocent lived in a wealthier nation, one endowed with a system of emergency medical response, vascular surgeons, and well-equipped operating rooms, he would likely have left the hospital intact. But he was a poor boy in a poor village in a poor country, so he lost his leg. To these experts, the dearth of resources for health care in one of the world's poorest countries appears to be a reality that must be faced squarely.

Any assertion that vein graft surgery is possible in Malawi would strain the credulity of those experts. In the health policy literature, the major debates focus on how to partition the meager pie of global health dollars: between prevention and treatment, between vaccines and drugs, between rural clinics and urban hospitals. Rather than exploring the political economy that denies the funding necessary to train vascular surgeons in Malawi, many health experts have instead critiqued the "sustainability" or "cost-effectiveness" of treating AIDS, multi-drug-resistant tuberculosis, and curable forms of cancer.[4] These writers seem to assume that they and their readers can do little more than optimize the paltry existing resources. They are engaged, quite deliberately, in a zero-sum game.[5]

Inadequate public-sector health-care funding, poorly trained medical staff, and outdated drugs and equipment are, in this formulation, a necessary consequence of a low GDP. The historian Randall Packard captures the essence of this idea, which he does not endorse, in the form of an implicit rebuke that runs beneath much of the global health literature: "It's Africa and India, what did you expect?"[6] The discourse that results is, inevitably, macabre. The tone of public-health literature is characterized by what the physician-anthropologist Jim Yong Kim has called "public health machismo"—that is, the idea that "someone has to make the decision who lives and dies."[7]

This presumption of scarcity is also pervasive in the historiography of social services in colonial and postcolonial Africa. The notion that economically impoverished regions are doomed to poor health services has long appeared in works of even the most careful scholars. To take just one example, in her 1958 report on a year of travels in British Africa, Labour Party activist Joan Wicken noted that each colony had a per capita income much lower than the United Kingdom's. "Given these figures," she concluded, "it is hardly surprising that Government officials constantly commented that certain things were desirable but not possible."[8] Here, Africa's "basic poverty" was sufficient explanation for governments' "difficulty in providing the most elementary public services."[9]

More recent historical scholarship has at times continued to accept at face value colonial officials' claims that resources were too scarce for robust social services, including health care. In these accounts, the causes of funding shortages take on the ring of the impersonal and inescapable, rather than being the result, at least in part, of discrete choices by policymakers. In a groundbreaking study of taxation in British colonial Africa, Leigh Gardner did not elaborate on her claim that postwar plans for improved social services in Northern Rhodesia and Kenya were stymied by "resource constraints." She did not say whether these resource constraints stemmed from the willful decisions of colonial officials or the inescapable poverty of colonial treasuries.[10] The anthropologist Hansjörg Dilger attributed the travails of African economies in the 1970s in part to "overfunded welfare systems." His was not a novel claim, but it is far from settled fact in the nascent literature on the economic history of Africa's turbulent 1970s.[11] Dilger neither elaborated on this assertion with evidence nor buttressed it with attribution.

These scholars were not unusual in tying aggregate income statistics to the quality and quantity of health-care services. The casual nature with which they make their causal claims is evidence only of the extent to which this equation has become common sense.[12] But is it so obvious that, in the past or in the present, poor patients in poor countries are fated to be denied the fruits of modern medicine beyond the barest basics? In other passages, some of the same scholars admitted that claims about the inevitability of scarcity were too facile. One reason to avoid equating aggregate poverty with necessarily dismal health-care services, they explained, was that it ignored the rapacious extraction of resources that could have benefited health-care systems. Wicken, for instance, explained that European investors in African mines and plantations extracted a massive share of the profits, while relatively little revenue went to the coffers of local governments.[13] Another reason to question the link was that health-care spending often increased not in response to economic growth, but in response to changes in political power. Gardner complicated her own acceptance of official claims of "resource constraints" when she explained that the extension of the franchise to Africans in Kenya and Northern Rhodesia just prior to independence gave them "greater bargaining power . . . and allowed them to lobby for fiscal transfers," including greater spending on health and education.[14] These effects of new political pressures during decolonization belied the claim that there was simply not enough money to increase spending on health and education. Thus, even as scholars sometimes accept official claims about the inevitability of dismal health-care services in poor countries, their own careful analyses call such claims into question.

How do we understand this seeming contradiction? One answer is that scarcity is, after all, a matter of degree. This book will not take a radically constructivist position by positing that scarcity is but a figment of the imagination. Scarcity is, at the extremes, inescapable for any material resource. Take Malawi: according to the International Monetary Fund (IMF), the nation had the second-lowest nominal GDP per capita in the world in 2016 (ahead of only war-ravaged South Sudan).[15] Clearly Malawi's strapped government cannot spend at will on anything and everything. It does have competing priorities, many of which—including education, agricultural supports, and social insurance—are essential for human flourishing. Furthermore, government spending requires revenue, which can be raised through tax collection, debt financing, or printing money. Each of these can have undesirable economic consequences, such as inflation and foreign currency shortages, when taken to extremes.

Still, only a myopic study of scarcity looks only at the domestic resources of a single nation, as if foreign flows of wealth did not exist. Throughout its history, Malawi has experienced the exactions of colonizers and international financiers, even as these individuals and institutions sought to obscure their own actions. The idea that national borders delimit the only relevant scope of analysis is, as we will find, another construction of scarcity that was refined during the colonial and postcolonial eras.

Furthermore, even after acknowledging the existence of inescapable scarcities, there is often a great distance between materially inevitable and socially constructed scarcities. This is evident in the fact that while Malawi has for so long languished with dismal health-care services, there are other places where per capita incomes remain low even as citizens are offered comprehensive health-care services,. The government of the southern Indian state of Kerala, which has a GDP per capita of only USD$3,100, offers both widespread access to primary care *and* free coronary artery bypass surgery to some poor citizens.[16] Another example is Rwanda, which devotes one-fifth of government expenditure to the health sector. The nation has achieved the steepest decline in under-age-five mortality rates in recorded human history. One government hospital provides cancer chemotherapy free of charge.[17] These examples, and others, challenge the supposedly inevitable trade-off between robust primary care and access to advanced biomedical services.

The political, rhetorical, moral, and economic dynamics that have worked to construct scarcity in popular imaginaries have still not been sufficiently subjected to rigorous historical analysis. Instead, the study of colonial and postcolonial spending priorities has taken moral and historical relativism as its lodestar. Reliance on government archives has led, insidiously, to accepting at face value favored explanations of colonial and postcolonial officials. These rationalizations, formulated in attempts to fend off demands for greater social service spending, have come to be understood as self-evident rationales rather than self-interested rationalizations.

Some justifications for neglect in Malawi were more naked than others. Throughout its period as a little-remarked corner of the British Empire, Nyasaland (today's Malawi) was known not as a colony but as a protectorate. The imperial construction of the "protectorate" is a fairly obvious simulacrum, yet it is one that continues to color historians' perceptions of the possible in health-care services for colonized peoples. A protectorate is, by definition, an autonomous part of a sovereign state. This was another piece of the social construction of scarcity in Malawi's history, for officials contended that protectorates had even less claim on imperial treasuries than colonies. The contention that Nyasaland's chiefs had asked for British protection voluntarily (rather than at gunpoint) and subsequently been allowed to rule autonomously (without onerous demands for taxes and wartime manpower) has by now been thoroughly debunked.[18] But the idea, stemming from this fiction, that the metropole could not be expected to ensure that Africans had health-care services anywhere comparable to those enjoyed by British citizens or even subjects of proper colonies has endured. The claim here, made by colonial apologists or historians who accept the construction of the protectorate, is that it is ahistoric to compare British metropolitan standards of medicine to those of Africans in a protectorate.[19] But nothing could be further from ahistoricity than to ignore the medical officers and Colonial Office officials who were scandalized by the conditions in Nyasaland's hospitals and clinics. It would be equally ahistoric to fail to mention the African intellectuals and colonial governors who placed little stock in the fiction of the protectorate, for they recognized the exploitation of Nyasaland's labor power (for migrant labor and the carrier service) and its resources (to repay misbegotten debts), all while the majority population and its titular indigenous rulers had little real power over their destiny. The protectorate concept was a social construct convenient to deflect demands for better treatment of colonized publics, but it should in no way dissuade historians from studying the deficiencies in health care or the foregone opportunities for its improvement.

A related construction of the colonial era that has perdured in histories of African social policy is the notion of "self-sufficiency"—that is, the UK Treasury's long-standing policy that colonies and protectorates had to pay for services out of their own domestic revenues.[20] Even after the metropolitan government began providing some funding for capital projects during the interwar years, it continued to insist that local revenues pay for noncapital health and education expenditures.[21] But the idea that colonized peoples were permitted to benefit even from those revenues extracted from them ignores the high costs they paid to maintain the apparatus of their own subjugation.[22] The construction of self-sufficiency also elides the socialization of costs and the privatization of gains in the colonial economy. African families were made to care for those left sick and disabled in colonial wars and by imperial industries. Meanwhile, absentee European owners of mines and plantations drew much of the wealth they extracted toward the metropole.[23] Studies attempting to measure the "profitability" of the colonies have generally found that most were a net loss for metropolitan treasuries, but such results should not be interpreted to demonstrate a net benefit to the colonized. Even if, in aggregate terms, the UK Treasury and taxpayers lost money to the colonial enterprise, sizable private profits were realized by well-connected financiers and industrialists.[24] These individuals, and their influence on colonial policy, still garner too little attention in colonial histories.

Other rhetorical tools in the armamentarium of neglect were less blatant but just as potent. Perhaps the oldest of rationalizations was that there simply was no money left for health after other, more urgent priorities. This line of argument was particularly ubiquitous during the Great Depression and the Second World War, but it was also used early in the interwar era (though as I will discuss, the claims often do not withstand scrutiny). For decades a massive share of Nyasaland's tax revenues was devoted to paying back a debt to a well-connected private financier for a railway line that local business enterprises did not want and would not use. In large part as a result of such arrangements, by 1937, 44 percent of Nyasaland's public expenditure went toward servicing the colony's debts. In that year, an additional 6 percent of Nyasaland's public expenditure was devoted to pension allowances for British colonial officials, while only 8 percent of government spending went to the Medical Department.[25]

Thus, little of the revenue that administrators collected (or often, forcibly extracted) in the form of hut taxes, poll taxes, income taxes, sales taxes, involuntary labor, and customs duties was spent on health, education, and social welfare. Those officials who did hope to spend more on social services were continually frustrated by the burden of the colony's massive debts, accrued through loans of dubious merit. Colonial administrators and doctors were well aware of these facts, and many highlighted them in reports calling for greater funding.

These were not the only means available to deflect demands. Economic theories were often deployed to justify forbearance on demands for health-care spending. During the 1960s, a number of economic advisers to African governments drew on modernization theory to counsel against "unproductive" social service spending. Later that same decade, the World Bank and a number of prominent foundations argued that population control constituted the only justifiable health-care program in poor countries, as "fertility control" should precede efforts at "mortality control." During the neoliberal era of the 1980s and 1990s, the IMF claimed that "macroeconomic stabilization" demanded an end to budget deficits and conditioned its loans on the implementation of fiscal austerity that drastically curtailed health and education programs.

At other moments, officials claimed that they would increase health-care spending if not for insuperable political obstacles. During the 1940s, some Labour Party leaders argued that colonial health-care spending was a worthy cause, but devoting great sums to health-care services for Africans would alienate key constituencies in the United Kingdom, thereby imperiling the party's chances of taking power. Later, during the decade-long Federation of Rhodesia and Nyasaland, officials in Southern Rhodesia claimed Africans in Nyasaland were already receiving more than their fair share of health-care spending, and in any case did not appreciate the efforts of the Federation government. What, they asked, would be the point of more health spending?

Thus the history of Malawi is rife with tools of neglect. Among these were excuses for delay, warnings of unintended consequences, assertions of more pressing claims on resources, and constructs that sought to mask power relations. At different times and for different reasons, this portfolio of rationalizations was used by the UK Colonial Office and Treasury, economic advisers, presidents, and international financial institutions to stanch proposed increases in health-care spending. Refined over decades, such rationalizations continue to pervade debates over health-care spending in the present.

While historians of colonial, postcolonial, or international health have tended to accept claims of scarcity at face value, scholars of other realms of public action have, in recent decades, contested them. Since the 1980s, the economist Amartya Sen has demonstrated that famine is rarely the result of a decline in available food. As a child in Bengal, he saw the devastation of a 1943 famine. UK prime minister Winston Churchill explained the death of one million Indians with neo-Malthusian logic (more precisely, that Indians were "breeding like rabbits"), even as he refused to organize relief.[26] Sen argued that the decisive factor in famine is not absolute scarcity, but rather inequalities in political power that lead to unequal distributions of "entitle-ments"—that is, the wages, welfare programs, or other means by which people acquire basic necessities.[27] Scarcity is often, in his telling, a political construction used to justify an existing distribution of resources that affords some an abundance while others starve.[28]

Inspired by Sen's studies, the Institute of Development Studies at the University of Sussex convened a meeting in 2005 on "the limits of scarcity." The collective statement of the assembled economists and sociologists coun-seled a general disposition of skepticism toward claims of scarcity:

> Scarcity . . . is not a natural condition. . . . Detailed sociological and political attention to what is actually happening on the ground has almost always located the causes of pressing social problems . . . not in an absolute scar-city but in socially generated scarcity arising from imbalances of power. . . . Moreover, the "scare" of scarcity has led to scarcity emerging as a political strategy for powerful groups.[29]

The statement asks researchers to denaturalize scarcity, to investigate the ways in which it is socially generated rather than immutably given. In applying this call to studies of health services, political scientist Ted Schrecker has called for research "at the interface of ethics and the social sciences that connects global-scale power relations and domestic political choices with the ways in which health-related scarcities are experienced differently, and the options for addressing them framed differently, by various protagonists on the ground."[30] Using archival and ethnographic research, I attempt to answer precisely that call in this book.

While historians of medicine in Africa have chronicled disease-specific campaigns and mission hospitals, detailed histories of government medical administration and practice are still few.[31] Those that do exist tend to focus on written plans—while tending to downplay the fact that few were ever brought to fruition—or to take a teleological perspective in which progress toward a robust system of lifesaving care was stepwise and steady. Even those histories that highlight the use of biomedical rationales for segregationist and economically exploitative policies generally do not explore the extent to which medical care was or was not a part of the daily lives of most Africans.[32] The result is a historiography that tends to emphasize either the *presence* of biomedicine over its absence (for the more celebratory narratives), or biopower and mass experimentation over neglect (in critical histories).[33]

The focus in this book on health-care budgets and political economy might strike some readers as retrograde. Since the postmodern turn, Africanists have written about scarcity in medicine, but they have been especially curious about how providers and patients have responded to difficult environments with feats of innovation, improvisation, appropriation, and hybridization.[34] This vein of inquiry has inspired rich literatures in both the history of medicine and medical anthropology.[35] Yet there are potential pitfalls to this approach. As Shula Marks observed, focusing the historical gaze on the inventiveness of bricolage in colonial and postcolonial Africa runs the risk of "forgetting that there is another history of actual morbidity and mortality."[36] Now, as in the past, the absence of strong biomedical and public health systems leads most often to suffering and death, not a stroke of genius.

Much of this book discusses the extent of commitment to Malawian public-sector health care of various colonial governments, national governments, and international organizations. There are a number of indicators for such a commitment, but reliance on any of them demands a number of caveats to guard against overly certain or outright faulty analysis. Looking for historical indicators in colonial and early postcolonial Africa, as anyone who has searched for them can attest, is a treacherous undertaking. Finding the assorted data in various archives can be difficult enough, but knowing what to make of them is even more challenging. Many of the problems are discussed at greater length in the chapters that follow, but a brief introduction to the paucity of statistical data is merited here. For example, GDP statistics, designed for use in industrialized economies, demand survey data that have never been accurately collected in many parts of sub-Saharan Africa. During the early twentieth century, population censuses in Malawi were scarcely more than back-of-the-envelope estimates. The most important indices, such as life expectancy, cannot be measured without vital registration, but births and deaths have never been systematically recorded and reported in Malawi; the earliest survey data that allow for some extrapolation of vital statistics were not collected until the 1970s.[37] Measures of disease prevalence were compromised by the limited reach of public health surveillance programs and by the poor diagnostic capabilities of health-care providers.[38]

The only category of data relevant to this study that was reliably reported throughout the colonial and postcolonial eras was government spending. Every regime that has ruled Malawi since the late nineteenth century, including the United Kingdom (1891–1953), the Federation of Rhodesia and Nyasaland (1953–1963), and Hastings Kamuzu Banda's long-lived dictatorial regime (1964–1994), was deeply concerned with government outlays. Most of the time this concern was impelled by a desire to limit spending on "uneconomic" activities such as health care. But a result of this miserly approach to governance was a careful accounting of expenditures. Using figures compiled under different regimes demands some faith in the comparability of data. Still, government spending figures represent the readiest, least compromised measure of the extent to which health care was a government priority at different moments in Malawi's history. A brief survey of changing public-sector outlays for health care will help to outline the history of government health care in Malawi.

Domestic public sector outlays for health care in Malawi have not, until very recently, reached a sizable share of the budget. Nor has such spending closely tracked aggregate government revenues. The share of government spending devoted to health care varied greatly over time. Figure I.1 charts the recurrent expenditure (that is, spending on recurring expenditures such as wages, drugs, and supplies rather than new buildings) in the Medical

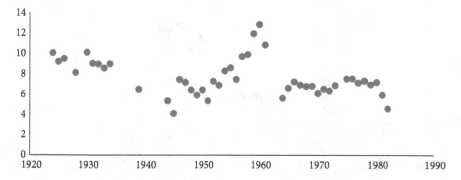

Figure I.1 Recurrent government health-care spending as share of total government recurrent expenditure, Nyasaland/Malawi, 1924–1982

Sources: Annual reports of the Medical Department (pre-1964); reports of World Bank Missions to Malawi (1964–1982).

Department between 1924 and 1982. This figure includes spending on curative medicine and public health. The graph shows that expenditure on curative medicine and public health never exceeded 13 percent of government expenditure during this period. The highest shares were attained during the 1920s, an era when almost all colonial health-care expenditure was devoted to the care of European officials, so it does not reflect a commitment to African health care. During the rest of the period, government spending devoted to health care was much lower than in contemporary Europe and the United States, and lower than the 15 percent pledge made by African ministers of health at Abuja in 2001.[39] But the share of government spending devoted to the Medical Department did not remain fixed. Analyzing the peaks and troughs can help to show when health care was treated as a priority by those in charge of Malawi's finances, and when it was not.

Spending can also be measured in terms of per capita expenditure. Figure I.2 shows recurrent domestic government health-care expenditure per capita in constant (inflation-adjusted) 2016 pounds sterling. This figure demonstrates that spending was always paltry; between 1924 and 1982, it never exceeded £7 in 2016 prices. As late as 2013, health-care expenditure per capita in Malawi (public and private, including foreign aid) was only £17.[40] The meagerness of this spending must be kept firmly in the foreground throughout this analysis. The degree to which it was simply inescapable,

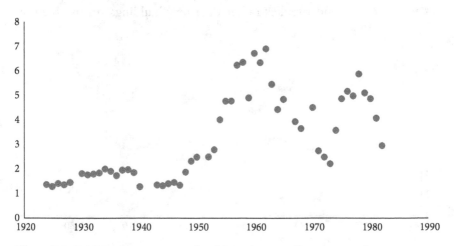

Figure I.2 Recurrent government health-care expenditure per capita, Nyasaland/Malawi, 1924–1982, in constant 2016 British pounds sterling

Sources: Annual reports of the Medical Department (pre-1964); reports of World Bank Missions to Malawi (1964–1982).

or instead the result of social action, is explored throughout. Figure I.2 also demonstrates that over the course of the twentieth century, there were moments of increasing per capita spending as well as periods of retrenchment. This book seeks to understand the factors that led to these of moments of increased and decreased expenditure. But the analysis also extends beyond domestic expenditures to include spending by "external" sources such as the UK Treasury, foreign governments, and international institutions.

While much of the history that follows concerns the construction of scarcity in Malawi, political inattention to health care was not total. Tactics of neglect were defeated, at brief and irregular intervals, with increased funding for facilities, supplies, and personnel. Given the extent of both materially and socially constructed scarcities, how did these increases in health-care spending occur? When and why did colonial medicine actually reach African subjects? The stakes invoked by these questions extend beyond the history of medicine in Malawi to more fundamental questions of causation explored by theorists of social and political change. Here I group the most relevant theories into three categories: those that attribute change to disruption, those that focus on the influence of elite reformists, and those that credit change to contingent events. In the following paragraphs I explore each of these schools of thought and begin to consider how they can be used to understand Malawi's history of medicine.

First were those theorists who considered social and political change a consequence of unrest. This idea was prominent in the more recent anarchist-inspired work of the political scientist James Scott, who contended that "most of the great political reforms of the nineteenth and twentieth century have been accompanied by massive episodes of civil disobedience, riot, law-breaking, the disruption of public order, and, at the limit, civil war. Such tumult not only accompanied dramatic political changes but was often absolutely instrumental in bringing them about."[41] A similar though not identical claim was made by political scientists Philip Klinker and Rogers Smith, who argued that advances in racial equality in the United States emerged from the exigencies of war mobilization and concurrent protests.[42]

The central concerns in this book are less often "great political reforms" than incremental changes in spending on social services, and I do not go so far as Scott in affording tumult singular motive historical power. At certain moments, though, civil disobedience, the disruption of public order, and war (global as well as civil) did prove to be important influences on the development of health-care infrastructure in Malawi and elsewhere.[43] For example, in moments of popular unrest during the Federation of Rhodesia and Nyasaland (1953–1963) and very early in Malawi's independence (1964), regimes imperiled by widespread protest touted health-care spending as evidence of concern for the public. The share of recurrent government expenditure devoted to medical care in Nyasaland and Malawi was higher during these eras of revolt than at any other point of the twentieth century (see figure I.1). This is not a coincidence. But even at these moments, unrest was not the only factor impelling health-care spending.

Other theorists saw social and political change—including increases in welfare spending—as a consequence of the moral commitments of elite decision-makers. Elite reformists were, in their histories, influential policymakers who proved adept at marshaling resources for the poor. One of the most prominent believers in the historical power of elite reformists was the philosopher Richard Rorty, who argued that social change was a result of the "sentimental education" of the powerful. In this process, those in a position to change things gained "an increasing ability to see the similarities between [themselves] and people very unlike [them] as outweighing the differences." Rorty understood the distaste with which many readers would receive his argument, which appeared "to hand our hopes for moral progress . . . over to condescension." Still, he insisted, we must accustom ourselves to "relying on those with the power to change things . . . rather than relying on something that has power over them."[44] This understanding of public policy looked not to the self-interest of elites (and the threats to these interests posed by unrest), but rather to their moral concerns, for the motive force in social and political change.[45]

Indeed, there were moments in Malawian history when elite reformists exerted significant influence on the scale of public-sector health-care spending in Malawi. They were not necessarily firebrands or revolutionaries; they may not have even believed impoverished or subject populations deserved government services at all comparable to those enjoyed by the rich. These officials often argued that the neglect had reached objectionable—or at least embarrassing—levels. They insisted that government health-care providers were made to practice in dismal conditions, with inadequate medicines and supplies. In making these criticisms, these actors were sometimes concerned with maintaining their own sense of professional standards or with avoiding international embarrassment should critics find out how they were treating their populations. But even these motivations are insufficient to account for all of their actions. Careerist concerns were powerful, but I argue that there were powerful sentimental commitments at play as well.

Examples of the influence of elite reformists in this book are many. The inclusion of public health as a focus of the 1929 UK Colonial Development Act (CDA) required the timely intervention of little-known members of Parliament (MPs) named Eustace Percy and Vernon Davies. Percy, a former parliamentary secretary to the minister of health, and Davies, a physician, had personal commitments to medical care and sought to broaden the act beyond its original purpose of simply increasing demand for British manufactures. During the 1930s, leaders in the Colonial Medical Service such as John Owen Shircore and Henry de Boer complained to the Colonial Office in London that health-care budgets in Nyasaland were so low as to be both professionally embarrassing and morally abhorrent. Malawians were elite reformists as well; during the 1970s, the obstetrician John David Chiphangwi risked his life by refusing to hide what he considered shameful overcrowding in a government maternity ward from Life President Hastings Kamuzu Banda during an official visit. At times such protests helped garner new resources. Working within discriminatory and exploitative colonial systems, these elites helped funnel resources down steep gradients of inequality to ensure some modicum of medical care reached subject African populations. Their advocacy was not primarily a response to social unrest, but rather the result of concerns about their own reputations as well as a product of deeply held moral commitments.

Other theorists of social change argued that the impetus for social change lay in particularities of social and political configurations. Rather than relying on any all-encompassing theory of change driven by single factors such as popular unrest or elite sentiment, these scholars sought to understand the interaction of the varied groups seeking to advance their interests in given historical moments. An exemplar of these scholars was Peter Baldwin, whose comparative historical analysis of welfare states in Western Europe challenged monolithic explanations, particularly those hinging on working-class mobilization. In detailed studies of France, Germany, Britain, Denmark, and Sweden, Baldwin sought to understand the risks faced by—and contests between—particular social groups, such as professionals, farmers, and factory laborers, at crucial moments in each national history of social insurance.[46] In detailing his approach, Baldwin said that while he was willing to make broad explanatory claims, he insisted on the value of the historian's "penchant for craggy detail."[47]

In this study, too, the importance of contingent social and political configurations is apparent. During the 1960s and 1970s, for instance, President Hastings Kamuzu Banda turned to foreign governments for funding to build new hospitals. In obtaining these funds, Banda exploited Malawi's unique position in major geopolitical struggles of the moment. As a black African state that condemned neither apartheid South Africa nor Portuguese rule in Mozambique in the early 1970s, Banda sought the rewards for his loyalty in the form of development aid. At the same time, Banda's use of the symbols of indigenous healing and the language of chiefly responsibility also left him vulnerable to claims on those responsibilities by physicians, like Chiphangwi, who claimed the government was not doing nearly enough. The idiosyncrasies of Malawi's geopolitical position and Banda's symbolism of rule helps, then, to explain the politics of medicine during the postcolonial era.

This importance of contingency in historical change helps to account for things that did *not* happen as well as things that did. Health-care spending in Nyasaland increased during some major moments of unrest, such as the First World War and the Federation of Rhodesia and Nyasaland. But it did not rise after the bloody Chilembwe uprising of 1915, nor after the anti-witchcraft movement of the early 1930s known as *mchape*. These were profound moments of ferment in Malawi's history, but they did not lead to increased health-care spending. The specific domestic and international circumstances in which these moments of unrest occurred helped to determine whether they led to increased spending or not. The official preference for a punitive response as opposed to a welfarist one (as in the case of Chilembwe), or a lack of concern with the consequences of unrest (as in the case of *mchape*), led, in these cases, to a decision not to increase health-care spending. These circumstances are explored in greater depth in the chapters that follow.

These schools of thought about the forces driving social and economic change are not mutually exclusive. The development of carrier hospitals in and around Nyasaland during the First World War, for instance, was a consequence of both wartime demands for labor and of elite concern with morally repugnant rates of mortality among the carriers. This historical moment lends credence to Scott's emphasis on disruption and to Rorty's focus on elite reformists. We need not subscribe to a monolithic theory of social change to see the value in the perspective each brings to Malawi's complex and conse-quential yet little-studied history of health care.

What Paul Farmer has called "the House of No," the omnipresent chorus of expert and official voices who claim that inescapable scarcity allows no more than threadbare health care for the poor, was built long ago.[48] Officials in the British colonial regime, Southern Rhodesia's Federal Ministry of Health, Malawi's postcolonial government, and international financial institutions of the neoliberal era all justified paltry health-care budgets with rationalizations about the inadvisability or—more often—the sheer impossibility of greater effort. The social construction of scarce medical care has, in Malawi, been under way for over a century.

But there is more to the story. Neglect is not always easy to sustain. It demands consistent political, rhetorical, and sometimes martial work, and sometimes this work failed or backfired. The inescapability of paltry health-care resources has often been challenged, by Africans and Europeans, colo-nized and colonizers, physicians and patients. For various reasons at various times, these challenges did sometimes prove successful in increasing finan-cial outlays for health from national governments, colonial treasuries, and bilateral and international aid agencies. In Malawi as in many other low-income areas of the globe, the archives are rife with disproven claims about the impossibility of doing more. The history of scarcity claims is, as Farmer explains, full of "confident statements about mutable situations."[49]

Recognizing that certain forms of scarcity are social constructions impels us to study the ways in which scarcity discourses become self-evident real-ities, how they produce human beings "socialized for scarcity," people who believe poor outcomes are inevitable. Such processes were the focus of a 1966 book by physician-sociologist Peter Berger and sociologist Thomas Luckmann entitled *The Social Construction of Reality*. Social constructions, the authors explained, are mental categories that groups create over time, in everyday conversations, to make sense of their shared world. These constructions involve arranging actions into categories in order to render the vast array of sensory stimuli in such a way as to allow decisions without end-less deliberation. As social constructions are passed from one generation to another, they are portrayed as natural and inevitable, rather than products of social, contingent mechanisms of understanding the world around us. Social constructions are legitimated by fields of knowledge and study, yet they are not indestructible. They can be challenged, disrupted, and tossed aside.[50]

According to Berger and Luckmann, there are three "moments" in the social construction of reality. In the first, "society is a human product." This,
in our case, is the process in which the idea of scarcity about health-care
spending and systems spread in everyday conversations and common parlance. The common invocation of scarcity is a theme in this book; in every
era of Malawian history, scarcity was one of the most common ideas in official correspondence and public proclamations. In Berger and Luckmann's
second moment, "society is an objective reality." In the case of Malawi's history of medicine, this part of the social construction of scarcity came when
the line between political priorities and unalterable realities became blurred.
Scarcity came to seem, in all cases, inescapable. Finally, in the third moment,
"man is a social product."[51] Health-care providers and policymakers became
socialized for scarcity, accepting it as unalterable reality. They themselves accepted as natural the idea that there was no more to spend and tried to make
do within the restricted bounds of the socially constructed possible.

This process of rendering the alterable into something that appears unalterable is familiar to social historians. As Marc Bloch observed, "Man spends
his time devising techniques of which he afterwards remains a more or less
willing prisoner."[52] A historical approach to scarcity in health care helps us to
better understand how assumptions are uttered, generation after generation,
in a pattern that eventually appears to repeat without human agency. But
archival research and oral histories also help us to see when and how these
assumptions have been challenged. Indeed, while the inevitability of threadbare health-care services came to seem like natural law to some officials, the
social construction of scarcity has always been an unfinished project. At no
point were all publics, providers, and policymakers wholly socialized for
scarcity. Even after enduring decades of neglect, patients and physicians and
even some colonial officials consistently demanded more funding. Many
wrote scathing critiques of the political economy of medical provision to
demonstrate that there was surely more money to be found. Many would not
accept arguments that only substandard care was possible. Further still, the
forces of neglect could, in brief moments, be overwhelmed. The boundary between the inescapable and the constructed did, in certain moments, shift. At
times, increased spending was propelled by political disruption or the threat
thereof. At other times, it was a result of the actions of a few well-placed elites
with a sentimental concern for the health of impoverished Malawians. And
at other interregna in the institutionalization of scarcity, particular social
configurations of group or national interests led to new spending. Delving

into this history allows us to denaturalize our inheritance, to understand the difference between inescapable and constructed scarcities, even to expand our moral imaginaries to include alternative, more just social worlds.

The arguments thus far have presented Malawi as a representative case of a larger historical process, one that has applicability to other parts of the colonial and postcolonial world. But of course Malawi and its colonial precursor, Nyasaland (1891–1964), are not in all ways representative. There are many peculiarities to the country, its history, and its systems of medical provision. I explore many of these particularities later in this and in subsequent chapters, but the main point I wish to make here is that Malawi remains an apt choice for this study because it represents an extreme example of what most would consider inescapable scarcities. As one of the British Empire's most destitute holdings, and today one of the world's poorest nations, the possibilities for health care seem, at first blush, severely constrained, not so much by the neglect of national and international policymakers as by a series of remote and unalterable misfortunes. Landlocked and barren of natural resources, Malawi is geographically ill-placed for prosperity. Ravaged by the Indian Ocean slave trade, it was war-torn even before Scottish missionaries arrived in the mid-nineteenth century. The vast majority of its people have remained poor semisubsistence farmers ever since. In contrast to Zambia's copper and Zimbabwe's gold and Botswana's diamonds, Malawi's main exports have been less valuable cash crops such as tea and tobacco. These exports garner Malawi's government relatively paltry resources, and they furnish self-interested capitalists few incentives to invest in a healthy, productive workforce.

Despite all of this, I attempt in this book to convince the skeptical reader that more robust health care in Malawi has long been possible. A wide variety of historical actors have argued, throughout the twentieth and early twenty-first centuries, that health-care facilities need not be so decrepit, that personnel need not be so hastily trained and inadequately equipped, and that even impoverished African patients need not endure standards that others would not tolerate. They are, I argue, largely correct. Instead of spending its (truly) scarce resources on health care, what financial resources Malawi did have were often extracted by colonial regimes and usurious creditors or ill-spent by a dictator. In spite of the profound material constraints facing policymakers in Nyasaland and Malawi, health care never received more than 13 percent of recurrent government spending between the 1920s and the 1980s, and it was usually much lower. Foreign aid for health care was usually extremely limited; these limits were the subject of numerous justifications, which are also explored in this book. If there remained considerable distance between inescapable and constructed scarcities in Malawi, then surely similar discrepancies can be found elsewhere. In other words, if more was possible in Malawi, then surely more could be done in other places with similarly dismal medical care but more available resources.[53]

This statement begs the question of what I mean by "available resources." I certainly include the funds in Malawi's public coffers. But available resources for health care include, in this study, not only domestic colonial and postcolonial state revenues. Some funds that could easily have been spent on health care never were, thanks in part to political decisions. Colonial officials who argued that there were simply not enough funds for decent social services for Africans had to ignore the relatively low portions of colonial budgets spent on such services, obfuscate about flows of wealth from the colonies to the metropole, maintain a hard line against releasing funds from the metropolitan treasury, and naturalize constructs such as the "protectorate" that elided exploitation while denying claims to equitable treatment. These claims were strategically deployed to deflect criticism and defend against any welfarist claims on public and private finances.

Health-care budgets were a function of decisions that at first glance appear little related to medical services. For instance, the history that follows discusses in detail the terms of an interwar railway loan, internal divisions within the Labour Party over postwar colonial development policy, and international debates over population control. I explore how these and other episodes had important effects on the availability of health care to millions of Malawians. The story of health care demands study not only of official records and memoirs of doctors within Malawi itself, but also of a geographically broader scope of social, political, and economic histories.

There are other particularities in Malawi's history that might lead some to question its generalizability. One that rarely goes unmentioned by imperial historians is the well-documented presence of missionary hospitals in Nyasaland. Documenting the inadequacies of government medical care might not elucidate the full story, these historians suggest, because privately run mission facilities have long had a significant role in the provision of medical care. Some historians have noted the prominence of missions in health-care provision in Malawian history.[54] There is much truth to this, particularly during the late nineteenth and early twentieth centuries. At least until the 1920s, medical care for Africans in Nyasaland was almost wholly provided by missions. Until the mid-1930s, missions were the only facilities providing training for African medical auxiliaries, who then staffed both mission and government facilities.[55] Yet while missions were, in the words of Harry Gear, "the early predominant medical force" in Nyasaland, few Africans could reach their facilities, and even fewer could afford the fees most charged for care.[56] By the mid-twentieth century government medical facilities had become a more frequent destination for sick Africans than missions.

To some extent the impression of Malawi as a heavily missionized space is a result of the rich historiography of missionary medicine in Malawi.[57] Missions were not especially numerous in Nyasaland, at least compared to other places in British southern Africa.[58] Colonial and postcolonial officials often highlighted the work of missions, perhaps because making them seem numerous absolved the government of responsibility for expanding health care. Aside from the particular strength of yet another social construction (Malawi as the uniquely missionized space), the mission experience in Malawian health care is not so unique.

Still, it is true that Malawi, like any colony or nation, had unique elements in the history of its health-care systems. This study focuses on what made Malawi's experience unique, for there is value in studying the political economy of health care at the level of a small nation. A granular study can illuminate, with precision and detail, the dynamics of neglect and their effects on the practice of medicine, the impacts of structural change as well as contingent events, of elites and popular politics, of military strategies and economic policies. The historiography of the institutions involved in colonial and postcolonial health care is growing, and scholars have done searching and revelatory archival research.[59] But the breadth (often global) and scope (usually, the entire development enterprise) of such studies leads, in most cases, to the elision of certain concerns. In particular, the real-world effects of policies on actual patients, nurses, and doctors are often recounted with a hefty dose of generality. Such histories also tend to accord great power to the heads of institutions, while focusing less on the midlevel managers and on-the-ground practitioners who sought to influence decisions and critique existing policies.

By focusing on a single colony and postcolony, I aim to demonstrate how both local and global discourses, decisions, and events have shaped the practices and rhetoric of delay and neglect in a specific place. And by extending this history of Malawi's health-care system *through* the colonial, Federation, and postcolonial eras, the continuities and discontinuities between these periods become more apparent. In particular, the social construction of scarcity becomes not the project solely of a colonial administration, a postcolonial dictator, or neoliberal international institutions, but rather a long-term endeavor. It was a problem that transcended any particular moment; it was not undone by independence, or the coming of multiparty democracy, or the shift to any new economic ideology.

To demonstrate the social construction and the consequences of scarcity in Malawi, this study draws upon archives in Malawi, the United Kingdom, and the United States. The documents in these archives detail both the varied rationalizations for health-care neglect as well as the effects of disruption, elite reformists, and particular configurations of political interests on that neglect. They also reveal the frustrations, complaints, and everyday realities of physicians, nurses, auxiliaries, caregivers, and patients in a perpetually underfunded health-care system. In the process of trying to heal and be healed with care that never reached contemporary European and American standards, these actors often recognized the socially constructed nature of the scarcity in which they operated. While some of these actors eventually became socialized for scarcity, many never accustomed themselves to it.

Each chapter of this book begins with a short story that highlights, in sometimes oblique ways, the consequences of this history of perpetual forbearance for the ethnographic present in Malawi. These vignettes demonstrate the impact of a century of socially constructed scarcity on people's health-care options, expectations, and outcomes. Though they are not as deeply analytical as in a work devoted wholly to ethnography, stories like Innocent's are intended to suggest, however briefly, the echoes and repercussions of the long project of neglect and constructed scarcity.

They are not intended to suggest that Malawi's past and present are identical.[60] The history of medicine in Malawi has long been dismal, but it has been marked by much change. Stasis is not the only theme; even regimes of perpetual delay and extraction used changing rationalizations and new forms of repression. Patients and health-care providers alike have responded with creativity, relying on networks of mutuality to make life possible even as they recognized the deadly consequences of official neglect.

I collected these stories during eleven months of fieldwork between 2011 and 2015 in two districts (Mangochi and Neno) in Malawi's Southern Province. Though at the time of my research I was a student in an MD/PhD program, I never took on any medical role in the villages, clinics, and hospitals I visited. I sought to befriend and interview the people I write about;

informed consent was obtained from each individual who appears. I originally chose to go to Mangochi due to its significance in early colonial African
history (when it was an important trading post) as well as due to its early
postindependence history (when it was the site of a short-lived rebellion
sparked in part by health-care user fees). I selected Neno because it has long
been among the poorest and most neglected areas of Malawi, where scarcity,
both inescapable and socially constructed, is an ever-present concern.

These stories form a "prelude" to all but one of the chapters; the remaining
prelude (to chapter 5) is a comparative history. The questions and issues
raised in each prelude are similar, though not identical, to those explored
in the corresponding chapters. The preludes, then, are intended to show
resonances and dissonances, to trace the lineaments of history in an emer-
gent present. I have changed the names of subjects (except for public figures)
and village names (but not district or hospital names) in the preludes to protect the identities of my interlocutors.

In order to demonstrate further what is particular and what is more gen-
eralizable in Malawi's history, I refer often to the secondary literature on
nearby colonies and postcolonies in British Africa. Most commonly I refer
to Tanganyika (since 1961, Tanzania), Uganda (independent since 1962),
and Northern Rhodesia (since 1964, Zambia). As nearby colonies in British
southern and eastern Africa, the government medical systems of these colonies had significant interaction with that in Nyasaland, as well as similar
administrative apparatuses. Each had its own particular historical trajectory,
with different demographics (Uganda had more European settlers as well as
more medical training for Africans), different levels of resources (Northern
Rhodesia had mining wealth from copper), and different ideologies postindependence (Zambia and Tanzania were led by "African socialists"). The
ferocity and persistence of neglect was particularly advanced in colonial
Nyasaland, in part because of how unimportant its population was considered to the metropolitan economy. Yet the same rhetorical, institutional, and
intellectual justifications for neglect were used in other colonies. Less frequent reference is made to medical care in settler colonies or Commonwealth
territories, as the dynamics of neglect (though powerful) were quite different
in these places.[61]

And so this book chronicles government medical care in Nyasaland and
Malawi, with a focus on the century between the First World War and the
second decade of the twenty-first century. It is not the history of one disease
or individual, but a political and social history of a government medical

system. The main actors are officials, health-care providers, and patients. Of course the government health-care sector was never more than one part of a plural medical system in Malawi, and it remains so today. For the vast majority of people in southern, central, and eastern Africa, care in times of illness is given neither by medical doctors nor by registered nurses, but by kin and neighbors.[62] This and other elements of the caregiving system—including missionary medicine, millenarian Christianity, and popular healers—enter the narrative, as they had significant effects on the history of government medical care. Yet a key point explored in this history is the *dynamism* of medical pluralism. The narrative details how Africans' care-seeking behavior changed over time in response to government policies, social transformation, and—in particular—novel therapeutics. Biomedicine itself was far from static; changes within the practice of medicine at "European" hospitals and clinics had profound effects on the demand for biomedical services. This work, then, is an attempt to follow the example of Steven Feierman and the call by Walter Bruchhausen for historically informed studies of patients' quest for healing.[63]

Reexamining the history of government health care—or lack thereof—in a former British protectorate does not necessarily require rehashing the same old questions about the nature of colonialism. At stake in much of the earlier literature on this subject was the beneficence or maleficence of an imagined unitary soul of colonialism. The battle lines were clear. On one side stood the hagiographers, and on the other the radical critics.[64] Already enough has been written to thoroughly rebut those who persist in extoling the supposed good works of British imperial rule, who see medical care as some kind of effective apologia for oppression.[65] But in the chapters that follow, the British colonial enterprise appears as what it was: simultaneously exploitative and unfree even as it employed many well-intentioned individuals.

There remains a need to cultivate a "willingness to be surprised," to question totalizing narratives, and to insist on inductive histories.[66] Even if, as this book shows, the deficiencies and discrimination inherent in colonial-era medicine did not end at independence, twenty-first-century global health care does not share all the sins of colonial medicine.[67] Nor were colonial doctors and officials simply handmaidens of economic exploitation. Even in the face of new rationalizations for spending less than was actually possible, some in the colonial service were vocal critics of neglect. After independence Malawi's own doctors would make their own stands against poor public-sector medical care, at significant professional and personal risk. The construction of scarcity was sophisticated, and although much work was invested in it, it was never quite perfected. It did have some vulnerabilities. Insistent moral claims, the exigencies of military or economic necessity, and changing geopolitical interests did lead to improved care at some moments.

The chapters ahead are organized chronologically. Each examines a different era to explore the various influences—internal and external—on public-sector health-care spending in colonial Nyasaland and postcolonial Malawi.

Chapter 1 draws a link between the conscription of hundreds of thousands of Nyasaland's Africans into the British military's carrier service during the First World War and the first efforts to provide some measure of government health care to rural colonial subjects during the 1920s. Prewar colonial civilian medical care was poor, but the wartime experience of medical care led to peacetime calls for better facilities.

Chapter 2 details both the political economy of interwar colonial neglect for social services and the crucial role of moral commitments on the part of a few MPs in puncturing this neglect. The imposition of a burdensome loan for an uneconomical railway gave many officials the excuse to resist increased funding for health care, but these excuses were challenged during the debate over the 1929 Colonial Development Act.

Chapter 3 demonstrates the recrudescence of neglect during and after the Great Depression. Although 1930s budgets remained static in Nyasaland, waves of unrest forced the Colonial Office and Treasury to raise levels of health-care spending elsewhere.

Chapter 4 explores how changes in political discourse within metropolitan Britain during and immediately after the Second World War altered debates about colonial medical provision. Enthusiasm for social protection in Britain, and the crisis of legitimacy that the war brought to imperial officials, led to increased interest in—if not always spending on—health care for the colonies.

Chapter 5 demonstrates how the newfound potency of postwar medical technologies made it ever more difficult for colonial officials to deny them to colonized publics. Rising attendance at government health-care facilities and a crescendo in civil unrest and repression drove an expansion in the health-care system in Nyasaland.

Chapter 6 examines the successes and failures of the work of neglect in Malawi's early postcolonial history (1964–1980). After a short-lived rebellion at the dawn of the new nation, Prime Minister Hastings Kamuzu Banda made health care part of his ideological platform, but despite some external funding, the health-care budget remained small.

Finally, chapter 7 explores how this history of neglect continued in the age of AIDS, only to be broken (at least temporarily) by the surge in global health-care spending beginning in the mid-2000s. In the 1970s and early 1980s, economic collapse and the dictates of international economic institutions hastened the collapse of the health-care system in Malawi in a moment when the AIDS crisis was just beginning. The future of health care in Malawi remains uncertain, even given the arrival of new global health funding.

This book, then, explores the rhetorical and political work required to sustain a regime of delay in Malawi's government medical care. The past and present of waiting for health care in Malawi is, in some ways, readily explicable. It is overdetermined that the administration of a backwater colony would deliver little health care to the colonized. But given that there was a rising demand for medical care among African publics as well as a burgeoning global discourse on welfare and social protection over the course of the twentieth century, forestalling improvements in health care required varied forms of rationalization and denial. The existence of rationalizations to spend less money may not be surprising, but the ways in which these arguments were deployed, defended, and (at certain moments) defeated have serious implications for health-care outcomes today.

Innocent's story demonstrates one of these implications. If Innocent had lived near a trained and equipped vascular surgeon, he would very likely have left the hospital with both his legs. Instead, he returned home with a stump and little hope of being able to afford a prosthetic limb. The process of training, employing, and equipping surgeons is no mystery. But it takes money, and money—as this book shows—is something Malawi's health-care sector has long been denied. Innocent's avoidable amputation was the product of a thousand decisions and omissions that left Malawi without the equipped and trained medical practitioners needed to salvage his leg. Because many of these decisions are quite remote in time and place from Innocent's village in 2015, they only come to light through an analysis that is both geographically broad and historically deep.

1

Drugs for the *Tengatenga*, 1861–1919

"They were always carrying the colonists," remembered "Francis," a forty-eight-year-old farmer in Nyanza, a lakeshore village near the town of Monkey Bay in southern Malawi. During five months in 2015, I rented a room in Francis's home, and I often asked him to tell me what he knew of the area's history. So, taking a brief respite from working his land to drink tea one morning in March 2015, Francis recounted some stories of the colonial era told by his parents and grandparents. He had heard from them that whenever a district commissioner traveled through the village on *ulendo* (tour) to meet with local leaders or collect taxes, villagers would have to carry his *machila* (hammock-stretcher) on their shoulders. "The people complained about it, a lot (*anadandaula kwambiri*)," he said.

Memories of carrying have even been etched into the names Malawians have given to the landscape. In the southwestern province of Neno, the poorest district in the world's poorest country, a schoolteacher explained the meaning of the name of a hill called Caliwoni near his home. It was not, he said, a Chichewa word. Rather, Caliwoni harkened back to an order uttered often in that place by a British official whenever he visited on tour. Villagers carrying the *machila* on which he rode would inevitably slow down when they reached the long, steep incline. "Carry on! Carry on!" the official would command. The villagers so associated that hill with this order that they Chewa-ized the phrase and named the hill Caliwoni.[1]

All kinds of forced labor remain vivid in Malawian memories of colonization. Still sipping his tea, Francis reminisced about the demands of *thangata* labor. *Thangata* was a system by which, in return for the privilege of living as squatters on the massive estates granted to European settlers by the colonial government, Africans were made for at least one month each year to perform unpaid labor as "rent."[2] During the colonial era (*ku nthawi atsamunda*), Francis remembered, people were beaten for refusing to perform *thangata* labor. They were sometimes beaten just because a settler found their work too slow for his liking.[3]

No More to Spend. Paul Farmer, Oxford University Press (2020). © Oxford University Press.
DOI: 10.1093/oso/9780190066192.001.0001

As bearers of European officials' *machilas*, as *thangata* laborers on European estates, and—as this chapter details—as carriers supplying troops in the East African theater during the First World War, African men and women were forced to work throughout the colonial era.

Personal memoirs written by former British officials and commentators tended to portray such labor as ennobling, even enjoyable.[4] Yet for many Africans, laboring for Europeans was often the stuff of bitter memories. Lewis Bandawe, a Lomwe immigrant from Portuguese Mozambique who would go on to serve as head clerk and interpreter in Nyasaland's High Court from 1934 from 1960, wrote in his memoirs that the British colonial government "was a terror to all people." To Bandawe, the iron collars used on prisoners, who were most often guilty of nothing more than defaulting on hut taxes, looked just like the ones he had seen on slaves in neighboring Mozambique.[5] Bandawe claimed (with perhaps some exaggeration) that "every European, with the exception of the missionaries, had a *chikoti*—a whip made of hippo's hide—which he used on his domestic servants and laborers."[6] Ending such practices was an animating force of anticolonial politics. For Francis, the most inspiring promise in the early speeches of Hastings Kamuzu Banda, Malawi's nationalist leader and first president, was his promise to end *thangata*.[7]

In 2015 Malawians did not suffer such overt systems of coercion. There remained, of course, plenty of work to do. The hungry season (December to March), when food from the previous harvest ran short but the work of tending to the next was hardest, was the busiest time. I lived with Francis and his family during this period and noted the daily routine. Five people (not including me) slept in Francis's home on most nights. Francis and his wife Edith slept in one room on a mat of woven banana leaves. Lucia, the couple's eight-year-old daughter, and Monica, their three-year-old niece, slept in another room. Samuel, the seventeen-year-old son of Francis's late sister, slept in a hut that doubled as Edith's kitchen.

Before daybreak, Francis's wife Edith was already awake, sweeping the house and the backyard with a broom made of twigs. She then walked one hundred meters to the nearest borehole, where she filled a fifty-liter basin. With little apparent difficulty, Edith lifted the basin and placed it on her head for the walk home. Walking into the dimly lit kitchen, a hut with no ventilation that would soon be filled with smoke, she packed branches into an earthen cookstove and started a fire to heat the water. Some of the water would be used to cook *nsima*, the maize porridge that is a Malawian staple. The remainder of the water was used for bathing and cleaning the dishes. Edith helped Lucia prepare for school, then tied Monica to her back with a *chitenje* cloth and departed to collect more firewood or to help Francis's elderly parents, who lived next door, with their chores. On other days she helped Francis and Samuel in the fields. Every evening she spent two hours preparing dinner.

Francis also rose before dawn, and during most days of the hungry season he walked two kilometers to the two-hectare field where he grew maize and groundnuts. There he carefully tended what would be the major source of his family's sustenance for the coming year. My rent helped Francis purchase a fifty-kilogram bag of fertilizer; this cost 16,500 kwacha (about US$40) at the nearest agricultural marketing board depot. Though fertilizer can increase yields by as much as threefold, it also added to Francis's workload. In addition to planting the crops and weeding the fields, he now had to apply fertilizer in a labor-intensive process. To me, Francis and Edith's exertions appeared unbelievable, especially because they lived on such a meager diet. Their daily *nsima* satiated hunger but furnished few calories.

For Francis and Edith, work abounded. The harvest rarely provided much more than subsistence. Still, Francis said he enjoyed farming. He was one of the few men in the village who did not spend every night in a canoe on the lake, fishing for *kampango* (catfish) or *usipa* (sardine-like fish) by the light of lanterns. The family was successful enough at farming to live a more comfortable life than others in their village. Their house was made not of wattle and daub, as were many others in the village, but of cement. Their floor was also cement, as opposed to the packed dirt many others had. Their roof was made of corrugated iron, not straw. Francis's family had even amassed wealth, which he stored in the inflation-proof, relatively illiquid form of livestock: ten chickens, four goats, and one pig.

Theirs was not a comfortable existence. If the annual rains did not fall at the right time and in the right amount, the family's exertions would come to naught. Like the rest of their village, they had neither electricity nor running water. Francis had a cell phone, but it had been broken for months. Still, the couple derived satisfaction from the fact that they labored on their own terms. Unlike their grandparents and great-grandparents, they were not colonial subjects. They were no one's beasts of burden.

Introduction

Malawian government health care was born of a war in which Africans were conscripted into labor by the hundreds of thousands. Whereas before the First World War the only sources of biomedical care for Africans in Nyasaland were the mission hospitals, the intense labor demands during the war spurred the construction of rudimentary government-run hospitals. In the aftermath of the war, experience with European medicine led native authorities, and the medical officers who interacted with them, to call for the construction of dispensaries around the country.

The decade that followed the war was the start of a period—which in many ways never ended—when Medical Department officials made incessant demands for additional funds from the territorial and imperial treasuries. As the colonial employees with the most frequent contact with rural Africans, doctors witnessed how the UK government's claims that it brought health, peace, and prosperity to the colonial populace were belied by quotidian realities. Africans, they argued, must be able to expect something in exchange for onerous taxation, forced labor, and alien rule. Colonized Africans in Nyasaland received very little government medical care until the era of the Central African Federation (1953–1963), but public-sector health care was born during this earlier era, after a Great War that claimed the lives of thousands of the colony's inhabitants.

Before the Great War, medical care for Africans in Nyasaland was sparse and almost wholly provided by missions. Mission hospitals had been established at Cape Maclear in 1875, Bandawe in 1881, Livingstonia in 1894, and Zomba in 1896. They were important not only for the care they provided, but also because they educated and trained the African medical auxiliaries who later worked in both mission and government facilities.[8] Indeed, missions were responsible for almost all of the European settlers' early efforts at educating Africans: In 1927, Nyasaland's fourteen missions accounted for ten times more spending on African education than did the government.[9]

Missionaries used medicine to demonstrate goodwill and secure legitimacy, especially during moments of strife and uncertainty. The Scottish missionary physician David Livingstone, who lived in present-day Malawi with members of the Anglican Church from the Universities Mission to Central Africa (UMCA) between 1861 and 1864, claimed medicine was an "aid in convincing the people that we were really anxious for their welfare."[10]

Medicine, Livingstone believed, was an important display of the beneficence of European civilization.[11]

This first UMCA mission ended in disaster. Malaria, famine, violent confrontations with Yao slave traders, and disillusionment led surviving members of the team to abandon the post for Zanzibar. Missionaries would return in the decades that followed, with similar plans to use medical care as an entrée for evangelism. Such was the case for the Free Church of Scotland Livingstonia mission, which was originally established at Cape Maclear in 1875 before moving north to Bandawe in 1881 and then to Khondowe in 1894.[12] At these stations, another Scottish physician, Robert Laws, performed surgeries on African patients. In his biography of Laws, William Pringle Livingstone attributed the early support the mission garnered among the surrounding African population to Laws's medical work:

> The natives were quietly taking stock of the white men, observing all their actions, and reading their character. . . .What chiefly won them was the medical work of the Doctor. Stories of his skill and kindliness were carried by the few whom he attended and retold in the villages, and one after another they ventured to the Station for medicine.[13]

The biographer's appraisal of the effectiveness of Laws's practice was surely influenced by his own concerns. William Pringle Livingstone was a journalist for religious publications and a committed evangelist, so it fell to later historians to note that only a few Africans ever sought European medicine from the early missionary physicians, who were mainly focused on keeping fellow missionaries alive.[14] Still, in his account of Laws, Livingstone captured some of the motivations driving many missionaries in what would become Malawi. The work of educating and providing medical care for Africans formed an important part of the self-identity of the missionaries. After its initial abortive attempt to establish a mission in the 1860s, the UMCA returned in 1880 to set up a new outpost on Likoma Island. Following his arrival there in 1899, Dr. Robert Howard built a network of clinics staffed by European nurses and African medical assistants along the shore of Lake Malawi (then, Lake Nyasa).[15] In 1875, the Church of Scotland established the Blantyre Mission in the Shire Highlands, and in 1896 Dr. Neil Macvicar began training some of the mission's best-educated Africans as medical assistants at a newly established African hospital.[16] The Livingstonia mission began its own small training program for African medical assistants in 1904.[17]

These institutions have been well-chronicled in works that often highlight physicians' sacrifices and heroism, on the one hand, and their use of health-related rationalizations for racial segregation, on the other.[18] Yet we should be careful not to paint a picture of medical plenty during this period. As late as 1940, the first year in which the government reported figures for mission clinic attendances, less than 4 percent of Africans in Nyasaland visited a mission outpatient clinic over the course of a year.[19]

Part of the reason for the paucity of medicine in Nyasaland stemmed from the fact that, like many other colonial regimes in Southern and Central Africa (including Northern and Southern Rhodesia, South Africa, Mozambique, and the Congo), it began as a for-profit, private enterprise. Established in 1891, the British Central African Protectorate was originally a public-private venture funded by Cecil Rhodes's British South Africa Company (BSAC). Rhodes did not think the territory would ever be very profitable and paid His Majesty's government to administer it on a shoestring budget of £10,000 per year (£1.16 million in 2016 prices). He agreed to fund the establishment of the "protectorate" in part to advance his dream of British rule "from the Cape to Cairo," and in part because the British government had agreed that in return for the BSAC's funding of Nyasaland, it would secure the sole rights to exploit gold fields in Mashonaland (in present-day Zimbabwe).[20] The imperative from the start in Nyasaland (so renamed in 1907) was to spend as little as possible while maintaining a modicum of order and aiding the few European planters to run estates profitably. The ethos of extreme economy continued to affect access to medical services even after the Nyasaland administration's formal ties to the BSAC were severed in 1911.[21]

Before the First World War, the government medical service was devoted almost entirely to the care of European officials and to scientific research. In this era, British medical officers came to Africa to build reputations as researchers, to discover new pathogens, and to enter the bacteriological pantheon of Koch and Pasteur, rather than to provide medical care.[22] Such was the case with Dr. Hugh Stannus, stationed at Fort Johnston as a medical officer to the King's African Rifles (Nyasaland's military force) from 1905 to 1910. Stannus built a pathology laboratory, started a medical library, and authored publications on sleeping sickness, yaws, blackwater fever, and albinism.[23] From the perspective of the metropolitan government, the role of medical officers in Nyasaland before the First World War was to protect the few Africans, Indians, and Europeans involved in the threadbare administration of the new territory. Almost a quarter-century later, in 1913, Nyasaland's

Medical Department had only twelve medical officers (doctors) and five nurses.[24] In 1914, the only government hospitals providing care for Africans were small facilities at Port Herald (four beds), Zomba (forty-six beds), Fort Johnston (five beds), and Karonga (two beds).[25]

For their part, Africans found their care among a variety of practitioners, including but not limited to missionaries. Indeed, the historian Markku Hokkanen has pointed out that one way to understand the pluralistic medical culture of late-nineteenth- and early-twentieth-century Nyasaland is to view missionary doctors and nurses as "marginal practitioners (although with an expanding practice) in a medical culture where local healers and midwives formed the medical orthodoxy."[26] Africans in the region have long availed themselves of diverse providers, with divergent epistemologies and different technologies. Even when European biomedical providers conceived of their own work as a contest with "witch doctors" and "traditional medicine," their patients proved much more comfortable with an eclectic mix of providers. As anthropologists would later discover, decisions about care-seeking were often driven by trial and error as well as by lay understandings of the etiologies of various illnesses.[27]

The imposition of colonial rule disrupted precolonial public health measures extant in African societies, including those in Nyasaland. Variolation against smallpox, a practice in which fluid from smallpox scabs was rubbed into superficial scratches made on the skin in the hopes of conferring immunity after a mild, protective infection, had been performed for centuries in many parts of the continent. The colonial government outlawed variolation in Nyasaland in 1908.[28] Population displacements from the wars of imperial conquest led many to flee to the bush, where they were susceptible to sleeping sickness (human trypanosomiasis). Colonial officials also forbade their subjects from setting controlled fires around villages to rid areas of the tsetse flies that carried the disease.[29] The widespread nineteenth-century practice of hedging risks against drought through the cultivation of crops with different moisture requirements was replaced by the colonial governments' insistence on growing a select few crops.[30] Thus, many precolonial public health and social protection practices did not survive the decades following the late-nineteenth-century "Scramble for Africa."

Those public health measures that were instituted during the early years of the twentieth century were martial in nature and ill-suited to securing the trust of peoples so recently conquered, often by force. A July 1903 ordinance aimed at limiting sleeping sickness required Africans seeking to cross district borders to enter only at specified government stations, where they would be made to submit to a medical examination. These exams would begin with palpation of the cervical glands (in the neck); if enlarged, the traveler's glands might be punctured for diagnosis. If huts were believed to lie within the range of the tsetse fly, officials could order the abandonment of entire villages.[31]

Though smallpox vaccination campaigns garnered trust at first, eventually the harsh measures of limited efficacy bred social resistance. African medical assistants from the Church of Scotland Blantyre Mission used scalpels and calf lymph to vaccinate the surrounding population during a short-lived epidemic in 1899–1900. The brevity of this outbreak seemed, to government officials, to confirm the utility of native vaccinators.[32] The colonial administration began to pay the wages of the native vaccinators and purchase supplies of lymph.[33] Africans willingly presented (and paid) for vaccination at the Livingstonia Mission.[34] Nearly a decade without a serious smallpox epidemic in Nyasaland bred confidence among both missionary doctors and the colony's chief medical administrator that the vaccination program was effective. In 1907, Principal Medical Officer Henry Hearsey confidently declared, "epidemics of smallpox, such as were common in the protectorate some years ago, do not now occur."[35] When outbreaks struck Nyasaland the very next year, the colonial administration issued the Vaccine Ordinance of 1908, which made vaccination compulsory. By 1913, the government reported that the African assistants administered 143,502 vaccinations in that year alone.[36]

These campaigns may have been less effective than advertised. Even Hearsey doubted the accuracy of the vaccinators' returns. The few medical officers in the employ of the government did little to verify them. Doctors also recognized that their lymph was often stored so long that it lost its capacity to stimulate immunity. Some of the vaccinators' efforts seemed worse than useless. In 1909, a district resident reported that the high frequency of severe ulcers on the arms of the recently vaccinated might be attributable to a particular vaccinator's wont to use a blood-soaked, dirt-stained scalpel to carve gaping wounds into patients' arms.[37]

These campaigns were, however, effective at demonstrating to African subjects the similarities between public health and the recent wars of colonial conquest. In 1899 the nascent colonial administration responded to a smallpox outbreak in the Ntcheu District village of Ntonda by burning houses and enforcing a cordon sanitaire with soldiers. Even missionaries joined in the arson. Dr. Walter Elmslie of Livingstonia reported that after unsuccessfully "hunting for a case of small pox which is being hid away by the people," he "burnt down several houses where we knew he had been, so the stupid people may begin to see their own interests and help us."[38]

The frequent recurrence of smallpox in coming decades, and the often-unexplained brutality of measures taken in the name of disease control, would spur a backlash against smallpox vaccination campaigns. [39] Vaccinators lamented villagers' refusal to cooperate during a 1936 outbreak.[40] Resistance would take on special importance in the late 1950s, when the Federation government claimed that the leadership of the opposition Malawi Congress Party had frightened the people into rejecting vaccinations.

Thus, coercive public health measures, not curative medicine, were the only introduction most Africans received to government health-care provision before the Great War. Unless they lived near a religious mission, most Africans never saw a doctor or nurse. The burning of villages by armed police resembled nothing so much as the battles only recently fought by some of Nyasaland's peoples against British and BSAC troops during the 1890s.[41] The most profound impact of European occupation for most Africans was annual hut taxation; these levies compelled thousands of men to leave their villages in search of wage labor on plantations and in mines.[42] When migrants reached the mines of South Africa in the first decades of the twentieth century, they did not experience many wonders of modern medicine. Instead, they lived and worked in such squalor and died at such high rates that embarrassed government officials in the Transvaal temporarily banned recruitment of workers from Central Africa.[43] Curative medicine was not, then, a meaningful part of the experience of being governed.

"Invited to Die for a Cause Which Is Not Theirs"

For many Africans in Nyasaland, introduction to European curative medicine came during a period of profound upheaval. The First World War or, as it was known to many in the region, the *nkhani chiwaya* ("war of the big gun"), has long been remembered as a time of forced labor and mass death. William Berry, a medical officer in Nyasaland during the 1930s, recalled an aphorism coined by "an observant Bantu chief," who described the chronicity of the European presence in Africa: "First the missionary, then the trader, then the gunboat."[44] Indeed, it was a gunboat that heralded the start of hostilities between the United Kingdom and Germany in East Africa. On

August 8, 1914—four days after Germany invaded Belgium, prompting the British to declare war on Germany—British warships fired on a railway station at the German East Africa capital, Dar es Salaam. On August 13 the war reached Nyasaland; sitting in port on the shore of Lake Nyasa, the German ship *Hermann von Wissmann* was incapacitated by a shot from the British gunboat *Guendolen*. This was no great battle, as the German captain had not even been alerted to the outbreak of war.[45] Still, that moment opened a new theater, one that would be fought in Nyasaland as well as in all of its neighboring colonies: German East Africa (today's Tanzania), Portuguese East Africa (today's Mozambique), and Northern Rhodesia (today's Zambia).[46]

If Africans in Nyasaland did not immediately feel the most terrible exactions of war, eventually they would toil, and die, in droves. Opposition to the war surfaced early. In an unpublished letter to the *Nyasaland Times* in January 1915, the preacher John Chilembwe, who had returned to Nyasaland after a seminary education in the United States, decried the lot of Africans in "this present world." They were, he declared, "invited to die for a cause which is not theirs."[47] As it happened, this would prove a dramatic understatement. Africans were not so much invited as forced to join the war.

Chilembwe would not live to see the worst of native conscription. After leading a short-lived armed uprising calling for an "Africa for the Africans," he was shot dead by colonial police in February 1915.[48] This episode fostered among officials a reticence to extend education to the general African population. Their major concern, in the words of a commission of inquiry, was "a tendency to extend the field of teaching to the detriment of its quality, and to establish schools which cannot be properly supervised."[49] Subsequent limitations on mission education and paltry government spending on African education would make it far more difficult to find suitable candidates for medical training for decades after.[50] This was perhaps the most important effect of the Chilembwe uprising on the future of Nyasaland's health-care system. And though later episodes of unrest would lead to greater health-care spending, this one did not. Government health care for the general African population was not yet a part of the political imaginary of either African subjects or officials. This would change within the span of a few years, after the war introduced the notion of more widespread government medical provision.

In the aftermath of Chilembwe's bloody, abortive uprising, British officials were reticent to arm the newly restive African population. This changed later in the war, when the demand for reinforcements led to the conscription of many African soldiers (*askari*). But British commanders were far more desperate for human carriers than armed troops. Food, munitions, medicines, mail, and even whiskey were supplied via a route that demanded vast quantities of human labor.[51] Ocean, river, and rail transport from South Africa only reached as far as Blantyre (along the main supply line) and Livingstone, Northern Rhodesia (on a subsidiary route). Pack animals could not survive in the tsetse-infested regions, as they were quickly killed off by trypanosomiasis.[52] So all along the 120 miles from Blantyre to Fort Johnston, along a 700-mile route from Livingstone to Fife in Northern Rhodesia, and up mountains and through the dense brush of German East Africa, African carriers were the British army's beasts of burden. Among Africans the carrier service was known as *tengatenga*; *kutenga* means "to take" in Chichewa, and *tengatenga* translates roughly as "to take very far." The pay for carrier service was not sufficient to draw Africans into the service; carriers were paid six shillings per month, the same amount white settler volunteers earned in a single day.

In February 1916, Brigadier General Edward Northey arrived as commander of the Nyasaland-Rhodesian forces to find his troops desperately short of food. *Askari* and carriers were receiving "starvation rations" of 1.25 pounds of maize each day, as supplies ran short near the front lines.[53] Northey made constant demands for additional carriers from Nyasaland governor George Smith. Smith set quotas for each of the chiefs. Some who failed to meet them were whipped.[54] When this system proved insufficient, the administration pursued and conscripted Africans who were delinquent on the hut tax. When defaulters went into hiding, police kidnapped their wives until they surrendered. But these conscripts were also insufficient to meet the demand for labor. Police began nighttime raids to kidnap any able-bodied men they could find.[55] The intensity of these campaigns was assured by the administration's policy that police who failed to conscript sufficient carriers had their pay withheld.

Carrier labor was not new to the region. Since at least the fourteenth century, long-distance trading networks in eastern and central Africa had relied on human porters.[56] During the early colonial era, private transport companies and government officials hired—or sometimes forced into service—tens of thousands of carriers to move food and other crucial goods along otherwise impassable roads.[57] But the war did bring something new, as both the scale of the demand for porters and the ferocity of coercion were unprecedented in the region's history. A total of 169,000 men, women, and children in Nyasaland—8 percent of the total population—worked in the carrier service during the war.[58] *Tengatenga* brought extreme privation; even the *Nyasaland Times*, then essentially a mouthpiece of official propaganda, reported that maize was "ground up, husks and all, and then issued as rations."[59]

These carriers were worked harder than precolonial-era porters. For instance, whereas nineteenth-century porters carried no more than twenty kilograms, First World War porters carried an average of twenty-seven kilograms.[60] Carriers were beaten with whips by conductors—including missionary priests—and left to die of exposure and exhaustion.[61] They succumbed to dysentery and pneumonia, smallpox and plague. Francis Baily, a convoy officer in German East Africa during the war, recalled the experience:

> A carrier is one of the lowest forms of life . . . and he is always more or less in a state of misery . . . he takes no interest whatever in the war. . . . The mortality among carriers was extremely high, because, contrary to the popular idea, the native is no more immune to local diseases than anybody else, and goes down with malaria, dysentery and diarrhea very much the same as a white man.[62]

Even Governor Smith, who had orchestrated the brutal recruitment campaign of carrier labor, estimated that the mortality rate for carriers was 4–5 percent during 1917–1918.[63]

In a final stroke of suffering, survivors of carrier service returned home to two more scourges: epidemic and famine. Thousands who had survived carrier service died on the walk home at the end of the war during the 1918–1919 global influenza pandemic.[64] Then, in April 1919, villages across the protectorate found themselves without food. According to Nyasaland governor Hector Duff, the famine was due in part to the failure of the early grain harvest, but he admitted the cause was "chiefly the fact that immense quantities of stored native grain had been requisitioned for the use of the troops and that scores of thousands of able bodied natives had been withdrawn from their homes to serve as military porters." Thus, the effects of the war on health rippled far beyond even the hundreds of thousands compelled into labor.[65]

In addition to widespread death, the war brought something else. It was the moment many Africans had their first exposure to European curative medicine. Attempting to maintain supply lines, and partially in response to metropolitan critiques of the brutalities of carrier service, the British military set up "carrier hospitals" near the front lines in German East Africa. In some accounts these medical facilities appeared quite impressive. The official history of the First World War, commissioned by the UK government, claimed "the supply of medical stores and drugs, ordnance stores and comforts was ... sufficient for the needs of the force." Medical care for carriers was provided at "twenty-eight mixed rest stations, five casualty clearing hospitals, and seven carrier hospitals."[66] In August 1917 these facilities were staffed by "80 medical officers, 3 sub-assistant surgeons, 14 Roman Catholic priests, 23 nursing sisters, 24 dispensers, and 123 British other ranks."[67] The history did mention an "excessive death-rate" among the carriers but attributed this primarily to "the poor physique of the African native."[68]

More recent histories have challenged this portrait of a robust carrier medical service. As Melvin Page explained, official lists of hospitals, personnel, and medical supplies were often never realized in practice. A missionary without any medical training who treated many of the carriers remembered that most of his medicines were looted from a German mission, but he could not read German and was therefore unable to understand the labels. He mostly gave sick patients "salts, Livingstone's rouser pills [an antimalarial pill containing quinine and a mixture of purgatives], quinine, boric powder and dressings and bandages." Even those hospitals with trained nurses were overwhelmed by sick carriers. "Our hospital is so crammed that patients sleep on top of one another," remembered a Catholic nun. At another hospital in Mwenzo, the facilities were so small that many cases were turned away.[69]

Within Nyasaland the war left medical services more threadbare than ever. Seven of the twelve doctors employed by the government were seconded to the front in German East Africa: "Owing to the extreme shortage of staff it was not possible to keep open more than three civil stations, namely, Port Herald, Blantyre and Zomba."[70] Another hospital remained in operation at Fort Johnston, but it was under military control. Even obtaining medical staff for Nyasaland's troops proved extremely difficult.

Despite the shortcomings of medical care for carriers and *askari*, more of Nyasaland's Africans came into contact with government-run British medical facilities during the war than at any time previously. "For the first time," claims the historian Colin Baker, "hundreds of thousands of Nyasaland Africans had access to Government medical services."[71] This might be an overstatement, depending on one's definition of "access" and "medical services." As explained previously, the quality of care available to those carriers who made it to these "hospitals" was poor. But Baker is correct when he contends that this experience "was bound to lead to pressure—whether voiced or not—to extend medical facilities after the war." Popular memories of carrier hospitals, and officials' desire to maintain some semblance of attention to Africans, impelled the construction of dozens of dispensaries throughout Nyasaland during the early 1920s.

Bringing Medicine Back from the War

In 1921, three years after the war's end, Nyasaland's principal medical officer, Dr. Henry Hearsey, drafted a circular and sent it to the chief secretary in Zomba for comment. Hearsey, who had occupied his post since 1902, wrote: "A not unimportant part of the scheme for providing medical aid to the native population is the provision of Rural Dispensaries in areas distant from stations where Medical Officers and Sub-Assistant Surgeons are posted." Since government provision of medical care in rural areas had not previously been a part of peacetime medical policy, Hearsey sought to justify the departure from past practice. "That there is an urgent need for such Dispensaries was forced on my mind when I closed down those which had been erected on Lines of Communication during the late War. Various Headmen and others enquired of me what they were now to do with their sick who needed treatment." Even though the carrier hospitals had been sparse, poorly equipped, and staffed with minimally trained personnel, Africans remembered them as one of the few parts of the war experience worth keeping. In response to the inquiries of native authorities, Hearsey announced his plans:

> It is my intention to indent this coming year for a quantity of concentrated stock mixtures for easy dispensing, which together with simple dressings, etc., would be supplied to these dispensaries. They would be placed in charge of intelligent native Hospital and Dispensary Attendants who had received some training and experience in our native hospitals.[72]

Hearsey's circular asked each of Nyasaland's district residents to send him locations appropriate for these new dispensaries. The criteria he proposed were the density of the population in that area and the distance from a mission health facility for natives. Hearsey sought to situate the dispensaries not to serve areas of commercial activity or military importance, but rather to reach the largest population possible.

Only two weeks later, when the chief secretary sent a copy of Hearsey's circular to district officials, he heavily edited both its content and tone. No longer did the circular open with a declaration of the importance of medical care for Africans. The chief secretary's language was less enthusiastic: "I am directed to inform you that a proposal has been put forward by the Principal Medical Officer for the establishment of dispensaries in rural areas." The chief secretary's revised circular added another criterion for the site of rural dispensaries, namely that "accessibility to the medical headquarters of the District should also be taken into consideration." By prioritizing sites with ready access to administrative centers, the chief secretary had compromised Hearsey's ideal of serving populations in areas remote from extant health-care services. In another curtailment of Hearsey's vision, the chief secretary added that "not more than four sites in your district should be reported upon."[73]

Similar stipulations would become a recurring theme in the history of Nyasaland's medical service. Medical officers laid out proposals for expanded or improved services, pointing to popular demands or professional imperatives. Their superiors demanded cost containment. Directors of medical services and medical officers were almost always encouraging more health-care facilities, more rapid expansion, and more spending, while administrators holding the purse strings in Zomba and London tried to deflect these demands.

When Hearsey had sent his proposal to the chief secretary in 1921, there were already plans afoot, and funds allocated in the budget, to build seven health facilities for Africans. Recognizing the extreme economies under which the colonial budget operated at the time, Hearsey admitted that his plan might have to wait. Still, he believed that with the information provided by the districts, he would be able to gradually expand the dispensary system "as opportunities occur," eventually building sixty-four new dispensaries.[74]

Initially, prospects for Hearsey's proposal seemed poor. The Treasury Department in London demanded Nyasaland cut its proposed 1922–1923 budget in order to achieve an operating surplus of £80,000 (£3.52 million in 2016 prices). This surplus would permit Nyasaland's government to cover expected losses on the privately owned Trans-Zambesi Railway, whose profits Nyasaland had been compelled by officials in Whitehall to guarantee in 1919. In order to meet these demands for austerity, Acting Governor Richard Rankine cut £39,000 (£1.72 million in 2016 prices) from his 1922–1923 budget, including £500 (£22,000 in 2016 prices) he had originally allocated for construction of the new dispensaries.[75] Upset at being forced to make these revisions, Rankine lodged a protest with Winston Churchill, secretary of state for the colonies. He complained that although "it has not been possible in the past to provide to any extent for medical attendance of natives," there remained "a great need for this," particularly "if we are to prevent the large waste of human life and energy which goes unchecked at present among the natives."[76]

Undersecretary of State for the Colonies Gilbert Grindle passed this plea to the true arbiter of budgetary matters, Chancellor of the Exchequer Robert Home. In his memorandum, Grindle added that slow population growth and poor health among natives underscored "the urgent need for increased medical attention to the native population."[77] Eventually the Treasury relented, if only slightly, in its demand for economy. In doing so, they cited a forecast by a Treasury official, who predicted that Nyasaland's tariff and tax revenues in 1922–1923 would be higher than originally estimated.[78] Controller of Supply Services George Barstow informed Grindle that the Treasury was prepared to allow the reinsertion of one-third of Rankine's proposed cuts.[79] Ultimately, Nyasaland's 1922–1923 budget did include £768 (£33,800 in 2016 prices) for dispensary attendants' salaries, £580 (£25,500 in 2016 prices) for supplies, and £500 (£22,000 in 2016 prices) for dispensary construction.[80] An enthusiastic Hearsey reported that he had already begun recruiting attendants.[81]

The significance of this new funding should not be overstated. The first year's indent for the new attendants' salaries (£768) represented less than 1 percent of the £100,000 (£4.40 million in 2016 prices) collected from African subjects through the annual hut tax.[82] Even in the principal medical officer's initial plans, the dispensaries were to be austere facilities. Each would consist of two huts of wattle and daub, one for the dispensary itself and another for the attendants' living quarters.[83]

Still, this new funding did represent a change. Why, aside from the changed revenue forecast, did the UK Treasury agree to the dispensary construction? Beyond the lingering memory of carrier hospitals, there were other forces impelling the British administration to pay slightly more attention to the health of natives. Historians Richard Rotberg and Colin Baker both note that British missionaries complained often to government officials about the inadequacies of medical care for Africans, while European landowners began to see the potential for greater output from healthier laborers.[84] The demand for labor during the interwar years made state health-care interventions appear more and more a necessary ingredient for efficient production. There was also a newfound focus on social service provision in the major treatises and justificatory doctrines of the British Empire. The historian Joseph Hodge has argued that the new rhetoric was part of an effort to establish "a new moral basis of trusteeship" in response to metropolitan critics of empire as well as to voices within the Colonial Office itself. These commentators argued that the moral basis would be buttressed by expanded access to health and sanitation services among indigenous populations.[85] As former governor-general of Nigeria Lord Frederick Lugard, architect of the principle of indirect rule, explained in *The Dual Mandate in British Tropical Africa* in 1922, "The white man was at first engaged in consolidating his own position, and making the tropics healthier for Europeans engaged in their own development. He has now accepted the principle that they must be made more healthy for the native population."[86] This principle was less rigorously followed than Lugard's statement would indicate, but there was a shift in rhetoric and (to a far lesser extent) budgets during the early 1920s.

Nyasaland was not the only colony in British Africa where the medical administration sought increased facilities and medical training for natives in the years after the First World War. In 1922, Dr. John Gilks, Kenya's principal medical officer, wrote of his department that it was "no longer considered merely as an organization maintained by Government to facilitate administration by maintaining the personnel of the executive in health, but as a Department of Government responsible for the carrying out of the most important function for which Government itself is established, namely the maintenance in health of the general population of the country and the improvement of the conditions under which that population lives."[87] In 1924 a government-run training program for African medical assistants, who would follow curricula similar to those used by European medical schools, began at Makerere in Uganda.[88] In response to demands by chiefs for curative medicine, Tanganyika began rural dispensary construction in 1926, though these dispensaries were paid for by the share of hut tax revenue kept by local native authorities.[89] During the 1920s, medical officers authored plans for health-care services for African populations in rural areas across British Africa, including Nigeria, the Gold Coast, and Bechuanaland.[90]

Unsurprisingly, the visions of healthy, well-served native populations evoked by this rhetoric remained far from daily realities. At the few native hospitals in Nyasaland during the early 1920s, medical officers wrote scathingly about the conditions in which they were made to practice. A 1921 annual report authored by Dr. Raymond Busy, the senior medical officer in Blantyre, declared:

> The present position of the Native Hospital is unsatisfactory from all points of view. . . .There is only one ward, which has to be used for all classes of cases. . . .Government should build a proper new Native Hospital . . . with separate wards for medical, surgical and female patients and with good rooms for outpatients and for operations.[91]

Busy's proposal was not approved. Three years later, in a new post as Nyasaland's principal medical officer, Busy sent the chief secretary another complaint about Blantyre's native hospital, this one written by A. G. Eldred, his successor as Blantyre's senior medical officer. Eldred's report was even more vivid, describing the hospital as "one large ward, in which all patients, prisoners, and the general native public have to be herded." Lacking even a room to treat outpatients, "the dressing of wounds and ulcers is at present performed practically in the main road." [92] In 1925, citing the hospital's "disrepair," F. E. Whitehead, Nyasaland's new director of medical and sanitary services, shuttered the building and paid the Blantyre Mission Hospital to treat African inpatients referred from government dispensaries.[93]

Though a few African auxiliaries in government service had completed courses at mission hospitals, there was no formal instruction for dispensers during the 1920s.[94] These trainees were recruited from among the small cadre of young African males who had received some education at mission schools. The recruits were then apprenticed for a few months under mission-trained African staff, including Thomas Cheonga and Daniel Gondwe, at the native hospital in Zomba before being sent out on their own.[95] When they reached rural outposts, the new dispensers did not draw in droves. Patients were, in theory, to be given quinine to treat "fever," bandages for dressing wounds, and various mixtures for helminth infections such as hookworm and tapeworm. Frequently they lacked even these supplies.[96] Attendance figures belied the Medical Department's claim that dispensers were "giving the natives confidence in European medicine."[97] In 1927 the average dispensary saw only four patients a day.[98]

Though dispensaries and African hospitals made a modicum of care available to the general population, members of the colonial administration did not take great pride in them. In 1925, of the fourteen government "hospitals" for natives (the administration counted the government-subsidized Blantyre

Mission as one such hospital), only seven had a medical officer. The other seven were overseen by subassistant surgeons; this cadre, usually brought in from British India, completed the same curriculum as medical graduates in Great Britain, but they could be employed at much lower cost. At two hospitals the subassistant surgeon in charge was present only two or three months each year.[99] These facilities were not very popular. As Nyasaland governor Shenton Thomas lamented in a dispatch to the Colonial Office in 1930, native hospitals were so poorly maintained that "Africans of the better type flatly refused to enter."[100]

Part of the reason for the low attendance was that there were few diseases for which European medicine was thought, among the African population, to be effective. During the early 1920s, the new native dispensaries joined mission hospitals in attempting to cure yaws, a treponemal infection closely related to syphilis, though spread via nonsexual contact.[101] Yaws was not a fatal infection, but it caused disfiguring and often debilitating ulcers that could erode skin, tissue, and even bone. The dispensaries and hospitals initially used "Castellani's mixture," a combination of tartar emetic, sodium salicylate, and potassium iodide that had been used by David Livingstone in the 1860s. But the treatment was "disappointing," as relapses were common and advanced cases were rarely cured.[102] In 1925 medical officers in Karonga and Dedza introduced an intramuscular injection of sodium bismuth tartrate. It appeared to demonstrate some efficacy as a treatment for yaws; six injections over three weeks halted the ulceration (though, unbeknown to the investigators, this suppression would usually not be permanent).[103] The injections were intramuscular (not intravenous, as were other treatments such as salvarsan), so some of the dressers who staffed native dispensaries were permitted to administer them by themselves.[104] The injections proved modestly popular. Outpatient attendances for yaws climbed from 479 in 1925 to 2,227 in 1928.[105]

Still, few Africans had access to what was generally believed to be the safest, most effective yaws treatment available. Yaws symptoms could be quickly suppressed by injections of neosalvarsan, a drug discovered by German physician Paul Ehrlich in 1912 and used in Europe as a treatment for venereal syphilis.[106] A few missions and native hospitals in Nyasaland began using this injection during the 1920s for both syphilis and yaws. The drug proved fairly painless, and within weeks of treatment most patients' outward manifestations had disappeared. But the Medical Department deemed neosalvarsan too expensive for "general use."[107] In 1921, a missionary in Tanganyika reported that neosalvarsan cost him 10 shillings per dose.[108] Five years later, writing in the pages of the *Lancet*, John Owen Shircore (then Tanganyika's director of medical services), reported that with that amount of money, he could prepare over three hundred doses of the (less effective) bismuth injection.[109] In addition, because neosalvarsan had to be administered intravenously, it was used only at stations staffed by medical officers.[110]

Despite the popularity of yaws treatment, most Africans did not seek care at government or mission facilities for other serious illnesses. As Terence Ranger explained, "there was remarkably little of the predicted carry-over effect. Readiness to come for yaws treatment did *not* break down a more general 'mistrust of European methods.'"[111] I argue in chapter 5 that Nyasaland Africans were skeptical empiricists in their therapy-seeking behavior, and they evaluated the efficacy of individual treatments, rather than "European medicine" as a whole. In the late 1920s European medicine seemed effective at treating yaws, though even here the popularity of injections would abate as lesions reappeared in previously treated patients.[112] As John Christopherson, a missionary physician working in Tanzania, declared in 1921, "the native only judges by results."[113]

European medicine had not yet demonstrated an ability to cure many other illnesses. The number of African and Asian outpatient attendances did rise during the 1920s (markedly after the construction of dispensaries, from 19,089 in 1921 to 96,088 in 1923, then more slowly, to 168,181 in 1928). By 1928 there was still barely one outpatient admission per year for every ten Africans in Nyasaland.[114] Christopherson may have been right when he claimed "every case cured is placed in the native mind to the credit of the government," but in the 1920s these cases remained few and far between.[115]

Conclusion

Government medicine was not the most pervasive fact of colonial rule for African subjects in early colonial Nyasaland. During the early 1920s, a flat hut tax of 6 shillings was due from the inhabitants of each hut every October 1. Default carried a prison term of six months, hut demolition, and even the seizing of the defaulter's wife as a hostage until payment was made.[116] As late as the mid-1930s, tax defaulters imprisoned in Mlanje were made to remove buckets of feces and urine from the latrines in the homes of Europeans.[117]

Beyond the conscription of wartime carriers and punishments for tax defaulters, the government was known among Africans for its neglect during times of want. During a deadly famine in 1922–1923, British administrators set the price of imported maize at more than two times the rate the government had ever paid to peasant producers, and it refused to release stored maize from granaries.[118] So while the principal medical officer succeeded in garnering some funds to make government medicine for Africans more widely available, this was a small departure from colonial policy of the era.

Whereas before the First World War the only sources of biomedical care in Nyasaland were the mission hospitals, the intense demands for African labor during the war spurred the construction of government-run hospitals and dispensaries. These ill-equipped facilities were tasked with the care of the hundreds of thousands of "carriers" forced to carry munitions, rations, and other supplies. Many conscripted carriers and soldiers had their first contact with hospitals during the Great War, even if these facilities were not nearly so well-equipped as described in the UK government's official account of the conflict.

In the aftermath of war, experience with biomedicine at these hospitals led native authorities and colonial medical officers to call for the construction of additional health-care facilities. These facilities were staffed by poorly trained African auxiliaries and operated under extreme economies. According to colonial officials of the 1920s, these health-care facilities had not secured the confidence of most Africans. But the hospitals and dispensaries owed their very existence to the even more threadbare carrier hospitals that inaugurated the era of biomedical care for Africans in Nyasaland. Persistent advocacy by the director of medical services, who invoked the recent war, helped prompt the construction of rural dispensaries around the colony. The feverish demand for labor during the Great War had indirectly helped bring medical care to Africans even in rural areas, but the work of neglect had been stayed only briefly.

2

"Territories of Vast Potentiality,"
1919–1930

Prelude

It was finally clear to me why he had insisted on arriving so early. The clinic was already full of waiting patients. I had offered to accompany Chisomo, Francis's father-in-law, to the clinic one morning, as he was having trouble with his indwelling urinary catheter and had pain in his lower abdomen. By the time we dismounted the bicycles and paid the cyclists who had taken us the twelve kilometers from Chisomo's home to the Monkey Bay hospital, there was already a long line in front of the clinic door. In the outpatient department of this hospital, renovated with funds from Iceland's government a decade earlier, approximately thirty other people were waiting to be seen. They sat along the wall of a long hallway, mostly in silence. Some squeezed together on benches with their heads in their hands. Most of the women were sitting on the floor, their legs stuck out ramrod straight.

The medical assistant arrived at 8:30, a half hour late. A young woman in a white coat, she had a tired, harried expression. As soon as she unlocked the door, there was a mad dash to follow her inside. The line in the hallway was not so much the agreed order in which the patients were to be seen as it was a starting line for a race that recommenced every time the door opened. The visits were incredibly short. Each patient spent two to three minutes in the room, then exited to enter another crowd of patients seeking to fill prescriptions at the pharmacy.

Chisomo eventually cajoled and cornered his way into the room and invited me to join him. He did not wait for the medical assistant to ask him a question. Instead he handed over a tattered yellow booklet. This booklet, which Malawians called a "passbook" (a relic, perhaps, of the passbooks blacks were made to carry in Southern Rhodesia and apartheid South Africa[1]), contained Chisomo's medical history and was required of him whenever he presented

No More to Spend. Paul Farmer, Oxford University Press (2020). © Oxford University Press.
DOI: 10.1093/oso/9780190066192.001.0001

for care at any government facility. Chisomo explained that he needed a new urinary catheter. Looking at his passbook, the medical assistant could gather as much. The book contained cursory notes, each no more than two or three lines long, scribbled during past visits. The last one, from six weeks earlier, read, "BPH, catheter change, return 2 weeks." Chisomo excused his tardiness by saying he had been in too much pain to walk and did not have other means of transport until I offered to pay two young men to take us to Monkey Bay by bicycle.

The medical assistant stepped out of the room to gather a new urinary catheter set from the equipment room. She returned, asked Chisomo to lie on an exam table, and proceeded to replace the catheter without keeping the tubing, or her gloves, sterile. When she finished, Chisomo sat up and pulled up his pants. The medical assistant wrote a prescription for ciprofloxacin in his passbook. This was, she counseled, to treat a urinary tract infection that he had all but certainly developed from having the catheter in his bladder for so long. She told him to return in another three weeks.

To any health professional from a wealthier place, this scene would seem highly unusual. Benign prostatic hypertrophy (BPH), a condition in which the prostate enlarges, is common in older men around the world. It is almost never a life-threatening condition; its main effect is to render urination more difficult by blocking outflow from the bladder into the urethra. In the United States it is often treated with medicines that allow urine to flow more readily. If symptoms do not improve, surgery to remove some of the prostate tissue might be indicated. In some cases, a catheter is placed directly into the bladder—this is known as a suprapubic catheter. But aside from significantly impaired elderly patients, few people in the United States use Foley catheters (which are inserted in the urethra and forced up into the bladder) for periods longer than a few months. As the medical assistant noted, such treatments almost invariably lead to urinary tract infections, which can damage the bladder and the kidneys.

Another curious feature of Chisomo's management was the ready assumption, at all of his visits, that BPH was his diagnosis. Difficulty passing urine in an elderly male does not automatically indicate that he has BPH. There are other, more worrying diagnoses, including kidney stones, prostate cancer, or bladder cancer, that can cause similar symptoms. The notes in Chisomo's passbook detailed no prior workup to rule out these diagnoses. The persistence of Chisomo's pain, which often left him in agony, and the high prevalence of *Schistosoma haematobium*, a well-established cause of bladder cancer, on the southern shores of Lake Malawi, rendered unjustifiable the assumption that his only diagnosis was BPH.

A complete workup might have required a referral to one of Malawi's central hospitals, but the clinical encounter might have been conducted differently even in the outpatient setting. For instance, a rectal exam can help differentiate between BPH and prostate cancer. No such exam was noted in Chisomo's passbook. With only two years of training after secondary school, the medical assistant might not have known the full differential diagnosis for Chisomo's presenting complaints. More important, she was overwhelmed. The reasons were obvious. By the time Chisomo's visit was complete—unlike the other patients that morning, his took all of ten minutes—the line for the outpatient department had grown to sixty people. The medical assistant was the only provider in the department that day. She expected to see about one hundred patients, as she did on most days. She clearly wanted out. During our visit, the only question she had for me was whether I knew of any scholarships for training in the United States. Thus, for want of staff, training, and equipment, a sick man was given a cursory exam and inadequate treatment for a condition he may not even have had.

Still, Chisomo reported feeling better in the days after his clinic visits. Like many Malawians I met, he found government medicine valuable, if hard to access and not at all adequate. He returned home with one of the tales of relief (albeit partial and temporary) that led many of Malawi's sick to form long lines outside clinics every morning. But a week after his visit, I found Chisomo again lying on the ground outside his home, writhing in pain. Once again, he could barely pass any urine.

Better care was on offer nearby, for those who could pay. After one of Francis's neighbors, an elderly woman named Dalitso, complained of diffuse abdominal pain, I offered to accompany her to the Catholic Mission at Nankhwali and to pay her fees. The mission was about six kilometers from Nyanza village on a windy dirt path. The mission maintained a beautiful campus, thick with foliage. As we walked up the hill to the clinic on a Wednesday morning, congregants could be heard singing hymns inside the majestic church. The walls of the clinic were painted white and sky blue. The paint looked new. The floors had just been cleaned. Only one other patient (a mother with a baby) was waiting to be seen on the bench outside the immaculate exam rooms.

Patients at the mission clinic were seen by a clinical officer, a cadre of provider that received three years of training (while medical assistants received only two).[2] The clinical officer, named Paul, admitted that his job was easier than any commensurate public-sector position.[3] The fees, he explained, kept many sick people away, so he ended up seeing no more than twenty patients a day. The limited volume allowed him more time with each patient. After having her vitals taken by a kindly attendant, Dalitso was examined by Paul. Rather than simply listening to a chief complaint and scribbling in her passbook, Paul asked for a history before he performed a thorough physical exam. Finding symptoms consistent with intestinal amoebiasis, he prescribed erythromycin. The visit and the medicine cost 1,500 kwacha (roughly £1.50), much more than Dalitso, who lived alone in a decaying wattle-and-daub hut with a leaky thatch roof, would ever have paid on her own.

The disparity between the care available to those who could pay to attend the private clinics and those who had to attend the public-sector clinics came to mind when I heard the slogan for a USAID-funded, Johns Hopkins–run, behavior-change campaign. In brightly colored lettering, a poster affixed to a wall near the hospital dispensary in Monkey Bay read *Moyo ndi mpamba, samalireni!* The literal translation from Chichewa is "Life is precious, take care of it!" The campaign's purpose was to encourage Malawians to prevent diarrheal disease by washing their hands and treating drinking water with chlorine packets. No Malawians I asked had ever heard the aphorism before the *Moyo ndi mpamba* campaign began running radio advertisements three years prior. But the mantra "life is precious" seemed to encapsulate much of the experience of being both ill and impoverished in Malawi. Unable to pay for the superior care at private clinics and missions, most relied on a perpetually underfunded public sector, where overworked, underpaid staff struggled with Malawi's massive disease burden. Few Malawians doubted that greater appreciation for the preciousness of their lives would help them. They needed no ad campaign to convince them of the most obvious fact of Malawian life. The mantra, repeated in posters plastered on the walls of crowded hospitals, seemed less an exhortation than a cruel joke.[4]

Introduction

During the interwar era, the main adversary of colonial physicians and African medical assistants was not microbes of the gut and blood but the parsimony of the UK Treasury. Nyasaland was an extreme example of this insistence on austerity for health-care services, particularly after the colony's inhabitants were saddled with a huge debt for a railroad they did not want and would rarely use. Working in these circumstances, officials and politicians seeking to increase staff, supplies, and facilities in Nyasaland's Medical Department could do so only through the deft manipulation of political and administrative processes. Such manipulation occurred during the passage of the 1929 Colonial Development Act (CDA). This legislation was the culmination of a long-standing project of Conservative colonial secretaries Alfred Milner and Leo Amery. Their intent was to coax funds from the Treasury Department to build railways, roads, and bridges in the colonies, thereby increasing trade and employment both in Britain and its dependencies. Much of the history written on the CDA has focused on evaluating the extent to which this act fulfilled these aims. But this literature has largely overlooked what is the focus here, namely the subversion of the law's original intent by British politicians and colonial administrators with an interest in improving colonial health-care services. A handful of little-known MPs amended the CDA to allow the fund to be used to improve and expand health-care services.

After the law's passage, the Colonial Office sought to use the new funding to build hospitals and health centers. A colonial physician and administrator named John Owen Shircore wrote a critique of the low quality and poor reach of Nyasaland's extant health-care services and described a plan to improve them. His report helped garner funding sufficient to fund the construction of twelve new district hospitals and thirty-six additional dispensaries. This chapter recounts both a history of constructed scarcity and a brief moment when that construction was broken.

The Yoke of Debt

After the construction of Hearsey's rural dispensaries, few additional steps to expand or improve medical provision for Africans in Nyasaland were made during the rest of the 1920s. This paucity of government medical provision only began to change in the early 1930s, after Nyasaland became a major beneficiary of the CDA. Most histories of colonial development in Africa tend to downplay the significance of this act. Its passage did not lead to any wholesale change in UK Treasury policy toward African colonies, particularly after the Great Depression led to even more stringent budget controls.[5] But for Nyasaland's Medical Department, funding from the CDA was a major windfall. Many of Malawi's present-day district hospitals were first constructed with funds from this act. In large part, the government health sector in Nyasaland received a disproportionate share of the act's funding because of the persistent advocacy of its medical officials. They were, in this instance, elite reformists driving increased medical expenditures on subject African populations.

To fully appreciate the profound departure that CDA funding represented for Nyasaland, it is first necessary to understand the fiscal history of the protectorate during the interwar years. In 1919, UK colonial secretary Lord Milner and chancellor of the exchequer Austen Chamberlain agreed to guarantee debt taken on by the Mozambique Company, a private corporation funded by British investors, for the construction of a railway line. The line, which was known as the Trans-Zambesi Railway (TZR), was to run entirely outside Nyasaland, from the port of Beira to the southern bank of the Zambesi River in Portuguese East Africa.[6] Ostensibly its purpose was to link landlocked Nyasaland to the Indian Ocean, but its route was too long to transport goods for a reasonable price. The proposed railway was unnecessarily uneconomical, since it was longer and costlier than another possible route terminating further north, at Quelimane.

The route was, in fact, so costly that the Mozambique Company failed to raise private capital sufficient to finance its construction.[7] But Libert Oury, the Mozambique Company chairman, lobbied hard for British government financing. Crucially for him, a line commencing at Beira, a town built on company-owned land, would increase his profits.[8] Not for nothing was Oury known as "the other Rhodes." The British consul in Mozambique called him "a financial spider sitting in the midst of his web in London."[9] Oury plied a former Nyasaland governor, Sir Alfred Sharpe, with partnerships in a few of his firms.[10] Sharpe, for his part, had friends in the Foreign and Colonial Offices and was a member of the St. Stephen's Club, a famous Westminster watering hole for Conservative Party politicians. Though he could not secure the support of European settlers in Nyasaland—who foresaw that they would ultimately bear much of the cost of the inevitably unprofitable venture— Oury did not despair. He knew that the final decision would be made not in Nyasaland but in London. There he helped organize a dinner which, though ostensibly held to honor a hero of the Great War's East African theater, General Edward Northey, focused on the need for Oury's preferred railway line. Sir John Rees, a Unionist MP and former civil servant in India, claimed the line was necessary to rescue Nyasaland, a "Cinderella of the colonies."[11]

These displays helped render the railway line—and the loan guarantee—commonsensical among officials in Whitehall.

Indeed, by 1919 Oury had convinced Colonial Secretary Milner to support his plan. In a decision with grave implications for Nyasaland's future finances, Milner decided—without consulting the Nyasaland administration—to guarantee private railway investors an annual rate of return of at least 6 percent for twenty-five years. Initially, Milner claimed the UK Treasury would underwrite the guarantee. But the Treasury refused and decreed that Nyasaland must guarantee the debt with its own coffers. If Nyasaland's government proved unable to cover the losses from current revenues, the protectorate would be forced to take out loans from the Treasury at 7 percent interest.[12] So without the consent of Nyasaland's governor, much less its subject African people, the colony was made liable for ensuring high rates of private metropolitan profit for a railway that was too impractical to be of any real use.

Sure enough, the railroad quickly racked up operating losses.[13] As early as 1921, a junior Treasury official gave a pessimistic appraisal of the line's prospects and blamed the Colonial Office for misunderstanding—and even misrepresenting—the project. After insinuating that Lord Milner had deceived it about the line's future profitability, the Treasury dismissed the Colonial Office's plea that the imperial exchequer should assume responsibility for payments that would otherwise be a tremendous burden on Nyasaland's budget.[14]

Nyasaland's government suddenly faced a future of inordinate payments on the loan guarantee. After a 1921 agreement between the Colonial Office and the Treasury, Nyasaland was made to devote half its annual revenues over a protected "standard revenue" of £275,000 (£11.1 million in 2016 prices) toward the loan guarantee. While the railway extolled its venture in promotions aimed at metropolitan audiences (see figure 2.1), Nyasaland's governors wrote London to complain about the burdens of the arrangement. Specifically, they pointed to the impediments it placed on sorely needed increases in expenditure, including spending on the Medical Department. Treasury officials most often responded with calls for further tax increases and spending cuts.[15] By 1928 the protected "standard revenue" had been raised only to £300,000 (£16.9 million in 2016 prices).[16] As Harold Philips, who had worked as both assistant district commissioner and financial secretary in Nyasaland, remembered, "Treasury control [was] a horrible thing . . . they couldn't spend a penny unless it had

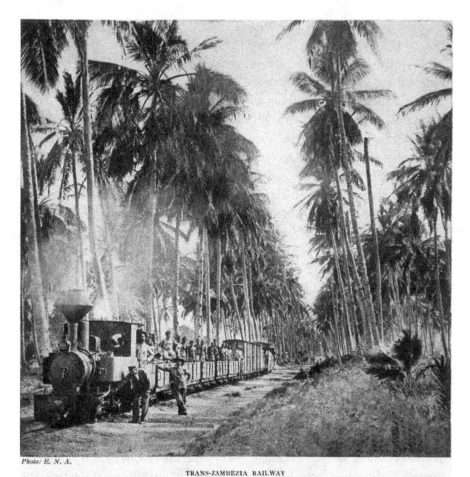

Photo: E. N. A.

TRANS-ZAMBEZIA RAILWAY

Not only has this railway inaugurated a new epoch of economic prosperity for Nyasaland by providing it with direct access to an ocean port, but it has also opened up a region of great forests, a sportsman's paradise wherein the elephant, the lion, the rhino and the antelope have roamed since the beginning of Time.

Figure 2.1 Trans-Zambesi Railway poster, 1925

Source: Exclusive News Agency, London. Reproduced with permission of Alamy Stock Photo.

first been approved by some backroom boy in London [who] didn't know a thing about it."[17]

In July 1928 Colonial Secretary Leo Amery complained to Chancellor of the Exchequer Winston Churchill that Nyasaland's "social services are at a scandalously low ebb" and the "death rate is disgraceful." Recounting a meeting between his subordinates and lower-level Treasury officials, Amery remembered, "We asked for some little mitigation. But we were turned down by the Treasury pretty stiffly." Churchill's Treasury offered a slight increase in the protected revenue to £325,000 (£18.4 million in 2016 prices) but demanded in return increases in customs duties on "native" goods such as matches, salt, and beads as well as an increase in the hut tax. John Sidebotham, a budget official in the Colonial Office, pointed out this would burden African subjects. Negotiations reached an impasse.

Nyasaland's Africans seemed doomed to remain impoverished, indebted, and without any robust social services.[18] Such was the assessment of Parliamentary Under-Secretary Ormsby-Gore, who lamented, "The Treasury have for years resisted . . . any attempts to get Nyasaland out of the slough of despond." After mentioning the desperate need for "wise expenditure on public health, scientific agriculture," and "education," Orsmby-Gore declared, "The history of all grant-aided, i.e. Treasury-controlled, dependencies in the last thirty years has always shown the starvation of these life-giving services."[19]

The 1929 Colonial Development Act

Nyasaland's budget and health-care sector only began to emerge from the "slough of despond" in 1930 thanks, strangely enough, to rising unemployment in Britain. The coming chapters recount moments when Nyasaland's health-care spending increased in response to crises, both nearby and far-flung. Such was the case at this moment, when, as the historian Rudolf von Albertini notes, "Economic crisis . . . brought these proposals into public discussion."[20] In the months leading up to the 1929 UK general election, the governing Conservative Party searched for ideas to include in its platform. The campaign, its leaders knew, would be fought largely on the issue of unemployment. Statistics published by the Board of Trade every month showed the number of Britons registering for unemployment insurance rising in late 1928, from 1.37 million in August to 1.57 million in December.[21] Particularly in northern industrial constituencies, both Conservative MPs and the Unionist MPs in their governing coalition worried about voter discontent over unemployment.[22] Only two years earlier, in 1926, the entire nation had ground to a halt for eight days during a general strike in which millions of workers took to picket lines. Although labor unrest had quieted significantly, and though joblessness was not nearly as grave as it would become in the early 1930s, the rising unemployment figures in late 1928 and early 1929 seemed likely to bolster the electoral prospects of the Labour Party, particularly if workers mobilized once again.

This potential for renewed militancy among the perpetually precarious factory and mine labor of the metropole spurred leading Conservative politicians to seek measures to shore up the demand for employment. In discussions of policies they might propose, Amery reproposed an idea he and his predecessor, Lord Milner, had been advocating since 1922: to spend Treasury funds to build transportation networks in colonial holdings. Financed by a "colonial development fund," this measure would combat domestic unemployment in two ways: First, road and railway construction paid for by the fund would spur orders for factories in Britain, and second, the resulting transportation infrastructure would open new markets for British producers.[23] A memorandum circulating in Whitehall in October 1928 promised that orders of millions of pounds of railway materials would reduce "industrial irritation" that could otherwise affect "the Ballot Box to the detriment of the government in power."[24]

Other prominent Conservatives were not so enthusiastic about this idea. Prime Minister Stanley Baldwin was at first noncommittal. Churchill adamantly opposed the departure from the long-standing policy restricting colonies from accessing UK Treasury funds that such a colonial development policy would entail.[25] Churchill proved so obstinate that Amery even asked Baldwin to remove him from his position. Amery did not conceal his derision for what he saw as Churchill's myopically martial understanding of imperial governance: "If Winston could only be induced to go away and wage war somewhere something might perhaps be done."[26]

But eventually Amery secured the support of other cabinet members and Conservative leaders. In February 1929 John Davidson, chairman of the Conservative Party and a close confidant of Baldwin's, wrote to the prime minister that a large-scale policy of colonial development would demonstrate their party was "still full of energy." It would, he continued, "fire the imagination of the country." Amery and Davidson eventually won over their colleagues. By early April, even Churchill reluctantly conceded.[27]

On April 18, 1929, Baldwin opened the campaign with an address before an audience of Conservative and Unionist Party loyalists in London. While laying out his party's plan to fight domestic unemployment, he included a call for a colonial development fund (CDF):

If you sum up what our ideal is—to find permanent employment—you may sum it up in this way, I think: that it is the modernization of industry at home and the multiplication of markets overseas. And that has caused us to look once more at the development of our own Colonies. . . . Overseas, and particularly in Africa, we have territories of vast potentiality, and we want them to develop . . . and so we shall provide out of our imperial funds such sums as are required . . . to pay the interest in the initial years of unfruitful schemes which otherwise must be postponed.[28]

The Conservatives included the CDF in their general election manifesto. During question hour in the House of Commons, Amery predicted that the fund would be used to build roads and railways in British Africa.[29] These projects would, he hastened to explain, require British goods produced by British workers.

While the Labour Party did not include a CDF in its own election platform, such a fund would come into existence under the new Labour government. The Conservatives met defeat in the May 30 general election, as Labour won 151 new seats and secured a plurality. Within weeks the Labour government adopted the Conservative idea of a CDF as an immediate response to unemployment. This was largely the work of "Jimmy" Thomas, a former railway labor organizer and colonial secretary who had been tasked by the new prime minister, Ramsay MacDonald, with coordinating the new government's response to unemployment. In the first postelection meeting of a committee set up to address unemployment, Thomas made the link between development spending in the colonies and job creation at home.[30] He did this again in a speech to the House of Commons on July 4, when he previewed an upcoming bill to authorize up to £1 million (£56.7 million in 2016 prices) in annual spending for colonial development.[31] On July 12, Thomas moved a resolution to establish a CDF as well as an advisory committee to assist the Treasury in judging the merits of applications submitted by colonial governments.[32]

The Fascist vs. the Pedant: The Debate over Health Care in Colonial Development

In their public comments, Thomas, Amery, and Baldwin had always stated that physical capital projects—and in particular, roads and railways—were to be the main beneficiaries of the new colonial development funding. Such projects, they promised, would entail large orders of goods from domestic factories, while the resulting transportation networks would decrease shipping costs for primary products from the colonies. Health care was not a central feature of either the Conservative or Labour Party leadership's original visions for the CDF. Yet a curiously large share of the funding made available by the CDA (16 percent between 1929 and 1940) went to health-care projects.

Why was such a sizable share of funding originally intended to build railways and telephone wires used instead to construct hospitals and clinics? To some historians, the use of the CDF for health care is evidence of a certain sort of failure. In his five-volume *Official History of Colonial Development*, D. J. Morgan writes of the period after the passage of the 1929 act that "the subsequent move away from emphasis on economic toward concern with social projects serves to confirm the fact that viable economic openings were just not abundantly available in the Colonial Empire as a whole."[33] Yet this characterization overlooks the fact that during the 1929 debates over the CDA, vocal backbench MPs worked to ensure that the "promotion of public health" was an explicitly authorized purpose of the new funding. The subsequent use of the CDF on health-care projects was less a failure than a skillful subversion of Amery's and Thomas's original intent to address unemployment in the United Kingdom. Because CDF health-care spending would soon prove so important for Nyasaland's Medical Department, the political maneuvers that effected this subversion are related here.

When the Colonial Development Bill of 1929 was first discussed on July 12, a number of MPs urged that "medical services" should be included in bill's list of "means" by which the fund could be used to further colonial development. Five days later, when the bill was discussed again, Under-Secretary of State for the Colonies William Lunn sought to allay these concerns, promising the MPs that health care would be available to those Africans who worked on the infrastructure projects funded by the CDA. Past experience, Lunn claimed, had shown "the wisdom of giving attention to the health conditions of those who labor in these great enterprises."[34] Lunn then attempted to move on to other matters.

But one MP was unsatisfied with this clarification. Lord Eustace Percy had served as a Conservative MP from Hastings since 1921. Though not a particularly prominent member of the Conservative Party, he was deeply interested in health and education. In the previous decade, he had served as parliamentary secretary to the Ministry of Health (1923) and president of the Board of Education (1924–1929).[35] Percy argued that the bill, as written, seemed to indicate to future officials that health-care projects were not a legitimate purpose for the CDF. If, Percy continued, grants for development of the health services "are to be permissible under the Bill, [they] will be admissible under Section I (I, 1)—'any other means.'" But, he insisted, "If you mention 'any other means' and specify one of those other means, as is done in the paragraph in the words 'including surveys,' we run very great risks of finding that health will be excluded."

Sir Oswald Mosley, a Labour MP who helped coordinate the new government's employment policies alongside Jimmy Thomas, tried to answer Lord Percy's question. "I hope," he said, "I can give some more encouragement than he found in the bill, because the governing words are—aiding and developing agriculture and industry. . . . It should be clear that, where you are dealing with the promotion of industry, the health of those engaged in industry is of primary concern."

Yet Percy—who, according to a biographer, had a reputation for being "pedantic" and "always ready to magnify small differences"—persisted: "I am afraid that, grammatically, I do not find comfort in those words."[36]

Mosley tried to quell Percy's concerns: "It would be a very narrow and very mistaken reading of the purposes of this Bill if the great human element, upon which, after all, all industrial efficiency rests in the first degree, was excluded from its purview."

Here, the physician and Unionist MP Vernon Davies entered the fray.[37] "Why not include [health services] specifically?" he asked Mosley.

Mosley was not known for his tolerance of criticism; within three years, he would leave the Labour Party to found the British Union of Fascists. By the late 1930s, he was best known as Adolf Hitler's chief British apologist. On this day, Davies's challenge brought Mosley to exasperation: "I have been trying for some five minutes to explain that it was included."

Davies, though, remained as unconvinced as Lord Percy: "With great respect to the honorable Baronet [Mosley], I do not agree with him."

Aided by Davies, Lord Percy pressed ahead, calling for amendments that would include the promotion of health and education in the explicitly listed purposes of the CDF. It was not enough, he added, to improve the health of laborers working for European employers. Improving the health of the entire "native community" had to be an explicitly stated aim.

When debate recommenced on the bill the next day, Mosley addressed Percy's request. Mosley acceded to the insertion of "the promotion of public health" as a purpose of the fund. But, he contended, the phrase "native community" should not be included because it might exclude "white settlers," "Indian settlers," and "Arabs." Mosley also argued that education "does not really fall within the scope of this bill." Education was, he explained, "a most important matter, but it falls under the ordinary colonial administration." These amendments passed without further discussion. The entire bill was approved by the House of Commons and the House of Lords and received the royal assent on July 26.

The Commons debate has been recounted here because health funding under the CDA would become an important part of the subsequent development of Nyasaland's government health sector. In contrast to the previous three decades of colonial rule, the number of government health-care facilities for Nyasaland's Africans expanded rapidly after the passage of the 1929 act. But this funding was made possible only by the persistent objections of a "pedant" (Percy) and a physician (Davies) in the House of Commons. The debate reveals how a few persistent politicians partially transformed a measure sold by Conservative and Labour leaders as an answer to domestic concerns into a fund that would aid the construction of hospitals in the colonies. In 1929, British unemployment was a crisis capable of overcoming the resistance to colonial spending in the UK Treasury. With this "emergency measure" virtually assured of passage, Percy and Davies were able to add health services to the law's original, more politically potent justification. With a few well-timed remarks, two little-known backbench MPs used their knowledge of the mechanics of power to help increase the availability of health care in far-flung corners of the empire.

Opening the Purse, Slightly

Officials in Nyasaland jumped at the opportunity to secure additional funds. In the autumn of 1929, Nyasaland's acting governor, Wilfred Bennett Davidson-Houston, wrote to Lord Passfield, the Labour government's secretary of state for the colonies and a prominent socialist reformer. The governor informed Passfield that he hoped to submit proposals for funding to the newly established Colonial Development Advisory Committee (CDAC), the group tasked with deciding on the merit of submissions to the CDF.[38]

At first prospects did not look good; the CDAC was already considering funding for a rail bridge over the Zambesi River, thereby connecting the port of Beira to Nyasaland by a continuous railway line.[39] But Nyasaland's new governor, Shenton Thomas, a former schoolteacher less than three months into his first Colonial Service assignment, insisted that the bridge was not enough. Thomas wrote to the Colonial Office on January 30, 1930, explaining why Nyasaland remained so poor, and what it would take to increase production:

> Money is necessary for development and the money has not been forthcoming. And, until the money is forthcoming, the country will not develop. . . . Roads in themselves will not produce crops; crops cannot be grown without skilled and systematic agricultural supervision; and that supervision will only be partially effective *unless it is exercised over a healthy population*.[40]

Governor Thomas's main request was to use the CDF to allow for an increase in Nyasaland's "standard revenue" from £300,000 (£17.1 million in 2016 prices) to £450,000 (£25.7 million in 2016 prices) for ten years (1930–1939).[41] The ability to devote domestic revenues to domestic expenditures would, Thomas explained, allow him to increase recurrent expenditure on priority areas such as health. In a February 24 debate in the House of Commons, Amery spoke approvingly of Thomas's proposal:

> Nyasaland has been a Treasury controlled territory, conducted, as such territories are apt to be, on the absolute minimum of expenditure . . . If we are to open up Nyasaland and its resources by this new connection with the sea [the Zambesi Bridge], it would be well worth while at the same time relaxing a little that extreme rigour which limits its medical services, its sanitary services, and its general educational and administrative services.[42]

In March 1930 the CDAC approved Thomas's proposal and urged expedited negotiations with the UK Treasury, which still held sole power over Nyasaland's standard revenue arrangement. In an April 11 letter to Treasury Secretary Philip Snowden, Under-Secretary of State for the Colonies Sir Samuel Wilson argued for a clean break with the parsimony of the past decade:

The natives are underfed and under paid ... such important social services as medical and sanitary work ... have been so restricted as to fall far below the standard normally attained by backward British Dependencies. ... The Protectorate should at least be maintained in a condition to avoid the grave public discredit which would attach to His Majesty's Government, both in this country and abroad, should the present scandalous state of Nyasaland attract attention.[43]

This time the Treasury agreed. Nyasaland's standard revenue was increased to £450,000, freeing the colonial administration to spend more of the taxes raised within the protectorate on domestic services. Nyasaland's recurrent expenditure on health rose immediately, even as the world entered a crushing economic depression. After barely moving during the 1920s—rising only from £29,804 in 1924 (£1.62 million in 2016 prices) to £33,191 in 1928 (£1.87 million in 2016 prices)—it increased to £42,496 in 1930 (£2.43 million in 2016 prices), then to £49,138 in 1934 (£3.17 million in 2016 prices).[44]

Even more important for the health sector was the development expenditure—that is, spending on new buildings and durable equipment—made possible by the CDF. During the campaign to raise Nyasaland's standard revenue, Governor Thomas had prepared a set of plans for CDAC consideration. In late 1929, he sent a circular to each of his departments—including the Medical Department—asking for proposals consistent with the aims of the CDA.[45] The Medical Department proposal included a request for £80,596 (£4.57 million in 2016 prices), with funding to be split roughly equally between the renovation of existing hospitals and dispensaries and the construction of new facilities.

These proposals were included in the governor's January 30, 1930, memorandum to the CDAC and were considered at a meeting on May 7.[46] While most of Nyasaland's other proposals were approved at this meeting, the CDAC asked Nyasaland to submit a more ambitious program of medical and sanitary improvement that reflected the expanded possibilities of the new standard revenue. This encouragement to request *more* funding for health care was unprecedented in Nyasaland's relationship with Whitehall and would scarcely be repeated again.

This enthusiasm for colonial health-care spending was in large part a result of the CDAC leadership's special interest in health. The chairman, Sir Basil Blackett, was a Calcutta-born son of missionaries who had worked for decades as a finance expert in the British civil service. Blackett had served as president of the British Social Hygiene Council, a government-funded body known before 1925 as the National Council for Combating Venereal Diseases.[47] During his tenure on the CDAC, health-related projects made up a large proportion of the grants awarded. In fiscal year 1930–1931, health accounted for 18 percent of grants approved by Blackett's CDAC. In 1931–1932 this figure rose to 44 percent.[48]

The CDAC's request that Nyasaland spend more on health care also had the support of other prominent figures in the Labour government. On June 26, 1930, Under-Secretary of State for the Colonies Thomas Drummond Shiels, a Scottish physician known for his sympathy for black African nationalist politicians and trade unionists, spoke in the House of Commons about the need for CDF support for health services in Nyasaland:

> The terms of reference of the Fund were broadly drawn, and it has been found possible to include ... schemes to develop and assist the public health service. ... There is no doubt that we have been hampered, especially in certain Colonies, such as Nyasaland, because of the former parsimoniousness of the Treasury, but we are now hopeful that in Nyasaland and other parts we may be able, with the help of the Colonial Development Fund, not only to assist in public health but also in the training of subordinate medical personnel and of midwives and in other ways to meet the very real need to which honorable Members have called attention.[49]

Even Snowden's Treasury echoed this encouragement, suggesting that Governor Thomas should submit "a complete scheme of development within the additional funds that will be available." Among the priorities set out by the Treasury for the development scheme were "measures to improve the physical condition of the natives" so as to facilitate increased production.[50]

By this point neither Shiels, Blackett, nor even the Treasury felt compelled to demonstrate any proof that colonial health schemes would aid employment in Britain. With the CDA passed, and the funds authorized, the Colonial Office felt free to pursue development as it saw fit.[51] In 1930 the CDAC complained, in its first interim report, that the schemes being submitted were too paltry. The Colonial Office responded by setting up a special committee to deploy public health specialists to the colonies to devise bolder plans for the CDAC.[52]

The Shircore Report of 1930

Seeking a new, more robust plan for Nyasaland's health services in short order, the Colonial Office requested the assistance of Dr. John Owen Shircore, the director of medical services in Tanganyika. By 1930 Shircore was an experienced hand. The son of a captain in the Indian Medical Service, he had studied in Edinburgh, London, and Cambridge before joining the Colonial Service in 1908. Shircore had begun his work as a medical officer in northern Nyasaland before joining the East African Medical Service during the First World War. During the 1920s, Shircore oversaw the establishment of a network of rural dispensaries staffed by "tribal dressers" in Tanganyika.[53] He also launched massively popular voluntary chemotherapeutic campaigns, treating more than 374,584 cases of yaws and 72,377 cases of syphilis with a preparation of bismuth sodium tartrate and soamin (an arsenical) that he had devised himself.[54] Shircore's work in Tanganyika demonstrated that though he was not blind to persistent Treasury demands for cost containment, he was unwilling to let fiscal concerns dictate all of his policies. He argued against using tryparsamide monotherapy to treat sleeping sickness, since in high doses the drug often caused atrophy of the optic nerve (and consequent vision loss) or even death. Shircore also advocated individual examinations of the sick over "wholesale blood examination of village populations," which "tends to destroy the confidence of the people . . . [and] results in obstruction and the concealment of cases."[55]

Shircore arrived in Zomba on August 9, 1930. Over the next forty days, he covered more than one thousand miles by motorcar, visiting native hospitals, European hospitals, and rural dispensaries. In his report on Nyasaland, submitted on September 20, Shircore was resolute about the need for far more spending. "Little progress has been made," he reported. "The department is merely in embryo."[56]

Shircore rendered bleak assessments of existing conditions. European hospitals were "adequate for their purpose," but African hospitals offered only 170 beds for an estimated African population of 1.4 million.[57] The quality of African facilities was, in his telling, desultory. Patients were housed in a wattle and daub hut in Chikwawa and in "dilapidated" buildings in Fort Manning and Kota-Kota. The accommodations for patients came in for particular criticism:

Drugs are adequate, but medical and domestic equipment, such as beds, blankets, sheets and pillows, require thorough overhauling. . . . Africans, unless dangerously ill or destitute, will not apply for the treatment as in-patients or stay in hospital unless reasonably well provided with food and comfort.[58]

Shircore called for substantial increases in facilities, staff, equipment, and training over the four-year period covered by the report. He proposed seventeen new African hospitals, to be equipped with adequate surgical supplies and diagnostic equipment, including X-ray machines. He recommended that thirty-six new dispensaries be added to the existing eighty-three.

Shircore also recommended more than doubling recurrent expenditure on personnel. This would allow for an increase in the number of medical officers from eleven to eighteen. The number of subassistant surgeons was to be increased from eight to twenty using recruits from Bombay. A bacteriologist was to be hired and a properly equipped laboratory constructed. The Sanitation Branch was to be expanded to two European health officers and eighty African sanitary inspectors.

Shircore's most ambitious proposal for personnel concerned the cadre of African hospital assistants. Over ten years, he planned to have hospital assistants replace the existing dispensers, who, he claimed, possessed "no knowledge of drugs and merely dole[d] out stock mixtures."[59] Instead of cursorily trained dispensers, Shircore envisioned at least one hospital assistant at every health facility, and at least one health facility for every twenty thousand people. Even assuming zero growth in Malawi's population, this ratio required the cadre of African hospital assistants to grow from eight to seventy. To reach this figure, Shircore proposed a government-run medical training school similar to one he had already established in Tanganyika.

Shircore's report was not a radical document. His total request for development expenditure was £110,325 over four years (£6.25 million in 2016 prices), exceeding Governor Thomas's original request to the CDAC by roughly £30,000.[60] Though he called for improved facilities and staffing at African hospitals, he did not propose to alter the status quo, in which the cost of inpatient care on a per-day basis was more than two times higher in European hospitals than in African hospitals.[61]

The CDAC approved most of Shircore's request, allotting £101,410 (£5.75 million in 2016 prices) to Nyasaland's Medical Department.[62] But during the depths of the Great Depression, the imperial Treasury scaled back the CDF, and Nyasaland's development plan with it.[63] As the Depression dampened revenues throughout the empire, calls for ambitious schemes turned to demands for cuts. Ultimately, the Treasury approved CDF expenditures for Nyasaland's Medical Department of only £78,284 (£4.61 million in 2016 prices).

Nevertheless, CDF spending represented more infrastructure funding than Nyasaland's Medical Department had ever received before. By 1938, twelve new or renovated hospitals had been completed. The total number of hospital beds had tripled since 1930. The funding proved sufficient to build thirty-six new rural dispensaries and three new maternity and child-welfare clinics.[64] The newly constructed Zomba African Hospital was opened, staffed by two medical officers, two nursing sisters, and a pathologist, and equipped with a new laboratory and X-ray machine.[65] Personnel remained the largest bottleneck to expanded access. The number of medical officers rose from eleven in 1930 to fourteen in 1933, but it would not exceed fifteen until after the Second World War. The number of subassistant surgeons on the government payroll rose from eight in 1930 to ten in 1933, but increased no further during the decade. Though the government-run Medical Training School opened in Zomba in 1936 with training programs for nurses, midwives, sanitary inspectors, laboratory assistants, and dressers, Shircore's plans to train a large cadre of hospital assistants at the school were, for the moment, unrealized.[66]

The new development funds and increased recurrent spending changed the quantity and quality of medical care at government hospitals.[67] In the early 1930s, medical officer Walter Gopsill was deployed to Cholo, a district in Nyasaland's south. Before 1930, the station had only a small outpatient dispensary for a district of fifty-three thousand people. Nyasaland's Public Works Department used the funding to erect a one-hundred-bed hospital. Gopsill was also heartened that "the native staff at the hospital had considerably increased and improved." He worked alongside "well trained dressers, and dispensers, [and] nurses."[68] Still, some aspects of care remained poor. Funding to feed hospital patients was so paltry that Gopsill required inpatients with venereal diseases to supply their own "bags of mealie meal."[69] He ruefully observed that his hospitals were only provided with sufficient bed sheets just before the governor's official visits.[70]

Conclusion

The impoverishment of Nyasaland's medical department by the 1919 TZR loan guarantee has postcolonial parallels. Multilateral and bilateral aid agencies have consistently favored large, capital-intensive projects over health and education. Muckraking exposés and confessional memoirs have depicted loans from the World Bank, USAID, and other agencies to build dams, roads, and railways in poor countries as ploys to profit European, American, and (more recently) Chinese manufacturers and financiers, prop up puppet dictators, and entrap poor countries in debt.[71] The pleas of Colonial Office officials to the Treasury to lessen the crushing burden of the TZR loan guarantee on Nyasaland's population also find echoes in the moral obligations invoked by the international debt relief ("Jubilee") movement of the 1990s and 2000s. Neither set of campaigners would accept the claims of scarcity that their critics used to justify inaction.

A railway loan might seem tangential to the history of health care in Nyasaland. Admittedly, portraying the loan as a part of the story of neglect in the history of health care in Malawi does involve a kind counterfactual reasoning. It suggests, implicitly, that if Nyasaland had not been burdened with the debt, officials may well have chosen to invest some of the available funds in health services for Africans.[72] There is no way to prove that they would have done so. But this "road not traveled" was quite plausible, particularly given the number of officials in Zomba (e.g., Shircore, Thomas) and Whitehall (e.g., Ormsby-Gore, Amery) who expressed embarrassment at the "scandalous" level of health-care spending during the 1920s and early 1930s. Even more convincingly, as soon as the burden of Nyasaland's debt was relieved, even slightly, by the CDA of 1929, health-care spending increased much more quickly. In any study of budgetary priorities, it is necessary to look not only at a single line item such as health, but also at those line items that claimed significant shares of available resources. The loan severely constrained the resources of the government of Nyasaland. But officials recognized that it was not, in fact, truly impossible for Nyasaland to spend more on health care, for the railway loan was a choice, and not a necessary one. For this reason, the origins of the TZR loan remain an indispensable part of the history of health care in colonial Nyasaland.

The parliamentary and bureaucratic histories demonstrate the influence of deft, timely, and dogged maneuvers by elite reformists to secure greater expenditures for the colonized. As the following chapters demonstrate, a number of doctors in the colonial and postcolonial eras were not satisfied with the standard of care they were able to offer patients, and they insisted on more. In some moments their complaints went unanswered, but at others they did result in new facilities, new equipment, new drugs, and more staff. Events in the 1920s and early 1930s were the first such demonstration of the power of elite reformists.

3

"We Have to Wait for Riots and Disturbances," 1931–1941

Prelude

Nicotine was dead. The news spread quickly among the crowd gathered on the dirt road outside Monkey Bay District Hospital. The normally bustling shop stalls hawking sodas and *mandazis* (fried dough) had been shuttered. Policemen and soldiers stood guard inside the hospital gate. Huddled together in small groups, the adults spoke in hushed tones, their eyes downcast. No one wailed with grief, not yet. Those loud lamentations would come two days later, at Nicotine's funeral. Incongruously, a girl skipped in the road in front of the hospital, her face alight with an unknowing smile. A young man chided her: "Simuli ndi chisoni?" ("Have you no sympathy?"). The girl stopped, looked about, and quickly adopted the somber expression evident on all the other faces.

Nicotine was the nickname given to a good-natured man in his early twenties who always seemed to have a cigarette in his hand. This was unusual in Malawi, where although tobacco remained the country's leading export, few could afford a cigarette habit. Nicotine lived with his grandmother and had recently received an impressive score on the national secondary school examination. One bystander reported witnessing Nicotine being beaten by a policeman; another recounted seeing blood pouring from his nose.

When I arrived in town, the action was already over. From the beachfront hostel where I had been spending a weekend relaxing, I had heard gunshots. After waiting for a few hours to ensure there were no more shots, I walked into town to ask what had happened. Earlier that day, I was told, people from the fishing village of Masasa had gathered outside a local government building, where they had heard that their local hereditary chiefs and elected officials were holding a secret meeting with a representative from Mota Engil, a publicly traded multinational corporation based in Portugal with over $2 billion in revenue in 2014. During that year, the Malawi government and Mota Engil

No More to Spend. Paul Farmer, Oxford University Press (2020). © Oxford University Press.
DOI: 10.1093/oso/9780190066192.001.0001

had been in talks about plans to build a five-star resort hotel.[1] In the words of one Mota Engil promotional article, it would be a "ranch-style resort, with a beautiful pool, a golf course, and an inlet connecting the pool to the lake," to be operated by "a world-famous brand name hotelier."[2] The planning process had become complicated a few months earlier when Masasa residents had obtained a copy of closely held plans showing that the resort would displace their entire lakeshore village.

After months passed with barely any official response to their complaints, Masasa residents were angry. Most had already been displaced seven years earlier when the government had seized their verdant plots to make room for housing for employees of another company. Since then the displaced had built thatch-roofed huts on a beach, where most eked out a living by fishing. Few believed the politicians who promised a resort would bring jobs. Already an exclusive $400-per-night lodge was operating on a peninsula visible from their village. But signs on the outskirts of this retreat warned residents that trespassers would be shot, and it employed only a handful of locals. The soon-to-be-displaced had been promised monetary compensation, but the plot where they suspected they would be moved was suitable for neither fishing nor farming.

When the region's "traditional authority," Nankumba, left a meeting on the afternoon of February 3, 2015, he was met by an angry crowd. The assembly had been stoked to a furor by a rumor that he was planning to sign away their land. What happened next was the subject of much debate among local Malawians and in cursory press reports (none written on the basis of first-hand knowledge or detailed research). The account that follows is the consensus view of most of the dozen people I interviewed in Monkey Bay.

The Masasa protesters destroyed Nankumba's car, which was rumored to have been given to him by Mota Engil. Nankumba was bloodied but not gravely injured by protestors. After being pelted with rocks thrown by some of the protestors, the police opened fire on the crowd using live rounds. The bullets struck at least seven people. Nicotine died from his injuries, while the others survived. Some of the victims were not even involved in the protest. Nicotine was not even from Masasa.

During the shooting the protestors fled, but they were far from done expressing their displeasure. A few men ran into town and ransacked a local bar owned by Ward Councilor Bulireni. Bulireni had once been a local favorite. He had run for office unsuccessfully twice before winning over the voters in his last campaign with displays of generosity, such as letting constituents use his truck for funerals. But he had fallen out of favor when it was rumored that he was among those who signed away Masasa residents' land to Mota Engil.

This episode included all the outrage and David-and-Goliath drama one would expect from a muckraking magazine article. But even in the Malawian press the coverage was sparse and one-sided. A Chichewa-language broadcast on the independent radio station Zodiak FM that evening featured an interview with Mangochi's police inspector. None of the protestors were interviewed, nor were other witnesses. Newspapers quoted statements from local politicians following the "fracas," but no reporters interviewed the villagers threatened with displacement or even the victims of the police shootings.[3] The foreign press did not report on the event at all.

Not that it would have been easy for reporters to discern what had happened even if they had come to Monkey Bay. No one I talked to around Monkey Bay admitted being involved in the protests. Fearing police reprisals, the men of Masasa found shelter outside their village that night. In later statements, Mota Engil disclaimed any interest in building the lakeside resort, explaining that it was more of a favor to the government. A great conflagration had erupted, then disappeared from view. The episode barely registered in the media; as in the 1930s, Malawians were seen by many outsiders as essentially placid.

Still, the protests had lasting effects. Two months later a leading daily newspaper published an op-ed criticizing the protestors for throwing up "disincentives to investment" and denying themselves "thousands of jobs."[4] There would be no compensation paid, by either Mota Engil or the government, to Nicotine's family or to the six who had been injured. Yet despite the scarce and biased media coverage, Mota Engil canceled its planned $50 million project. Malawian president Peter Mutharika continued to plead with the company to reconsider.[5] The protestors had proved surprisingly powerful.

Introduction

Officials in Nyasaland had yet to spend their last CDF dollars before they began to face backlash from London. The perception in both the Colonial Office and the Treasury was that the Medical Department had expanded more than enough. This perception became more prominent in the years after Basil Blackett, the chairman of the CDAC and advocate for colonial medical and public health services, died in a car crash in August 1935.

Intra-office debates about the need for further expansion had begun even earlier. Each side deployed its favored statistics to paint a drastically different portrait of Nyasaland's health services. In May 1935 a Colonial Office official in London sent a letter to the Treasury arguing that because Nyasaland's number of medical officers compared favorably with neighboring colonies on a per capita basis, increases in recurrent expenditure could be stopped.[6] Writing in dissent, Nyasaland's director of medical services argued that Nyasaland remained an impoverished colony with much lower per capita recurrent health-care expenditure than other British colonies in southern and eastern Africa.[7] Governor Harold Kittermaster added that on a per capita basis, Nyasaland's government spent less on health care (7.4 pence per capita) than any other dependency in East Africa.[8] Still, Colonial Office staff persisted in depicting Nyasaland as a colony amply served by medical services.[9]

The Colonial Office's argument that enough had been done for Nyasaland marked a decided change in focus from just five years earlier. By late 1935 Lord Passfield was no longer colonial secretary, and the UK government was run by a coalition of Labour, Conservatives, and Liberals. Two downturns in global demand (one in 1929–1933 and another in 1937–1938) led to plummeting prices for the region's mineral and agricultural commodities, leaving colonial treasuries with lower revenues. Nyasaland's African population found less of the wage labor that helped them pay hut taxes.[10] These political and economic shifts drastically changed the appetite for colonial development funding in London. The Colonial Office began demanding spending cutbacks. Marcus Greenhill, who had spent sixteen years at the Colonial Office in London, complained that government medical provision had expanded far too quickly. "Nyasaland," he opined, "has a service far in advance of its present stage of development including a large number of hospitals and clinics, etc. which it cannot use to the fullest extent."[11]

The de Boer Report

Not everyone agreed with the call for spending cuts. Once again, the rebuke came from a veteran member of the colonial medical services. Henry Speldewinde de Boer became Nyasaland's director of medical services in

1938. Born in Ceylon, he had studied medicine in London, then served in the Royal Army Medical Corps during the First World War. He had already spent twelve years as a medical officer and medical administrator in Kenya, Northern Rhodesia, and Uganda, and was known for his expertise in malariology as well as maternal and child welfare.[12] Immediately upon his arrival in Nyasaland, de Boer set off on a tour of the protectorate. In his subsequent report to the Colonial Office, he opened with blunt language:

> The present services are completely inadequate to touch even the fringe of our medical problem. They have not made true contact with the population as a whole, nor can they claim to have gained the confidence of any but a small section of the people. With our existing hospitals and dispensaries, it is doubtful whether [we] have made any serious reduction in the sickness and mortality rates.[13]

Africans, de Boer observed, did not believe rural medical services were efficacious. There were ninety dispensaries throughout the country, but de Boer argued that the dispensers were held in such low regard by Africans that "the average number of patients seen at most of our dispensaries does not exceed 15 a day," and most presented only with minor complaints.[14] "Can this be taken as an indication that there are no genuinely sick persons in our African villages?" he asked. "What little we do know goes to prove the contrary!"

The answer to these deficiencies was not, de Boer argued, a halt in the construction of new facilities. In fact, he called for a rapid increase in hospital beds and new dispensaries.[15] But he also focused on improving the training of medical staff. Noting that the hospital assistant training program envisioned by Shircore had not been undertaken, de Boer renewed his call, aiming for an increase in the number of African hospital assistants in government service from 15 in 1938 to 116 by 1947. He also proposed significant increases in the numbers of medical officers (from 14 to 20) and European nursing sisters (from 12 to 30). His proposal called for additional capital expenditure of £122,766 (£7.55 million in 2016 prices) over eight years and a doubling of annual recurrent expenditure by 1947.

De Boer proposed fiscal measures to fund his program. These proposals reflected his understanding of Nyasaland's role as a labor reserve for southern Africa.[16] He suggested that industries benefiting from migrant labor take on additional responsibilities for the health of Africans remaining in or returning to Nyasaland: "Every batch of returning natives includes one or more individuals bringing back . . . diseases that may flare up and affect adversely the balance of nature that has existed. Our Africans are generally admitted to be our country's only important asset. Can we say that it is not a wasting asset?"[17] In 1938 Southern Rhodesia remitted six of the twenty shillings it collected in taxes from Nyasaland's migrants to the Nyasaland government; de Boer suggested that the entire amount be sent back to Nyasaland. He also proposed that the Union of South Africa levy a tax on Nyasaland natives living within its borders, to be remitted to Nyasaland. In addition, the Witwatersrand Native Labour Association (WENELA), a recruiting organization that drew recruits from Nyasaland for South Africa's mines, should be "asked to contribute £2 [£123 in 2016 prices] per head of labor recruited in Nyasaland."

De Boer knew that past proposals had not been fully implemented. He lamented: "The files of my department make for very sad reading." His predecessors' demands had "either been neglected completely or in approval so pared down and attenuated, that little progress eventuated."[18] Indeed, Nyasaland's recurrent budget for health care had been flat, in inflation-adjusted pounds sterling, since 1934. While the Medical Department had claimed more than 10.1 percent of the protectorate's total recurrent budget in 1930, this had dropped to 6.5 percent by 1939.[19]

The response to de Boer's report clearly demonstrated the conflict between Zomba and London over the quality of medical services that the population deserved. In a note accompanying de Boer's report in May 1939, Nyasaland governor Donald Mackenzie-Kennedy expressed his support for the plan, saying its enactment would "avoid a continuance of what can only be described as a sham and a pretense—hospitals and dispensaries, inadequately staffed and insufficiently supervised."[20] Officials at the Colonial Office, however, did not agree. Edmund Boyd, the principal private secretary to the colonial secretary, praised de Boer's "superabundant energy and enthusiasm" but dismissed his proposals as the unreasonable wishes of an administrator "coming fresh from Uganda, where medical and public health standards have reached a pretty high standard."[21] Arthur O'Brien, a member of the Colonial Advisory Medical Committee who had joined de Boer for part of his tour of Nyasaland, opined that de Boer's proposals for funding recurrent costs through charges on the governments of Southern Rhodesia and South Africa were not "practical." The only proposal in de Boer's report for which O'Brien offered wholehearted support was his call for improving housing and hospital accommodation for European settlers. The existing European hospitals,

O'Brien noted, were "disgraceful" and should be improved immediately. On the other hand, the expansion of African medical services could be "more gradual and spread over a longer period."[22]

Gerard Clauson, a Sanskrit philologist and a rising star at the Colonial Office then serving as head of the recently established Social Services Department, was more blunt.[23] He dismissed de Boer's proposals as "prohibitively expensive" before expanding on his view that Nyasaland's medical services for Africans were, in fact, too lavish:

> It seems to me fantastic to take a native who all his life has probably never slept anywhere except on the ground or a few boards and [when] he gets into the hospital to put him into a bed with blankets, sheets and other appurtenances and wait on him hand and foot. The solution seems to be to imitate the French who provide much humbler accommodation at their hospitals, [in] which the patient can be moved with his family and be nursed principally by them, the Government providing treatment but not attendance and food.[24]

So while Nyasaland's director of medical services saw medical provision as "completely inadequate," and the governor thought it a "sham," Clauson argued that African patients were being pampered. Bedding, food, and professional attendance were, to his mind, more than any African patient in Nyasaland should reasonably expect. The answer was not more spending and more care for the sick, but rather less of both. De Boer thought African hospitals had empty beds because accommodation and equipment remained dreadful; Clauson thought patients in those hospitals enjoyed what was, to them, unbelievable luxury.

Doctors in Nyasaland did not share Clauson's opinions, particularly on feeding patients. Reporting on medical services in 1939 after a cut to the recurrent health-care budget, de Boer complained that it was "becoming more difficult to provide patients admitted with a satisfactory diet. In a country where the average inhabitant suffers from defective nutrition, good feeding is an important part of curative medicine."[25] Medical officers saw patients' kin nursing and feeding the sick in their hospitals each day. Though grateful for such caregiving, medical officers considered this a complement to, rather than a substitute for, trained nursing and hospital feeding.[26]

Clauson penned his critical response to the de Boer report on August 8, 1939. Less than a month later, on September 1, Germany invaded Poland.

In response, the United Kingdom and France declared war on Germany. It had been difficult to secure finances for expanding medical services before the war began; it proved impossible to do so during the war. As one official remembered, the war brought with it a new "disease" called "Algef" (*après la guerre est fini*; "after the war is over"), a refrain that became the "customary direction on nearly all new proposals."[27] Not until after the war did Nyasaland's health services become an imperial priority once more.

To what can we attribute Whitehall's distaste for health-care spending in Nyasaland during the mid- to late 1930s? Surely the Great Depression and the advent of the Second World War were significant factors, but as will become apparent in the next section, health services in other colonies garnered far more attention during this period. Clauson and officials in Whitehall rebutted de Boer's report so readily in part because Nyasaland was seen as politically placid. While Northern Rhodesia and British West Africa and the West Indies erupted in strikes and riots, Nyasaland's officials reported no episodes of great concern. In an era when health care was used as a political palliative, Nyasaland's Africans seemed to issue no cry worthy of response.

This is not to say that Nyasaland's Africans were, in fact, quiet. In 1932 an anti-witchcraft movement spread rapidly across the protectorate. People were made to drink a concoction known as *mchape* (a derivation of the word *kuchapa*, which means "to wash"), which *mchape* leaders claimed would harm only practitioners of sorcery. The movement spread like wildfire, in part because it helped discontented young men, who often led the *mchape* sessions, counter the authority of their elders.[28] But while officials took note, they were not terribly concerned.[29] Indirect rule continued to function, and production on European estates was not much affected. This was not the kind of unrest that would spur increased health-care spending.

Even when they encountered more explicitly subversive rhetoric, colonial officials remained unimpressed. In 1932 a government clerk named George Simeon Mwase sent officials in Zomba a manuscript that included a provocative biography of the revolutionary preacher John Chilembwe, as well as his own criticism of contemporary race relations and living conditions. But as historian Richard Rotberg has noted, Mwase "had long been regarded by many white administrators as an excessively opinionated, 'harmless,' compulsive writer of memoranda and tracts."[30]

In sum, leading colonial officials of the mid- and late 1930s were not nearly as devoted to colonial health as their predecessors had been and saw no imperative to spend more on medical care. During these years, political dissent and anti-witchcraft movements did not much concern them. European estate owners were the major economic power in the protectorate and were able to pursue profits unimpeded by unrest. Political legitimacy seemed assured.

Imperial Disquiet and the 1940 Colonial Development and Welfare Act

Elsewhere in the British Empire, officials did not share this sense of security. On the morning of May 29, 1935, the commissioner of Northern Rhodesia's Central Province called the colony's chief secretary to report a crisis. A thousand natives living in a town adjacent to the Roan Antelope copper mine in Luanshya District had marched to the compound offices. The commissioner begged for troops, but by the time they arrived blood had already been spilled. Local police—Africans led by white officers—attempted to disperse the crowd by charging into their midst. In response, some protestors hurled stones. The police superintendent attempted to frighten the protestors by firing shots into the air, but some of his subordinates interpreted the shots as an instruction to open fire. They sprayed bullets randomly into a crowd of miners, domestic servants, and local villagers. By the time the guns fell silent they had killed six and wounded twenty-two others.[31]

The Luanshya strike, and others across Northern Rhodesia's Copperbelt, shook the colonial administration. Governor Hubert Young commissioned a report on the "disturbances," which concluded that a major proximate cause of the strikes was news of a tax increase in the mining areas.[32] The entire incident stirred reformers to question what Africans in Northern Rhodesia received in return for their tax payments. Malaria, pneumonia, influenza, and intestinal infections were so rampant in the mines that Luanshya was known among Africans as "Death Valley." Despite the high morbidity and mortality rates, mine management had not built a hospital for Africans.[33] Shortly after the massacre, Colonial Office adviser and CDAC member Sir Alan Pim made Northern Rhodesia the focus of the last in a series of reports on financial administration in British Africa. His report, published in 1938, criticized the funneling of Northern Rhodesia's resource revenues to public coffers and private accounts in Britain and called for additional expenditures on health, education, and infrastructure.[34] Pim lamented that a development scheme for improvement of medical and public health services, submitted to the CDAC in 1936, had been awarded only £20,000 (£1.28 million in 2016 prices).[35] Health care was not yet a significant part of the response to burgeoning colonial unrest.

Subsequent episodes would lead to a shift in the role of health care in the metropolitan response. As Pim and others pondered the factors leading to riots in Northern Rhodesia, labor actions in British holdings in the Caribbean stoked even more concern about the direction of imperial policy. In June 1937 workers in the oil fields of Trinidad began a sit-down strike, demanding an end to racial discrimination in the workplace, unemployment insurance, workmen's compensation, and trade union recognition. Strikes proliferated around the island, growing to include dockworkers; laborers on sugar, cocoa, and coconut plantations; domestic servants; and some government employees.[36] In July laborers in Barbados rioted in Bridgetown and burned sugarcane fields in the countryside.[37] Fourteen people were shot dead by police. In October thousands of cocoa growers in the Gold Coast announced a boycott of "non-essential" European goods and a holdup of sales to buyers who had colluded to lower producer prices.[38] By the close of April 1938 the disquiet had reached Jamaica. Sugarcane workers on an estate of the West Indian Sugar Company went on strike during the harvest, protesting low and irregular pay and dismal lodging. Within two days, four protesters were dead and another thirteen were injured. Dockworkers and the unemployed in Kingston set fire to buildings, while firefighters threatened to join the strike unless their wages were increased.[39] The People's National Party, established by Jamaican attorney and protest leader Norman Manley in September 1938, campaigned on a platform of free universal secondary education and health care.[40]

Manley was not the only person in a position of influence who believed health and education would be of interest to newly restive colonial publics. Social services were foremost in the mind of Malcolm MacDonald, a thirty-six-year-old MP appointed to serve as secretary of state for the colonies in Neville Chamberlain's Conservative government in May 1938. MacDonald agreed with Labour MPs who demanded a royal commission be appointed to investigate the "disturbances" in the West Indies. In a memo calling for a royal commission, MacDonald argued that one necessary response to the unrest would be improved social services, financed in part by new imperial grants.[41] Labour MP Arthur Creech Jones also made this link between unrest and social service spending explicit in a speech before the House of Commons:

The truth is that until riots and disturbances occurred and we had unrest beginning to sweep from one end of our Colonial Empire to the other, very little was really being done [in social services]. . . . It is a sad commentary on our method of government when we have to wait for riots and disturbances to force us to do what is . . . right.[42]

Such rhetoric had already proven successful. By the time Creech Jones made this speech, MacDonald had announced that the prime minister and the Treasury had both agreed to his call for the appointment of a royal commission.[43] The commission's terms of reference—"to investigate the social and economic conditions [in the British West Indies], and matters connected therewith, and to make recommendations"—were broad and vague, but the members knew they had been tasked with finding an antidote to the recent unrest.[44]

Over the next eighteen months, as the commission did its work, MacDonald prepared to use its findings to announce a fundamental overhaul of the CDA. He and others in the Colonial Office believed that imperial grants should be vastly increased, from the existing £1 million per year to £10 million per year (£605 million in 2016 prices). And in contrast to the grants given under the existing CDA, MacDonald believed funding should cover recurrent as well as capital expenses for health and education.[45]

In 1939, as the specter of war loomed ever larger, MacDonald stressed the impact that development spending could have on Britain's standing in the world and, more practically, on its defense. MacDonald had been a labor organizer and knew how to foster a sense of crisis. He used these skills within the cabinet to argue for colonial development. As MacDonald asserted in a Colonial Office meeting on December 9, 1938, "It was an essential part of [Britain's] defense policy that her reputation as a Colonial power should be unassailable."[46] His efforts to drum up concern about colonial stability were aided by recent events. Over the summer, dockworkers had halted trade with strikes in Port Sudan (April–May 1939), Dar es Salaam (July 1939), and Mombasa (July–August 1939).[47] Few of the striking workers and rioting subjects throughout the empire had uttered slogans calling for health care and education, but MacDonald and others portrayed social services as an effective and economical palliative for political unrest.

For the moment, the prospects for actual colonial development spending remained dim. Two weeks after Britain declared war on Germany, a Treasury official chastised the CDAC for continuing to approve colonial development proposals: "We are not unmindful of the importance which your Secretary of State attaches to social services and economic development in the Colonies ... but first things must come first. ... We shall have to resign ourselves to stand still now."[48] MacDonald retorted that his approach to colonial development would avert costly unrest during the war. Even more important, it would improve Britain's standing abroad, particularly in the United States, thereby helping to ensure the empire remained intact in a postwar settlement.[49]

Treasury officials continued to object to the use of imperial funds for recurrent social service expenditures, which they believed would put "the Colonies on the dole from henceforth and forever." Still, MacDonald would not relent, replying that it was "essential to get away from the old principle that Colonies can only have what they themselves can pay for: they must have what a first-class Colonial power may reasonably be expected to provide." The Treasury finally yielded, agreeing in principle to the funding of both capital and recurrent expenditures.[50] The Colonial Office agreed that a single source of funding, voted annually by Parliament, should be capped at £5 million. The Treasury, for its part, had agreed to forgive £11 million of the total £15 million in debts owed by the colonies to the Imperial Exchequer.[51]

MacDonald had secured the necessary concessions from the Treasury. In a decision that angered Labour MPs, the prime minister's cabinet decided that the Royal Commission was so critical of British policy that it would not be published in full.[52] The report itself was not a revolutionary screed. It attributed some of the problems in the West Indies to the "moral standard" of the "negro population." The authors did, however, highlight the many grievances presented by members of the "negro" and "coloured" populations, including racial discrimination, the lack of support for peasant agriculture, and laws against strikes. In line with MacDonald's campaign for provision of social services, the report devoted many pages to the woefully inadequate provision of health care and education. Nevertheless, the report focused on the West Indies in its call for expanded auxiliary training, more rural clinics and hospitals, and far greater spending on preventive medicine. Increased spending on health services, according to the report's authors, was an integral part of any imperial response to unrest on the islands.[53]

Chamberlain's cabinet did permit MacDonald to publish the commission's summary recommendations alongside the "Statement of Policy on Colonial Development and Welfare."[54] The "Statement of Policy" was only six pages long, and the Colonial Office and Treasury had traded drafts in heated debate for months. The final statement announced a new colonial development policy, in which "assistance will be available not only for schemes involving capital expenditure necessary for Colonial development in the widest sense but also for helping to meet recurrent expenditure in the Colonies on certain services such as agriculture, education, health and housing."[55] The Colonial Development and Welfare bill moved uneventfully to passage, receiving the royal assent on July 17, 1940.[56]

The Colonial Development and Welfare (CDW) Act of 1940 was a dividend of disquiet. The labor unrest of the mid- and late-1930s and the outbreak of war furnished MacDonald with powerful political arguments capable of overcoming the long-standing objections of the Treasury.[57] Colonial Office reports and speeches by Labour MPs had stressed the need for social welfare in the colonies even before the "disturbances" in the West Indies, but the threat to imperial legitimacy that the unrest represented helped soften the objections of the Treasury and other skeptics.

Why did health and education spending seem a logical response to labor unrest? After all, investigations of the protests in Northern Rhodesia, Trinidad, Barbados, and Jamaica pointed to taxes, low pay, and poor working conditions as the causes, not the level of social service provision.[58] The historian Stephen Constantine argues that much of the answer lies in a spirit of imperial altruism. There was, however, a more self-interested motivation for the new departure. For officials in the Colonial Office, it was more politically palatable to propose increased health and education spending than to contemplate fundamental changes to an extractive and exploitative political economy. The sites of protest, such as the Luanshya mine and the West Indies Sugar Company plantation, were owned by companies registered in Britain that reaped tremendous profits from the mineral wealth and cheap labor available in the colonies. It was more acceptable to investors—British voters and, quite often, British politicians—to spend tax dollars on nurses and teachers than to lessen profits with higher wages.[59] Spending on social services was therefore an attempt to quiet colonized publics without making more fundamental changes to the imperial economic system.[60]

The fate of Nyasaland provides further support for this argument. Economically insignificant and comparatively unaffected by labor unrest, Nyasaland garnered only a small share of the debt relief and new funding made available by the passage of the CDW Act. The act only decreased Nyasaland's outstanding debt for the Trans-Zambesi Railroad loan guarantee from £550,000 (£32.4 million in 2016 prices) to £300,000 (£17.6 million in

2016 prices). Thus, Nyasaland was relieved of less than half of its debt, far less than the overall share of colonial debt forgiven by the Imperial Exchequer (more than two-thirds).[61]

At the start of the war, Nyasaland's medical officials struggled to even maintain existing programs. This was clear in the rapid demise of a government-run nutrition intervention. An ambitious nutrition survey began in three villages in Nkhotakota District in September 1938. Early results revealed that many people did not receive enough calories, particularly in the months before the harvest. In response, study director Benjamin Platt called for £10,000 per year (£605,000 in 2016 prices) for three years for "nutrition development units" (NDUs), multidisciplinary centers that would support agricultural diversification, fisheries, forestry, animal husbandry, maternity and child welfare centers, sanitation, and handicrafts.[62]

The plan foundered quickly. After the British rout at Dunkirk and the fall of France to the Nazis, officials in London drastically curtailed the budget, to £1,025 per year for three years.[63] As the war continued, officials in the Colonial Office and new leadership in Nyasaland made clear there was no more money for heady ideas. When the NDUs' three-year budget ran out in 1943, that program was also terminated and its staff reassigned to other duties.

The war depleted staff and supplies throughout Nyasaland's government medical system. Initially de Boer reported that despite the withdrawal of staff to aid the war effort, only three dispensaries had closed.[64] But in 1940, when Italy joined the Axis, another five government medical officers were released for military service in North Africa. Within two years the number of medical officers had fallen from eighteen to ten.[65] African hospital assistants were put in charge of daily operations at district hospitals in Chiradzulu, Chikwawa, Upper Shire, Ntcheu, Dedza, Dowa, Kasungu, and Nkhata Bay.[66] When the council of chiefs in Lilongwe District requested additional rural dispensaries in 1942, Governor Richards informed them that newly trained African auxiliaries were unavailable to staff any new facilities because they had been recruited to the military.[67]

Some remaining medical officers resorted to uncommon sacrifice. On the cusp of retirement, Shircore returned to Nyasaland in 1942. He wrote to the director of medical services, explaining that there was a "considerable population" in his district (Karonga) "for whom there are no immediate medical facilities." Sick patients in an area called Mlale faced an "arduous journey" to reach his hospital. Africans carried to the hospital were often so ill they died on the way or shortly after arrival. Shircore suggested renovating a building in Mlale owned by the estate of a European farmer. The building, he explained, could be used as a government dispensary.[68] Standard policy at that time was to deny requests for new dispensaries unless construction was financed out of the budgets of native authorities, who kept a small share of hut tax revenues. Mlale's native authority, Chief Kyungu, wanted to see the new dispensary built but said he lacked the funds to pay for it. Shircore donated £100 (£4,549 in 2016 prices) out of his own savings to pay for the building, in which he planned to live and to practice medicine.[69] Chief Kyungu and the governor gratefully accepted this offer. Neither Shircore's frustration nor his determination were unique. Chapter 5 explores further the unwillingness of medical officers to accept what they considered to be low standards of medical provision. Shircore's insistence on better care for Africans in his 1930 report might be interpreted as a manifestation of a professional imperative in a setting of heavy morbidity. Yet this episode points to another, deeper motivation: a sentimental commitment to the people of Malawi, a commitment that went beyond even the strictest of professional standards. Shircore was not only willing to complain about the inadequacies of care for Africans; he was also willing to devote his retirement and his savings to their remedy.

The dedication of European doctors proved all the more necessary because the Colonial Office was unwilling to train Nyasaland's African population in medicine. In fact, even when a remarkable young African proved enterprising enough to gain medical education outside the empire, Whitehall would not allow him to fulfill his lifelong dream of returning to Nyasaland to care for his countrymen. Born in a village outside Kasungu in 1898, Hastings Kamuzu Banda had left Nyasaland (or, as it was then known, the British Central African Protectorate) as a teenager to work as a janitor in a Southern Rhodesian hospital and a miner in South Africa. He secured a scholarship from the African Methodist Episcopal Church to study in the United States. After graduating from secondary school in Ohio, Banda began his undergraduate education at the University of Indiana before transferring to the University of Chicago. He then enrolled in medical school at Meharry Medical College, which he completed in 1937. Shortly thereafter, he left for Edinburgh to obtain the UK qualifications he would need to complete his stated goal of practicing in his native Nyasaland. After he had successfully completed this final task, the Livingstonia Mission—where he had planned to go—informed him in 1941 that he would not be able to work for them after all, because a group of white nurses insisted that they would not work with an African doctor. After much handwringing, the Colonial Office offered Banda a job as a medical officer in Nyasaland, but only on the condition that he not seek to interact socially with white doctors. Offended, Banda refused the offer, and instead took up work as a general practitioner—for patients of all races—in London.[70] The Colonial Office's concerns with the health of Africans did not, it appeared, surpass their trepidation about disturbing the racial order.[71]

Conclusion

As chapter 2 demonstrates, the Colonial Office used unemployment in the United Kingdom to garner funds for colonial development in the late 1920s. In the late 1930s the Colonial Office secured additional funds through the deft exploitation of metropolitan fears about colonial labor unrest. Yet while Nyasaland's Medical Department benefited from the 1929 CDA, a decade later Nyasaland was less of a priority. Both Shircore and de Boer wrote reports on the sorry state of its medical services, but they were received quite differently. When Shircore had been invited to write his report in 1930, he submitted his work to the sympathetic Basil Blackett at the CDAC. De Boer had no such support. Officials in Whitehall were unmoved by his apparently unsolicited report. In 1929 the special attention of a few key MPs rendered Nyasaland an object of imperial concern. A decade later the protectorate was known only for its relative political calm and economic insignificance. While other imperial subjects engaged in deadly riots and costly strikes, Nyasaland's Africans seemed to pose few commensurate threats. Health services would suffer for this seeming placidity.

This chapter and the previous one also demonstrate something else. The scathing tone of both the Shircore and de Boer reports provides further support for an emerging historiographic understanding of the differences between colonial doctors and other colonial administrators. Members of the UK Colonial Service have long been stereotyped as Oxbridge-educated white males, born into wealth, endowed with a penchant for sports, and with practical (if unexceptional) minds and adventurous spirits. In general, historians believed them to have shared a "world-view that was politically conservative, any more radical elements within it being silenced for the sake of preserving the status quo."[72] Yet Anna Crozier has demonstrated that medical officers hailed from a "more diverse social group" and trained at more varied institutions.[73] These biographical differences between doctors and other co-lonial officers help explain why Shircore and de Boer were so critical of the quality of medical services for Africans. Both had trained at leading med-ical schools in the United Kingdom (de Boer in London and Shircore in Edinburgh). Both had connections to South Asia. De Boer was born into a burgher family in Ceylon, and Shircore's father was in the Indian Medical Service, which enjoyed more resources and claimed greater prestige than the East African Medical Service.[74] Both de Boer and Shircore had practiced in other East African colonies, all of which spent more per capita on health care for Africans than did Nyasaland. Neither man was radical in his politics, and they, like all physicians in the Nyasaland government's employ, were white. But their backgrounds left them expecting more in the way of financial re-sources and dissatisfied with the state in which they found Nyasaland's med-ical services. Each wrote a scathing report that called for far greater spending on health care.

Such reports were not always sufficient to impel an expansion in Nyasaland's health services. Still, they reveal contests over budgets be-tween colonial medical officers and officials in Whitehall. These debates rarely appear in physicians' memoirs, which as Crozier notes, tended to "sensationalize Africa" while avoiding everyday struggles.[75] Yet as the next chapter demonstrates, sometimes the most bureaucratic prose can create the grandest sensations. In the midst of the Second World War, the writings of economists and reformers would expand expectations of medical provision throughout the empire.

4

Health in Wartime Development and Postwar Visions, 1941–1952

Prelude

Izeki was pressed for cash. Before his wife departed for the afternoon, she insisted she needed cloth diapers for their new baby. She expected Izeki to give her money to buy the diapers by the end of the day. She warned that she did not want find him still empty-handed upon her return.

At first, Izeki did not know what to do. He simply did not have the money. But all of a sudden, he had an idea. He walked from the porch of his mud-brick hut down the narrow path to the dirt road. There he tore small branches from a short tree. He laid the branches on the road, in two parallel lines separated by five meters. Between the lines he placed a small plastic bowl. Then he returned to his porch and sat down.

Soon this exercise had the desired effect. One passerby dismounted his bike when he came to the branches and walked between the two lines before remounting his bike after he passed them. Then another passerby—a man walking a goat—stopped to drop a few bills into the bowl. Two women also stopped to drop money into the bowl, then walked up the path to talk to Izeki. A few moments later, a man named Jakobo followed suit.

Izeki had made use of a local practice used to collect funds for an impending funeral. His neighbors were under the impression that there had been a death in Izeki's home. When Jakobo reached the porch, he rattled off a string of lamentations. *Nkani basi! Nyimbo basi! Azimayi watopa!* ("Enough of this news! Enough of this [funeral] music! The women are tired [of mourning]!").

Izeki, acting downtrodden, thanked Jakobo for coming. "What happened?" asked Jakobo.

"One of my children was hit by a car in town while walking to school," Izeki explained.

No More to Spend. Paul Farmer, Oxford University Press (2020). © Oxford University Press.
DOI: 10.1093/oso/9780190066192.001.0001

"Where will the funeral be held?" Jakobo asked. "In town? Or in the village?"

Tentatively, sensing he was a bit too far into the lie, Izeki answered, "Here, in the village."

"Well, in that case, I will bring the money to the *mfumu*," Jakobo offered. "He will organize the funeral, of course. That is his job."

"No!" yelled Izeki. Composing himself, he explained, "I want to plan it myself."

Izeki's wife soon returned and began sobbing inconsolably. Seeing the branches, the bowl, and the assembled mourners, she naturally assumed someone had died.

Unable to maintain his lie any longer, Izeki admitted no one had died. "I just didn't know where to find the money to buy diapers," he confessed. His wife stopped crying and joined the others in angry rebukes. Defeated, Izeki returned the donations.

The story of Izeki's spectacular failure is fiction. It was the plot of a Chichewa-language skit performed by the popular Malawi comedy duo Izeki and Jakobo. A video of this sketch, entitled *Matewera amwana* (Children's diapers), had nearly one hundred fifty thousand views on YouTube in the six years after it was first posted in January 2013.[1] The sketch resonates with its Malawian audience because it makes light of one of the most demanding community obligations in present-day Malawi: helping to pay for and attending local funerals. Izeki and Jakobo's sketches often draw upon anxieties about trust in impoverished village communities. In a more recent sketch, which garnered more than one hundred seventy thousand views on YouTube between 2013 and 2019, a crooked preacher was discovered to be pocketing money donated by his congregation in what he portrayed as a collection for the sick.[2]

In real life, the village chief is often the focal point of these anxieties about trust and expectations of protection. He (or sometimes she) serves as a tenuous link between the limited and patchwork support provided by the central government and the strained networks of support within kinship groups. Even though, as this chapter details, chiefs were lauded by colonial officials as wealthy providers for the needy during the colonial era, now (as then) they had neither much power to provide in times of need nor the social expectation that they could.

In Nyanza village, the chief did not cut a formidable figure. Chief Nyanza (the village is always an eponym of the chief) was an elderly man with the kind of face that looked stern even when he was being gentle. He had a slender frame, a prominent brow, sunken, slit-like eyes, and hollowed-out cheeks. At one meeting he wore a bright pink, button-down shirt, gray pants that were too short for his spindly legs, and old black sneakers. Like most chiefs in the Mangochi area, he wore a white *kufi* cap during official meetings. Though the chief was a Catholic, his chiefly garb had been influenced by the Yao Muslims, who had held sway in the region since they arrived from the south in the mid-nineteenth century.

Writing about fieldwork he had performed in the late 1940s in a village not far from Nyanza, social anthropologist Clyde Mitchell concluded, "A village headman may expect little material benefit from his position of authority . . . the position of headman is no sinecure."[3] The same could be said three-quarters of a century later. Chief Nyanza lived in a modest home. It was not the most well-appointed in the village, though its construction had been paid for by the owners of a resort lodge nearby. The lodge owners had sought to make a display of goodwill to counteract their reputation as a forbidding and miserly neighbor, and the chief had accepted the gift. At meetings, he almost always looked tired. Sitting on the porch of his home, he usually delivered an opening statement, then appeared as if he might be sleeping. Suddenly, and unprompted, at the close of each meeting he would open his eyes to offer closing words.

Still, he was trusted. Chief Nyanza had been born in the village but, this being a matrilocal area, he had spent most of his life in his wife's home twenty kilometers to the south. He became chief following the death of his brother in 2008, when he was summoned to return to Nyanza because he was reputed to be an honest arbiter and a strong advocate.

During one meeting when, once again, he seemed to be dozing, he perked up to make a point. The proceedings had thus far involved a lecture by well-dressed local bureaucrats from the Parks Department. They had driven to the meeting in a pickup truck to warn the residents of Nyanza that they would be fined if they were found illegally cutting down branches in the protected forest surrounding their village. The residents were annoyed by what they heard as condescension and unwillingness to consider their needs. They did not wish to contribute to deforestation, but none could afford gas stoves, and few could buy charcoal. How, they asked, were they to cook?

When the chief spoke, he channeled their frustrations. "We were here before this land was named a national park, and we will be here long after you have left your jobs," he told the officials. "The lodge has cordoned off so much of the land where we used to collect firewood," he continued. "We were not consulted about this, but now we have to go even further to find wood." He concluded with a barely veiled challenge: "We will do what we must to live."

Though his subjects appreciated these proud soliloquies, the chief could do little else to improve their lot. In an interview, he explained his responsibilities. First, he was a gatekeeper for some forms of public provision. He decided which of the households in his village should be given the limited number of coupons for fertilizer subsidies and which should receive food packages distributed during emergencies. Second, he was charged with allocating land to people moving to the village. Third, as Izeki and Jakobo's skit averred, he was responsible for organizing the funeral when anyone living in one of the village's three hundred homes died. Fourth, he adjudicated disputes within the village. This last responsibility, he said, was rife with difficulties (*ntchito wavuto*) that often involved verbal abuse by drunken combatants.

Chief Nyanza was not a rich man. He worried about money; like Francis, he had spent much of his income seeking a remedy for a family member in chronic pain. His wife had felt pain in her chest after meals for the past year. The hospital in Monkey Bay had prescribed cimetidine (a drug used to treat heartburn and peptic ulcers), but this treatment provided no relief. Her pain continued even after visits to the fee-charging clinic at the nearby Catholic mission and to the private hospital in Cape Maclear.

The chief and his wife had even traveled hours to see a famed *sing'anga* (traditional healer). The *sing'anga* had told the chief that his wife was dying because she had been taking on improper responsibilities. She had, he explained, been helping to manage the chief's relationship with his people, hearing stories she was not meant to hear. After that the chief tried to shield his wife from his official duties, but there had been little improvement. He hoped to go back to the *sing'anga* for another consultation but lacked the money for transport and fees. Like Francis, he feared that the maize harvest would be poor. Unlike Francis, he had no livestock to sell in times of need. Like Izeki in the sketch, the chief was trying to find money to meet his wife's needs. While his office held some vestigial authority, it was not a fount of power and wealth. Despite his intentions, he was no great provider for his people. He could not even salve his own wife's pain.

Introduction

Wartime visions of the welfare state circulated widely in the British Empire, forcing the Colonial Office to explain just how much social protection should be realized beyond the British Isles. Another set of ideas circulating during this period concerned social protection in the African village. The notion of "traditional" safety nets was repeated often by colonial officials, most frequently when they sought to justify the absence of robust welfare provision in the colonial state. These two understandings about the relationship between the state and the people would inform a debate, in Nyasaland and elsewhere, about imperial responsibilities for subject African peoples.

Both European and African expectations that governments could, and should, provide for their people began to change in Nyasaland during the Second World War. In contrast to the 1930s—when plans by Shircore and de Boer were frustrated by complacency in London—by the mid-1940s colonial labor stoppages and global conflict had engendered sufficient concern to spur increased funding for health-care programs. The craze in the United Kingdom over economist William Beveridge's plans for social security reforms—including the National Health Service—also increased attention to health policy in Britain's colonies.

Increased access to health services was the only facet of postwar social welfare policy that most officials agreed should apply even in rural Africa. Health services figured prominently in the colonial plans of the Labour Party, which came to power following a landslide victory in the 1945 UK general election. Arthur Creech Jones, a leading light in the Fabian Colonial Bureau and the new colonial secretary under Labour, promised the expansion of health services to support his larger declaration that "the old imperialism has come to an end." But at least initially, the rise of Labour did not seem to usher in any new era in colonial medical services. This new era would only begin, and then only tentatively, after another wave of strikes and riots, which swept across the empire in the late 1940s. Only then did the Colonial Office begin to increase spending on hospitals, clinics, and training institutions. Between 1944 and 1952 Nyasaland received some Colonial Development and Welfare Act of 1940 (CDW) aid for venereal disease treatment, and officials in Zomba finally began to improve and expand training of African medical auxiliaries. Still, scarcity remained the dominant paradigm throughout the war and in the early postwar years, as Labour's promises of an end to the "old imperialism" did not lead to much better health care for the sick of Nyasaland.

British Colonial Development discourse during the
Second World War

Debates over aid to the colonies for health and other social services did not abate with the outbreak of war. To be sure, the war effort did dampen imperial expenditures on social services and other development projects in the colonies. The 1940 "Statement of Policy" acknowledged that spending on the CDW Fund was not likely to reach the legislated maximum of £5 million per year "at any time during the war."[4] MacDonald's successor as secretary of state for the colonies, Lord Lloyd, added his own note of pessimism after the law's enactment: "Much that we had hoped to do under this Bill when it became law must wait for happier times." Though the law allowed for £5 million in annual spending (£294 million in 2016 prices), in the first year (1940–1941) the UK government spent only £177,802 (£10.5 million in 2016 prices) on CDW Fund schemes.[5]

At the same time, colonial treasuries were impelled to ship away both men and treasure to aid in the war effort. The transfer of financial resources could be substantial. Between 1939 and 1945, the imperial exchequer received monetary "gifts" from colonial governments, native rulers, and private groups and individuals in the colonies. Gifts from public and private sources in Nyasaland alone during the war years totaled £164,214 (£7.47 million in 2016 prices).[6] This sum represented nearly three times Nyasaland's recurrent budget for health in 1939. Other colonies sacrificed even more. In 1940 alone the protectorate of Basutoland so tightened its belt that revenues exceeded expenditures by £100,000 (£5.88 million in 2016 prices); the entire surplus was transferred to the imperial exchequer for the purchase of fighter planes. On the Zambian Copperbelt, chiefs proved so aggressive in following imperial instructions to collect funds for "charity appeals" such as a "Food for Britain" drive that local colonial officials grew concerned about the potential for rebellion.[7] Still, the official line was that these were acts of generosity and imperial patriotism, rather than compulsion. "The Bantu," declared the London-based Royal African Society in 1941, "are willing to give everything for victory."[8]

And give they did. The supply of men drawn from the colonies was even more impressive than the transfer of funds. By the end of the war, 473,000 soldiers in Britain's army hailed from the colonies. These soldiers made up a particularly large share of troops in battles against the Italians in East Africa and later against the Japanese in Burma. A government report after the war claimed that the "majority" of the troops from the colonies had volunteered, though some had been conscripted. Labor had also been conscripted in some colonies (including Nigeria, Kenya, Tanganyika, and Northern Rhodesia) during the war to increase production of agricultural and industrial products for the war effort.[9]

While the colonies gave blood and treasure throughout the conflict, they only began to receive substantial CDW funding after British officials became concerned about anticolonial sentiment in the United States. In April 1942, UK prime minister Winston Churchill and US president Franklin Roosevelt had "their first serious political argument." It concerned the future of the British Empire, particularly India. Indian nationalists had threatened to withhold support for the Allied war effort, so Roosevelt asked Churchill to make a firm commitment to grant Indians greater self-government. Churchill refused.[10]

Anti-imperial voices in the United States became an ever greater danger to British interests as it became clear that the United States would have the preeminent role in the postwar world. In May 1942, US under-secretary of state Sumner Welles announced that an Allied victory "must bring in its train the liberation of all people."[11] Vice President Henry Wallace urged the Roosevelt administration to advocate for immediate independence for colonized peoples.[12] In a May 1942 speech, Wallace predicted a "Century of the Common Man" that would commence after the war. The advent of this century would bring a rapid end to European empires:

> No nation will have the God-given right to exploit other nations. Older nations will have the privilege to help younger nations get started on the path to industrialization, but there must be neither military nor economic imperialism. The methods of the nineteenth century will not work in the people's century, which is now about to begin.[13]

Colonial development spending was, to apologists of British imperialism, a demonstration of beneficence directed not only at colonized subjects, but also at Roosevelt and other American architects of the coming postwar settlement. It was also a variant of Wallace's vision of a global New Deal, stripped of his call for an immediate end to colonial rule.

At the same time, Labour MPs and some quarters of the press began pointing to the discrepancy between CDW spending to that point and the originally publicized figure of £5 million per annum.[14] In response to pressures foreign and domestic, Churchill's government accelerated its approval of new CDW schemes. Up until October 31, 1942, after two years in operation, the secretary of state for the colonies had approved only 167 schemes involving a total financial liability of just over £2 million (£91 million in 2016 prices). Most of these plans were for possessions in the Caribbean, where memories of unrest were fresh and American attention was, by virtue of proximity, closely focused. But during the next two and a half years the secretary of state approved an additional 381 schemes involving liability of almost £14 million (£637 million in 2016 prices).[15] CDW schemes classified under the heading "medical, public health and sanitation" also increased after 1942. During the first two years of the CDW's existence, only thirty-five such schemes with an aggregate cost of £330,000 (£15 million in 2016 prices) had been approved. But over the next two and a half years, sixty-five such schemes were approved, involving costs of more than £2.6 million (£118 million in 2016 prices).[16]

Seeking a Colonial Policy for the Left

International pressures were not the only influence on wartime colonial development policy. During the war, the most prominent site in Britain for discussion and debate over how the government should improve living standards for the colonized was the Fabian Society. Given the society's history, this was an unlikely forum for such discourse. The Fabian Society had been established in 1884 to engage, according to the historian Mark Minion, in "a long and gradualist fight against the evils of late-nineteenth-century capitalism." At the same time, the society aimed to counter Marxists and radical trade unionists who called for social transformation by way of revolution. Instead, Fabians sought to achieve socialism in Britain through peaceful politics. Their membership, which included founders of the Labour Party, believed in democratic discourse.[17] Toward that end, the Fabians published essays, books, and pamphlets, primarily on domestic economic issues.

Disagreements within the society had long led its membership to steer clear of discussions of imperial policy.[18] Fabians had become slightly more vocal on colonial policy when Lord Passfield, a leading member, was appointed secretary of state for the colonies in 1929. But the society's reticence only really ended in 1940, when Rita Hinden, a thirty-one-year-old economist raised in South Africa and Palestine, suggested the establishment of the Fabian Colonial Bureau, a group that would be devoted to addressing problems in the empire.[19] At its first meeting, Hinden was elected secretary. To chair the bureau, the members chose Arthur Creech Jones, an MP who had long been the de facto spokesman for the Labour Party on colonial issues. The other founding members were an august group: evolutionary biologist Julian Huxley, Labour MP John Parker, former Labour MP James Francis Horrabin, socialist writer Margaret Cole, development economist W. Arthur Lewis, physician and former under-secretary of state for the colonies Sir Thomas Drummond Shiels, author and secretary for the Labour Party's Advisory Committee on Imperial Questions Leonard Woolf (better known, in many circles, as the husband of the writer Virginia Woolf), imperial historian Margery Perham, and historian of race relations William Macmillan. Their contacts with leading journalists were so strong that within six months of the bureau's first meeting they had published articles in the *Economist*, the *Manchester Guardian*, the *New Statesman*, *Time and Tide*, *Reynolds News*, the *Evening Standard*, and the *Daily Herald*. They had also recruited over a dozen MPs, who agreed to pose questions in Parliament or directly to the Colonial Office.[20] This was a small organization, but it was endowed with immense social capital.

Members of the Fabian Colonial Bureau produced most of the literature that defined the Labour Party's stance on colonial issues. Early in the war, bureau members tried to ensure that increased spending on colonial development and welfare was a major focus of Labour's rhetoric. In April 1940, Leonard Woolf's Advisory Committee on Imperial Questions issued the Labour Party's "Declaration of Policy for Colonial Peoples." Though the document did not say so explicitly, its promise to improve health care seemed designed to provide a justification sufficient to reconcile (for most Fabians) the contradictions inherent in socialist advocacy for the persistence of imperialism. In seeking to bring Britain's possessions to eventual independence, improving health care was a necessary and urgent step:

> Political self-government is not enough. It must be accompanied by economic independence and economic self-government. By economic independence we mean a new orientation of motive in colonial policy, putting first the satisfaction of urgent colonial needs (for instance nutrition and the conquest of the disease) and treating external trade as a secondary and auxiliary object.[21]

In September 1941, Woolf laid out, in greater detail, how this commitment to "the satisfaction of urgent colonial needs" would manifest in Labour Party policy, should it be handed the reins of government. In a memorandum on a postwar Labour agenda, Woolf argued that "much larger sums will have to be found" for economic development, education, and health "than is now usual in colonial budgets." But, he continued, lack of education and the low standard of health among the colonized caused poverty that limited colonial revenues. This "vicious circle" could be broken only with capital from Europe or the United States. Because resulting revenue growth would inevitably take time, this capital had to be provided on terms more generous than market-rate loans.[22]

Even within the Labour Party, Woolf's focus on social services found critics on both the left and right wings. On the left, longtime colonial commentator Norman Leys urged deletion of the section of the memorandum calling for "costly education and health services." He argued that land alienation, direct taxation of the poorest, and legal restrictions on free movement and political organization were the fundamental causes of colonial poverty. Leys discounted the importance of health care and education in the effort to stem endemic diseases, which "can be uprooted only as and when a general advance is made, that need not be slow but must be liberative." [23] To Leys, Labour's focus should remain on these causes, rather than on the social services that had so recently been the stated focus of Colonial Office policy under the Conservative prime minister Neville Chamberlain.

Farther to the right, Thomas Reid contended it was political suicide to advocate for increased colonial social service spending to a "groaning British taxpayer" besieged by war and want. Colonies had low "taxable capacity," so such "obviously desirable boons cannot be provided, unless we, or other altruists, finance the needs of about 500 million poverty-stricken people in the midst of our own bankruptcy." Woolf's proposed platform, Reid argued, was not only "generally impracticable" and "unjust to our own people," but "electorally disastrous to Labour, and therefore to the public and the world for whom a Labour Government in Britain after the war is a *sine qua non* of success for all." In any case, since "tropical people do not exercise birth control and breed up to the bare subsistence or below it as a rule," health and education spending would result in an increase in population rather than an increase in per capita wealth.[24] Labour, then, was not at all united in their visions for colonial development. Fierce critics of extractive economic policies mingled with neo-Malthusian colonial apologists, while still others tried to steer a middle course similar to the prewar policies pursued by the Colonial Office under Malcolm MacDonald.

Despite this dissension in Labour, members of the Fabian Colonial Bureau reiterated calls for social services. These calls grew louder after supportive words from an influential colonial expert, Lord Hailey. Hailey, a retired member of the Indian civil service, had become the preeminent public intellectual on colonial issues after the 1938 publication of the *African Survey*, a massive interdisciplinary study conducted under his direction. In a keynote address to the annual meeting of the Anti-Slavery and Aborigines Protection Society on May 28, 1942, Hailey suggested that the increasing expectations of state social protection within Britain should also change colonial policy. These expectations entailed a "conception of the State not merely as an agency for maintaining justice and equal rights, or for preventing abuse . . . but as the most active agency for promoting social welfare and improving the general standard of living." Judging the legitimacy of colonial government by the same criteria as domestic governance would "serve to justify our position as a colonial power to the outside world, and to mitigate some of the suspicion which now attaches to it."[25]

Hailey continued by calling for a statement outlining "our obligations to the colonial peoples . . . not as those of trustees, but as those incumbent on the modern state in regard to the improvement of the social services and the standards of living in its own domestic backward areas."[26] He said this statement should come in the form of a "colonial charter." This document, he explained, would be a supplement to the Atlantic Charter, a document signed by Churchill and Roosevelt in August 1941 to express shared aims in fighting the war. That document had included a "wish to see sovereign rights and self-government restored to those who have been forcibly deprived of them." Speaking before the House of Commons on September 9, Churchill said he felt compelled to clarify that the Atlantic Charter applied only to "the states and nations now under Nazi yoke" and did not address the "separate problem of progressive evolution of self-governing institutions in the regions and peoples which owe allegiance to the British Crown."[27]

Hinden, who noted the "disappointment" of peoples "in the colonies" upon hearing of Churchill's unwillingness to include them in the promises of the Atlantic Charter, quickly took up Hailey's call for a colonial charter. Within a week of Hailey's address, she had drafted a memo to members of the bureau to explain her thoughts on the politics and content of such a charter.

In a political stroke reminiscent of MacDonald's arguments to the Treasury a few years earlier, Hinden pointed to a particular colonial crisis to call for increased social spending. To Hinden, this crisis was the fall of British Malaya to the Japanese in January 1942. This defeat of mostly Indian and Malayan soldiers "seemed to indicate an apathy on the part of the colonial peoples to a British victory." She argued that one guarantee capable of increasing martial zeal in the colonies was a promise to improve social services.[28] She suggested that a colonial charter prepared by the bureau should include an imperial "responsibility" to "secure a uniform standard of social services."[29]

Enthusiasm for social protection swelled even more after the November 1942 publication of William Beveridge's *Social Insurance and Allied Services*. In 299 pages of text and tables, Beveridge's report painstakingly detailed a plan to expand and rationalize Britain's programs of social protection, including unemployment insurance, subsistence payments for the elderly and infirm, and children's allowances. He also proposed a government-run health-care system to be financed entirely by general taxation and provided free at the point of care.[30] Despite the report's dry prose and seemingly interminable tables, it was a sensation. Within two weeks of its release, nine out of ten Britons were telling pollsters they approved of it. Within a year, 600,000 copies of the report had been sold. [31] In 1945 the London correspondent of the *New York Herald Tribune* reported, "Beveridge has become almost a common noun in the English language. It stands for hope."[32] In seeking to fend off proposals that such policies be extended to Britain's colonies in Africa, official documents took to repeating a notion that African villages had their own robust, if primordial, forms of social security. The idea of village social protection was central to a 1944 publication written by Lucy Mair (a former student of Bronislaw Malinowski), who was then in the employ of the UK Ministry of Information.[33] Mair's report, entitled *Welfare in the British Colonies* and published by the nongovernmental Royal Institute for International Affairs, argued that in "traditional African societies . . . the aged and sick were cared for by their relatives."[34] Moreover, in the more centralized of these societies, people were protected by "a king or paramount chief" against disasters that threatened to overwhelm the resources of smaller kinship groups. Political leaders used the wealth garnered from the tributes of their followers to "store up a reserve of food against famine" or "offer hospitality to the many people who visited his fort."[35] Mair concluded that African societies offered "a complete system of social security provided for by the obligations of kinship."[36]

In April 1945, the Colonial Office echoed these arguments in a report entitled *Social Welfare in the Colonies*. The report claimed that prior to the imposition of colonial rule, the peoples of the British Empire "had worked out their own methods of dealing with social problems according to the resources at their disposal, often with remarkable success."[37] In Great Britain public provision of welfare was necessitated by the fact that there had been, until recently, little credence in the idea of a community as "an organic whole whose health and vitality depend upon the well-being of all its constituent members."[38] Lacking such a belief, the weak, poor, and unconnected were left without support in European societies. By contrast, the report claimed, in African villages notions of communal obligation had been widely accepted since time immemorial. European-style systems of social security were needed, then, only in urban areas, where the social norms of traditional life were threatened by "contact" with "industrial civilization."[39]

The authors of these works could turn to earlier ethnographic research to support their claim that African villages offered social protection sufficient to obviate the need for social security. But as John Iliffe has explained, anthropologists based their analyses of communal obligations on the testimony of chiefs, who during the colonial era had an interest in telling tales of "aristocratic philanthropy" to cement their own privileged positions in the contemporary system of indirect rule.[40] Missionaries and travelers in the nineteenth and twentieth centuries, on the other hand, often wrote of neglected orphans, abandoned epileptics, and discarded blind or mentally ill men and women.[41] But in the early decades of indirect rule, which afforded chiefs wealth and power while allowing colonial administrators to shirk responsibility for social provision, it was convenient for both groups to promote the mythology of a robust system of primordial social security.

Even when chiefs abandoned this idea, officials holding the purse strings of the budget kept repeating it. It is unclear whether officials really believed in the existence—and persistence—of primordial systems of social protection. Nevertheless, repeating the idea helped to justify the paucity of government social services and social insurance. Take, for instance, the official response to chiefs in Mlanje District in May 1949, who had asked "whether government through the Native Treasuries would agree to financial assistance being given to orphans." The provincial commissioner replied that he had rarely seen an abandoned orphan. The chiefs' requests grew more urgent in the coming months, as recent poor harvests heightened fears of famine. Chief Chikumbu argued that the aged, disabled, and orphaned were at particular risk for starvation. The African Council of the Southern Province proposed that three pence from each annual tax should be placed into a fund to aid the most vulnerable, but Nyasaland's financial secretary objected: "If any sort of arrangement was set up on the lines contemplated by the PC, the whole thing would snowball and become a crippling financial liability in a very short time." When, that same year, the Colonial Office adviser on social welfare wrote a report urging the Zomba administration to pursue social welfare with greater vigor, the chief secretary demurred: "The conclusions are to spend more money," he summarized, "and we have no more to spend."[42] While Southern Nyasaland hurtled toward a deadly famine—one in which officials would express their shock at widespread social abandonment of the aged, the disabled, and the orphaned—the Nyasaland government ruled that "special funds" for the aid of the vulnerable were counterproductive, as they "would lead to a further breaking down of the system of social security which has in the past been a feature of African rural society."[43]

Both during the war and in the years immediately following it, British administrators in Africa saw the need for government provision of social security as particular to wage labor. But for "subsistence economies," including most of Nyasaland, the colonial administration did not plan to provide the family allowances, disability insurance, and old age pensions then being universalized in the United Kingdom. The notion that Africans already enjoyed robust traditional social security was useful; as a 1944 Colonial Office report, entitled "Social Security in the Colonial Territories," insisted, "In subsistence economies . . . the tribe or the family still helps substantially to provide against old age, indigence and, to a more limited extent, sickness." The main point of this report was not to plot out progressive steps toward an African welfare state, but to argue that social security in the colonies was in no way a responsibility of the imperial exchequer: "In all cases the process must be visualized as one of an *internal* redistribution. . . . The importance of avoiding the establishment of a standard of minimum maintenance which may prove beyond the capacity of the community cannot be overemphasized."[44]

But the argument that African societies once administered their own robust, universal systems of social protection—and that they could do so again—was a myth. In fact, the historian A. G. Hopkins has a name for it: the "myth of Merrie Africa." It is, in his telling, the idea that precolonial Africa was a golden age of perfect harmony and communal values.[45] There were, to be sure, important mechanisms of social protection in precolonial Africa. For example, Steven Feierman, Michael Watts, and Elias Mandala have described systems of precolonial public works in which penurious subjects could work on chiefs' land in exchange for subsistence in Tanzania, Nigeria, and Malawi, respectively. But as each of these scholars is at pains to point out, these systems could be both exploitative and incomplete. Some people were inevitably left to die, particularly when disasters like droughts or disease were so generalized that they overwhelmed rulers.[46] And many systems of social protection did not survive the imposition of colonial rule, no so much because of the introduction of wage labor as because of the displacements of war, taxation, and colonial rule. Yet such nuance was not present in colonial officials' accounts of "traditional social security." By making these systems seem both resilient and fair, colonial regimes could reason away any governmental responsibility for social protection.

But even with this powerful myth at work, there was at least one piece of the postwar vision of social security that did figure in Colonial Office plans for non-wage-earning African populations. Increasing spending on preventive and curative health care had been a major part of the stated purpose of the CDW and continued to be included in colonial plans for postwar development. Lucy Mair may have extolled the virtues of "a complete system of social security" in "traditional" African societies, but she also argued that because disease remained widespread in these societies, "the importance of [government] medical work is particularly great."[47] The same Colonial Office reports that insisted that payments to the needy could only be financed by funds raised within the colonies also stated that colonial health and education were government responsibilities: "Even where the traditional organization is fully maintained, it is generally itself quite incapable of providing allied social services, particularly of public health and education, and the village or tribal social security provision needs to be systematically supplemented by extension of Government public health and education services."[48]

In his report, William Beveridge had called for universal access to health care, free at the point of care, in the United Kingdom.[49] Unlike some British citizens in the metropole, African subjects in Nyasaland did not have to pay for government health care at the point of service.[50] Still, health services were severely constrained, and their quality was dismal. The Beveridge Report, with its call for universally accessible high-quality health services, influenced official plans for Africans, even in rural areas. While bureaucrats insisted most colonized Africans would have to make do with traditional social security, no prominent members of the Colonial Office argued that such mechanisms could cure the sick as readily as antibiotic and antimalarial drugs.

Many officials in Nyasaland's colonial administration hoped that health services would be a significant focus of postwar CDW grants. Director of Medical Services Arthur Williams, who had studied at Cambridge and trained at West London Hospital before joining the Colonial Medical Service in 1912, offered a litany of complaints about the state of his department in the introduction to his 1944 proposal for postwar development.[51] While the hospital buildings were in fair condition, "the same cannot be said with respect to the standard of nursing, diagnostic facilities and transport services for the seriously sick and injured, and in the development of maternity and child welfare clinics at Government hospitals." Only a single hospital had an X-ray machine, which Williams insisted was "an essential part of the doctor's diagnostic equipment." Most of the hospitals lacked electricity. To those who doubted the hindrance this caused, Williams explained that "the difficulties of doing either surgical or maternity work at night with no illumination other than a hurricane lantern or temperamental pressure lamp have to be experienced to be appreciated." Nyasaland had only two ambulances, and both were intended primarily for Europeans. The personnel of rural dispensaries had poor diagnostic skills and—because most were not entrusted with intravenous injections or pills, which in any case were in short supply—few medicines capable of effecting cure.[52]

Preventive efforts fared little better. The existing contingent of fifty African "sanitary assistants" had little success in convincing rural African populations to submit to vaccination and sanitation campaigns. Instead of blaming the sanitary assistants, or the villagers, Williams criticized the miserliness of officials in Whitehall. Ignorance, he contended, was not the reason Africans built few cement floors or pit latrines; it was not the reason many did not use soap or wear shoes. Many Africans knew that these precautions were necessary to prevent hookworm and other endemic infections. Colonial Office bureaucrats were wrongheaded, he claimed, when they preached the virtues of prevention without helping penurious subjects pay for cement, or soap, or footwear.[53]

The historiography of "medical middles" has demonstrated that African nurses, medical assistants, orderlies, and public health workers were not passive receptacles of medical knowledge. Rather, the literature highlights the work these health-care providers did to transform European medical discourse and practice, creating hybridized systems that thrived in a variety of different social and ecological settings. Through creative bricolage, they adapted and translated multiple forms of medical knowledge.[54] But the sanitary campaigns, foiled for want of money, show the limits of adaptation in the face of material obstacles. In the absence of funds to buy raw materials for latrines and flooring, no hookworm campaign was going to succeed. The following chapters demonstrate similar failures with vaccines, which were either in chronically short supply or substandard in quality. Political economy and cultural history are not divorced, but depend on one another.

Williams consistently argued that the Medical Department's shortcomings could be addressed if he was given sufficient funding. Nyasaland's Post-War Development Committee, a body composed of officials and settlers, agreed. In 1945, the committee submitted a report requesting significant improvements in the quantity and quality of medical provision. Its ten-year plan even proposed an increase in the number of rural medical centers from just over one hundred to four hundred. The committee also proposed a concomitant increase in trained hospital assistants, which would be facilitated by an expansion of primary education and a new medical training school in Blantyre. The committee argued that most of the new funding should come from the UK Treasury, not domestic revenue. The committee's proposals (for health and all other departments) called for a total of £7.5 million (£292 million in 2016 prices) in capital and new recurrent costs between 1946 and 1955. The committee proposed that of this funding, £6.5 million should come from CDW Fund grants. The remaining £1 million, it suggested, should be paid for by "the Protectorate's surplus balances which have been loaned to His Majesty's Government during the war." Treasury had called these transfers "gifts" from the colonies, but Nyasaland wanted its money back.[55]

The prospects for such plans, in Nyasaland and elsewhere, appeared brighter following the July 1945 UK general election, the nation's first in ten years. Clement Attlee's Labour won in a landslide, increasing its number of seats in the House of Commons (a 640-seat body) from 154 to 393. With a sizable majority, Labour claimed a mandate to remake British society in the postwar dawn. They set to work passing and implementing the National Health Service (NHS). New social services spending seemed certain to reach the colonies, especially after Attlee named Arthur Creech Jones his secretary of state for the colonies in October 1946. In one of his first addresses as secretary, Creech Jones spoke before the Anti-Slavery and Aborigines Protection Society. His address was full of grand promises:

> So far as Britain is concerned, I think we can assume today that the old Imperialism has come to an end. . . . The past has left a legacy of trouble.

It has somehow to be dealt with in the progressive work we seek to do today. . . . We have to harness nature to the will of man and to safeguard the life of man and hold in check disease.[56]

A prosaic manifestation of this millenarian rhetoric came in the renewal of the Colonial Development and Welfare Act, passed in 1945.[57] Revisions included extending the CDW Fund's existence from 1951 to 1956 and increasing authorized funding to a total of £120 million (£3.71 billion in 2016 prices) between 1946 and 1956.[58]

Even before the 1945 election, the Colonial Office had sent development officers to the colonies to help draft new schemes.[59] Yet if these new deployments and Labour's victory seemed to augur a flood of new money, Nyasaland's administration would soon learn—as Shircore and de Boer had before—that recent unrest was a more powerful motivator for development funding than dismal indices of poverty and medical services. When the Colonial Office announced the CDW allocations for each colony in November 1945, Nyasaland was promised less than a third of its request.[60] Per capita allocations were much higher for Caribbean colonies that had experienced strikes in the 1930s. These islands were still seen as potential foci of strikes and riots, and as America's main vantage point on British imperialism.[61] Nyasaland was allocated £2 million, £1 per capita. By comparison, Trinidad received £1.83 per capita, Barbados £4.28 per capita, and Jamaica £5 per capita.[62] Following this announcement, Williams had to curtail his planned expansion of the medical services considerably.[63]

Labor Unrest, Once More

While an ideological commitment to welfare was not enough to significantly increase imperial spending for colonial health services, certain kinds of disruption could. In 1946 another wave of labor stoppages began; this time the focus was not the West Indies but British Africa. A range of workers, from dockworkers to domestic servants, organized general strikes in Mombasa and Dar es Salaam in 1947, while railway workers and miners went on strike in the Gold Coast.[64] In 1948 general strikes paralyzed both Zanzibar and the Southern Rhodesian city of Bulawayo.[65] Between 1946 and 1948 agricultural tenants, railway workers, and hospital orderlies stopped working to protest price controls, low pay, and poor working conditions in Anglo-Egyptian

Sudan.[66] Between the start of 1949 and the end of 1950, forty-six strikes in Nigeria resulted in 577,000 days of labor lost.[67]

Major grievances motivating these actions included shortages of consumer goods, inflation, low wages, and poor working conditions. But as had been the case during the late 1930s, health care figured prominently in the Colonial Office's response. In 1950 the CDW Act was revised once more, adding another £20 million (£637 million in 2016 prices) to the total fund.[68] In the House of Commons debate over this increased funding, MPs once more made the link between unrest and social welfare spending. Stanley Awbery, a former trade union leader and Labour MP, was the most explicit. He urged his colleagues to authorize far more than the £140 million (£4.46 billion in 2016 prices) planned for the fund: "A little help given two decades ago might have prevented the mountain of trouble we are experiencing today. Our record of omissions in this field of social welfare has proved fruitful soil for both unrest and Communism."[69]

Ultimately, the wave of labor action in Africa helped spur greater rhetorical *and* financial commitments to social services, including health care.[70] Between 1946 and 1955, the CDW Act approved £17 million (£541 million in 2016 prices) in grants and loans for health services schemes. The only category of funding that received a larger amount was education, which received £19 million (£605 million in 2016 prices).[71] Once again, though, many of the largest allocations went to postwar hotbeds of unrest. Between 1945 and 1960 the Federation of Nigeria was allocated £36.4 million, and Kenya was allocated £9.7 million, more than any other colonies in the entire British Empire. In part because Nyasaland became a center of unrest during the Federation period, it did receive more funding beginning in the 1950s. Between 1945 and 1960, Nyasaland was allocated £4.9 million (£127 million in 2016 prices) in CDW grants.[72]

In the end, what difference did it make to African patients in Nyasaland that Labour held power in Britain? Did the ideals of the Fabian Colonial Bureau actually impact decision-making in Whitehall? The existing historiography insinuates that in general, the Labour Party's rhetoric on imperialism masked a basic continuity with the policies of the previous half century.[73] But at least in health-care policy, Creech Jones's subordinates in the Colonial Office did advance some of his stated commitments during consequential deliberations.

Take, for instance, an episode in February 1949, when officials in the Colonial Office received news that UK manufacturers were declining to fill orders they had submitted because of instructions from other government ministries "that their output, or a large proportion of it, must be retained for the home market." Colonial Office employees became especially frustrated about export controls on medical supplies, namely "surgical dressings, surgical instruments, and electrical medical machinery." Limits on the export of X-ray machines to the colonies also garnered official attention. This technology had become crucial for tuberculosis diagnosis and monitoring as new chemotherapeutics (especially streptomycin) began to reach medical facilities in the colonies. But one British manufacturer of X-ray machines claimed that "he was allowed by the Ministry [of Health] a small quota merely to maintain his export connections," and that the company planned to export only one mobile X-ray machine in the next two years.[74]

Henry Wilkinson, comptroller of supplies for the Ministry of Health, confirmed that he had placed some controls on exports, but noted that even though orders of X-ray machines for the NHS were "seriously in arrears," he had "released" one unit to Tanganyika in 1948 and had promised another to Nigeria. Wilkinson also explained that, due to acute shortages and arrears in orders of gauze, lint, and bandages in the United Kingdom, only one-quarter of surgical dressings produced domestically were exported. He noted further that despite shortages of surgical instruments and streptomycin in NHS facilities, all colonial orders for these items were being met. All in all, he concluded, the colonies were "getting a fair share of the available supplies."[75]

At a March 28 meeting of the Cabinet Committee on Colonial Development, this issue became the subject of heated dispute. Wilkinson insisted he was "not willing to contemplate the diversion to export of anything which would endanger the health of this country." Hilton Poynton, an under-secretary of state for the colonies who had previously served in Sierra Leone, responded that Wilkinson's position was "not acceptable . . . as His Majesty's Government had an equal responsibility for safeguarding health in the Colonies."[76] Poynton and Wilkinson eventually agreed to a proposal put forward by the Ministry of Agriculture and Fisheries, in which the Colonial Office would provide other ministries "guidance on particular items which were for the time being of concern to the colonies." Poynton inserted the proviso that "colonial orders for these items should be treated on an equal footing with home orders."[77]

Shortly after this agreement was reached, Nyasaland finally received long-sought additional X-ray machines. Nyasaland's Postwar Development Committee had called, in 1944, for an increase in the Medical Department's supply of X-ray machines from one to eight. By the early 1950s, this figure had reached only three. In 1951 the Medical Department received its first radiologist, who in turn trained three African hospital assistants. The number of X-rays performed increased from 1,570 in 1950 to 2,956 in 1952.[78] Still, this expansion paled in comparison to the concurrent increase in X-ray units in the home market. Between 1950 and 1952 the NHS added 560 X-ray units across the United Kingdom.[79] Thus, the United Kingdom received more than 280 times as many X-ray units as Nyasaland, though the population of the former was only 17 times larger than that of the latter.

Nyasaland's Medical Department did enjoy increasing recurrent and capital budgets during the immediate postwar years. Between 1945 and 1952 recurrent spending more than doubled in inflation-adjusted terms.[80] New capital expenditures for the Medical Department came a few years later than requested, but between 1948 and 1953 totaled over £284,368 (£8.78 million in 2016 prices).[81] But the postwar expansion of Nyasaland's health sector was not as impressive as these numbers suggest. The postwar years in Nyasaland were marked by booming international prices for the commodities grown in Nyasaland as well as intensified tax collection. Both of these trends resulted in rising domestic government revenues, which increased from £1.2 million (£46.7 million in 2016 prices) in 1946 to £3.9 million (£152 million in 2016 prices) in 1952. Yet despite this windfall, the postwar governor, Geoffrey Colby, did not prioritize health care. When he requested additional CDW funding from the Colonial Office, it was not for health care but rather for roads, telecommunications, and electricity. Colby's only real interest in health, if we are to take his requests to the Colonial Office as an indication of his priorities, was in improving access to clean water.[82] The share of recurrent expenditure devoted to Nyasaland's Medical Department fell from 7.2 percent in 1947, the year before Colby arrived, to 5.9 percent in 1952.

Conclusion

This chapter recounts a contingent moment when various sorts of social welfare were considered in the British Empire. This era was a brief one. Still, the 1940s were a watershed, one driven in part by crises and changing expectations of government around the world. Debates about welfare during the 1940s, including calls for public-sector health care, subvention for agricultural inputs, and public pensions, have had lasting consequences for African

public policy. This shift in thinking about the role of the state in social provision would prove especially influential in changing the expectations of
African publics. The extent to which universalist health and social proteciton
policies devised for the metropolitan United Kingdom should also apply to
its colonies became a point of contention. In these debates, those who argued
against extending the newly expanded state responsibilities to the colonies
found support in ideas of "traditional social security" as well as well-trod
constructions of scarcity. As the next chapter demonstrates, the growing efficacy of biomedicine made expanded access to its therapeutics appear all the
more urgent in places. The politics of health care grew especially heated, in
large part because medicine became unprecedentedly popular.

5

"The Partnership Between a Rider and His Horse," 1953–1963

Prelude

In 1901, at the height of a campaign to control rebellious subjects in Madagascar, French military official Hubert Lyautey was reputed to have cabled his commanding general the following message: "If you can send me four doctors, I will send you back four companies." Lyautey was a leading proponent of what the historian Jim Paul has called "medical pacification." In his later postings in western Algeria and as resident general of the Protectorate of Morocco, Lyautey considered medical teams key components of any invasion or counterinsurgency campaign. The public demonstrations of goodwill he arranged were designed to silence critics of imperialism in Europe as much as to subdue African subjects. Concluding a speech before a medical audience in Brussels in 1926, shortly after his departure from Morocco, Lyautey described medicine not only as a tool of pacification, but as a moral vindication for the entire colonial enterprise:

> From the day when a notable, a *qaid*, or just some suffering devil decides to see a French doctor and leaves his office cured, the ice is broken, the first step is taken, and the relationship begins to be established. . . . Certainly the colonial expansion has its harsh aspects. It is not either beyond reproach or without blemish. But if there is something that ennobles it and justifies it, it is the action of the doctor, understood as a mission and an apostleship.[1]

This chapter shows how deployment of medicine as an antidote to political opposition and as justification for imperial rule was especially common during the late colonial era. Besieged by wholesale criticism of colonialism from prominent voices in Africa, Europe, and the United States, leaders of the Federation of Rhodesia and Nyasaland pointed to medical services as proof of the veracity of their promises of partnership and development.

No More to Spend. Paul Farmer, Oxford University Press (2020). © Oxford University Press.
DOI: 10.1093/oso/9780190066192.001.0001

Medicine continues to feature in debates over the nature of late colonial British rule elsewhere in Africa. In a letter to the editor printed in the *Guardian* in 2012 John Allen, a British veteran who had served in Kenya during the Mau Mau Revolt, objected to an assertion by columnist George Monbiot who, drawing on Caroline Elkins's historical work, wrote that "the British detained . . . almost the entire population of one and a half million people, in camps and fortified villages," where thousands were beaten or left to die of treatable illnesses.[2] Allen contended these settlements were not "gulags," as Elkins had called them, but instead humanely devised villages "where proper security could be provided." As evidence of British intent, he pointed to the "health centers" built by the British in those new villages, as well as "water supplies . . . sports grounds, markets and schools." The provision of health care was crucial to Allen's case. For him, the existence of clinics helped prove colonial officials were "fully dedicated to the wellbeing and advancement of the people they served."[3]

The most well-documented and dramatic example of the use of health care in postconflict reconstruction is Rwanda. In the decades after he led his rebel army in a campaign that put an end to the 1994 genocide—which had been, in the words of journalist Tom Burgis, "the fastest mass extermination in history"—Rwandan president Paul Kagame made health care a priority of his rule.[4] Writing in the editorial pages of the *Wall Street Journal* on April 7, 2014, the twentieth anniversary of the start of the genocide, President Kagame recounted the deliberate efforts his administration had made to integrate health care into the long process of reconciliation:

> In Rwanda, we are relying on universal human values, which include our culture and traditions, to find modern solutions to the unique challenges we faced in terms of justice and reconciliation following the genocide. . . . We chose to stay together. . . . We extended comprehensive health and education benefits to all our citizens.[5]

Facing ongoing threats to internal instability and external criticism of his rule, President Kagame made public-sector health care a showcase of his government's benevolence and seriousness of purpose. In the immediate aftermath of the genocide, the country was the poorest on the planet; political violence persisted, and physical infrastructure was in shambles. But long after health indices rebounded to pre-genocide levels, Kagame's government continued to achieve remarkable gains. Between 2000 and 2010 the maternal mortality rate declined 60 percent. Between 2000 and 2011 the under-five child mortality rate fell 70 percent. The decline in the crude mortality rate between 2000 and 2012 was the fastest in the world over that period.[6] The means by which these feats were accomplished—including high rates of health insurance enrollment, widespread vaccination coverage, and training of community health workers—have been well documented.[7] Crucially, by 2011 Rwanda devoted a higher share of its government expenditure to health care than any other nation in the African Union.[8] These changes are most explicable to those theorists who posit that such social change comes in the wake of political calamity.

But do health services achieve the aim of pacification? This chapter suggests that the interaction between public-sector health care and protest is more complicated. Unprecedented expenditure on health care could not prevent antigovernment forces from winning the public support and imperial acquiescence necessary to end the regime they so detested. But, as chapter 6 demonstrates, the new government of independent Malawi added kindling to an incipient rebellion when it tried to end the long-standing policy of free public-sector health care. Thus, the provision of health care has not always proven an effective measure to pacify ongoing unrest, but the denial of public-sector health care can foster discontent. Health services may not be a cure-all for political regimes facing crises of legitimacy, but political leaders neglect health care at their peril.

Introduction

"The native likes cough mixtures." So explained Nyasaland director of medical services Henry de Boer in a letter to the chief secretary in June 1941. This was both an observation and a lamentation. De Boer wished it were not so; he yearned for the day when prescriptions that were "actually necessary" were the same as those "desired by the patient." But given the distance between prevailing medical opinion and the expectations of African patients, de Boer found it necessary to instruct his staff to use drugs with "great care" and not exhaust scarce supplies simply to appease patients.[9]

De Boer's letter came in response to a request for medicines made a few weeks earlier. Two native authorities (Mbwana and Boghogo) in Chinteche District told the senior medical officer in Lilongwe that many of their people suffered from "coughing," while the nearest dispensary had no drugs to treat them.[10] The medical officer deployed Fred Nyirenda, a hospital assistant then stationed at Chinteche District Hospital, and a graduate of the Livingstonia Mission's training course in the early 1920s, to tour the villages.[11] Nyirenda reported he found "only coughs and colds," seasonal ailments that demanded no special treatment.[12]

Even if Nyirenda had found serious illnesses—he was likely worried about tuberculosis—the discord between patient and provider would not have been resolved. Through the late 1940s, the mainstay of tuberculosis treatment for Nyasaland's African patients was indoor bed rest. But as colonial medical officer John Goodall remembered, patients were loath to follow his instructions and preferred to "flock outside and lie in the sun."[13] The few tuberculosis patients who submitted to more heroic measures, at the hands of the colony's sole surgeon, had a procedure in which the affected lung was collapsed and the phrenic nerve crushed.[14] This treatment was invasive and was intended to relieve the worst of symptoms, not effect a cure.[15] While many patients sought cough mixtures, few submitted to long hospitalizations or painful surgical procedures.

But by the 1950s, the preferences of physicians and patients had both changed. With the arrival of novel drugs for a host of diseases, including tuberculosis, malaria, syphilis, and gonorrhea, European doctors and African hospital assistants had secured potent new therapeutics. Patients and providers alike had far greater confidence in the efficacy of these new drugs. For example, the number of patients voluntarily presenting for tuberculosis treatment increased from 366 in 1948 to 1,946 in 1958, following the introduction of streptomycin, PAS, and isoniazid. This pattern was repeated for a number of ailments. As a result, inpatient admission and outpatient attendance rose markedly in the first two postwar decades.

This chapter chronicles the consequences of the mid-twentieth-century antibiotic revolution in British Nyasaland. Patients began appearing at government hospitals and dispensaries in far greater numbers once drugs could meet expectations of efficacy. "The native only judges by results," the missionary physician John Christopherson had concluded in 1921.[16] John Lwanda has described how during the interwar era, comparative therapeutic efficacy in Chichewa was a discourse inflected with judgments about efficacy that were themselves tied up with race and class relations. *Mankhwala achizungu* (literally, "medicine of the whites") and *medicine achikuda* ("medicine of the blacks") were generally spoken of with respect; they could carry the power to harm or heal, but they were powerful. There was, however, a third category, known as *mankhwala achiboyi* ("medicine of the boys"). Here, "boy" was a reference to the hated moniker that Europeans gave their male workers, and the idea it carried was that this was the kind of medicine one would give to a servant, because it was less potent or even useless.[17]

It is telling that *mankhwala achiboyi* was a particularly common utterance during the interwar era. The fading of this term from common parlance was in part a result of the arrival of medicines many Africans considered useful in curing what ailed them. While yaws treatment of the 1920s had provided some temporary relief, and hookworm therapy of the 1930s could clear parasitic infestations, interwar European therapeutics could not cure Nyasaland's worst illnesses. Colonial doctors were all too well aware that news of their failures spread rapidly among Africans patients, their families, and indigenous healers.[18] But when more effective therapeutics entered public clinics after the war, so too did African patients.

Medical anthropologists have at times attributed to their subjects a logic of therapeutic evaluation that would appear irrational to the allopathic physician. In a study of the Mende of Sierra Leone, Caroline Bledsoe and Monica Goubaud concluded, "The most important elements of logical consistency that governed people's choices of medicines . . . seemed to be qualities such as shape, color, taste and consistency" of pills.[19] Bledsoe provided convincing evidence of the importance of locally specific beliefs about illness causation in health-care decision-making. Other less-evidenced ethnographic work has attributed the apparent skepticism of Western biomedicine among peoples in Latin America and Africa to "deep-seated mystical beliefs" or a "great lack of education."[20] But the history of biomedicine in Malawi demonstrates something quite different. Demand for the drugs and procedures on offer in government and mission clinics was a function of their efficacy in relieving symptoms and curing disease, rather than of cultural beliefs disconnected from biological realities. The mid-twentieth-century introduction of new antibiotics capable of curing previously fatal diseases led to a dramatic increase in attendance at government clinics.

Because few ethnographic studies of Africans' care-seeking behavior were conducted before the late 1960s, they mostly missed the changes resulting from the introduction of effective antibiotic therapies.[21] This chapter takes a different methodological approach, using colonial administrative data on disease-specific attendance.[22] Even with the necessary caveats about the accuracy of such data, this analysis demonstrates a rapid and significant increase in attendance at government facilities after the introduction of novel chemotherapeutics.

These findings are consistent with those of John Janzen, who, during the late 1960s in what was then Zaire, found that patients and their kin were empiricists. That is, patients were likely to be brought to the healer—biomedical or "traditional"—who had proven able to heal the sort of illness from which the patient seemed to be suffering.[23] The data are also consistent with a more recent review of the literature on medical pluralism in southern African history. In it, Anne Digby observed that African patients have long consulted a variety of healers, and many have held views on disease etiology that differed radically from those held by biomedical practitioners. Still, Digby contends, African patients' propensity to consult biomedical healers increased after they demonstrated greater rates of "therapeutic success" following the Second World War.[24] The evidence also demonstrates the profound *specificity* of African care-seeking behavior in midcentury Nyasaland. Patients began to present in greater numbers for a given disease soon after new, more efficacious treatments reached clinic shelves.

Historians of medicine have documented many shifts in health-seeking behavior impelled by the promise—rather than the proof—of better outcomes.[25] But this story is not one of overblown and unkept promises. With the arrival of new therapeutics, diseases were cured and suffering was relieved. The new drugs of the postwar era had demonstrable effects on mortality.[26] Nyasaland's Africans were not disposed to trust the promises of white officials during the late colonial era, a period of antigovernment popular mobilization and profound racial strife. The colonized found proof of medicine's efficacy not in official propaganda, but in the experiences of family members and neighbors. Medicine's newly demonstrated efficacy had profound political consequences, helping to impel the deeply unpopular Federation government to spend more on health care in Nyasaland than the British ever had.

Accounting for the Rise in Attendance

The use of medical and fiscal statistics in this chapter and the next merits at least a brief discussion of the circumstances attending their production. As explained in the introduction, budgets were so central to governance and so closely monitored that the veracity of revenue and expenditure figures can, in the main, be accepted. Even in the postcolonial era, the Malawi government under Hastings Kamuzu Banda was widely reputed to run an efficient and honest civil service; supporters and detractors alike considered budget figures accurate.[27]

Greater difficulties arise with statistics on patient attendance and diagnosis. Outpatient attendance figures were based on monthly reports filed by medical officers at hospitals and medical assistants at dispensaries. These figures were, to be sure, not entirely accurate, but there is little evidence to suggest any systematic bias that could account for an increase in attendance over time. Disease returns, on the other hand, reported the aggregated *diagnoses* made by medical providers. For diseases for which diagnoses were particularly uncertain—syphilis, tuberculosis, and malaria were famously difficult to definitively diagnose at midcentury—disease returns should not be read as the number of patients presenting with undeniable evidence of a given malady. In fact, after the Second World War, Nyasaland's directors of medical services were sufficiently doubtful of the accuracy of diagnoses at rural dispensaries that they did not include their disease returns in official statistics.[28] Thus, after 1940 the numbers presented in figures 5.6a and 5.6b include only those disease returns submitted by hospitals (though the total number of patient attendances was included in dispensary reports). But this actually renders the increase in attendance for certain diseases (e.g., tuberculosis, syphilis) after the Second World War all the more impressive.

Population statistics are among the most dubious, as censuses were infrequent and methodologically weak. Nyasaland's 1945 census was the last of the colonial era. Estimates for the next two decades were notoriously inexact. One official admitted that "the method of estimating the total population, in 1962, was to take the number of taxpayers [supposedly, all adult men, apart from those granted specific exemption for medical or other reasons], multiply by two to allow for those who avoided paying tax, and again by five to allow for dependents."[29] Figures are slightly more reliable after independence. In the 1966 census, enumerators visited all 1.5 million "dwelling units" in the country.[30] Censuses then followed roughly every decade, with one in 1977, and another in 1987.[31] In the following chapters I use population statistics to provide rough per capita figures. Though there is little evidence to indicate a systematic bias in these figures, they should not be regarded as accurate.

The dearth of statistics did not blind contemporary commentators to an undeniable trend during the 1950s and early 1960s. Writing in the *British Medical Journal* in 1960, Harry Gear, a consultant to the Federal Ministry of Health in Salisbury, marveled at "the insatiable demand for European medicine. Where less than a quarter of a century ago the large majority of Africans avoided European hospitals and clinics, they are now overwhelming them."[32] The situation had changed drastically since both Shircore (in 1930) and de Boer (in 1938) had lamented the sparse attendance by Africans at government hospitals and dispensaries. African outpatient attendance at government health facilities in Malawi increased rapidly, from 1.3 million in 1954 to 10.2 million in 1967. This increase far outpaced population growth; on a per capita basis, attendance increased from 0.45 in 1953 to 2.52 in 1969. African inpatient admissions rose as well, quadrupling between 1945 and 1965 (see figures 5.1, 5.2 and 5.3).

By the end of the 1960s, African outpatients attended government facilities far more often than mission ones. Figure 5.2 shows that in 1940, outpatient attendance was more than six times higher at government facilities than at missions. This ratio decreased to near-parity during the 1950s. But by the late 1960s, the figures were disparate once more; in 1969 government facilities treated more than four times as many African outpatients as the missions.[33] Data on inpatients, depicted in figure 5.3, indicate that government facilities and missions admitted similar numbers of patients throughout the 1950s and 1960s.

The parity between government and mission inpatient figures, and the disproportionate share of outpatients going to government facilities,

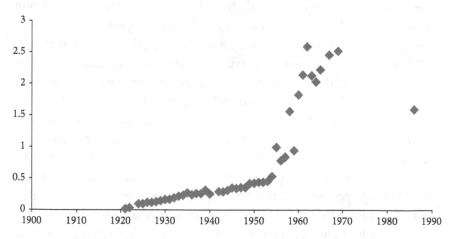

Figure 5.1 African outpatient attendance per capita at Nyasaland/Malawi government facilities, 1921–1986

Sources: Annual medical reports of the Medical Department (pre-1964) and reports of World Bank Missions to Malawi (1964–1986).

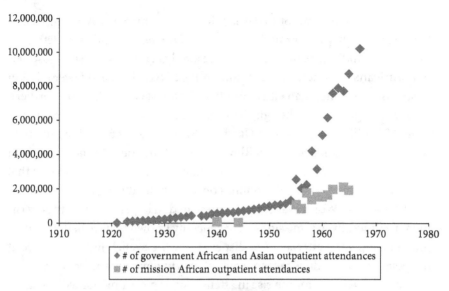

Figure 5.2 Government and mission outpatient attendance in Nyasaland/
Malawi, 1921–1967

Sources: Annual reports of the Medical Department (pre-1964); reports of World Bank Missions to
Malawi (1964–1982).

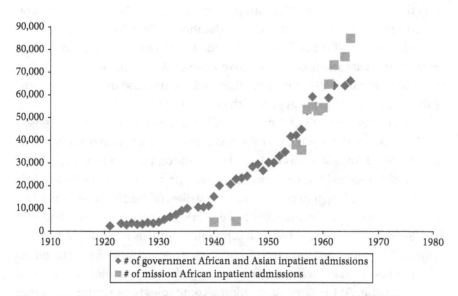

Figure 5.3 Government and mission inpatient admissions in Nyasaland/
Malawi, 1921–1965

Sources: Annual reports of the Medical Department (pre-1964); reports of World Bank Missions to
Malawi (1964–1982).

complicates the portrait of Malawi, still endorsed by many Africanists, as a land particularly rich in mission medicine. During the mid-twentieth century, Nyasaland's Africans were no more amply served by mission hospitals than Africans elsewhere in the region. In 1962 Nyasaland had fewer mission hospitals (sixty-one) than either Southern Rhodesia (sixty-five) or Northern Rhodesia (eighty), even though Nyasaland had an estimated African population (2.93 million) higher than Northern Rhodesia's (2.46 million) and only somewhat lower than Southern Rhodesia's (3.64 million).[34] Whereas early in the twentieth century government medicine for Africans was so absent that missions really were the only facilities open to them, during the two decades after the Second World War Africans presented in larger numbers to government facilities. Even if missions were generally known to have better-trained practitioners and better-stocked dispensaries, the availability of care free at the point of service drew far more outpatients to government facilities.

What can account for the rise in attendance at government medical facilities during the quarter century after the close of the Second World War? The idea that newly crowded hospitals were evidence of a turn away from "tradition" and toward "modern" European culture was often invoked by Southern Rhodesian officials during the Federation years. One of Gear's explanations for "the insatiable demand for European medicine" by 1960 was "the general acceptance of European culture and education."[35] It is true that the rise in attendance at medical facilities during the 1950s and 1960s was coincident with an increase in enrolment at government educational institutions. But the rise in medical attendance far outpaced the increase in educational enrollment, which barely kept pace with population growth.[36]

But it is true that tens of thousands of Nyasaland's Africans were exposed to European medicine each year via migration to work in mines and on plantations. Work in mines was dangerous, and though migrants had to submit to intrusive medical examinations, they were often not fully treated for their ailments.[37] This began to change after the strikes of the 1930s; seeking a less restive and more productive labor force, mining companies in the Rhodesias and South Africa began to tacitly accept, and eventually to publicize, the "stabilization" of African labor. Instead of being expected to come to the mines alone, mine workers were allowed to live with their families in improved mine housing. At the same time, mining companies began to provide more robust health services.[38] Still, such experiences could not explain the entire increase in overall attendance at government facilities beginning in the 1950s, which was far more generalized and abrupt.[39]

Furthermore, Africans living in Nyasaland had been exposed to Europeans for centuries, from the Portuguese traders and British missionaries of the nineteenth century, to the British and German troops of the First World War, to the employers and foremen in the mines and plantations.[40] The peak population of European settlers in Nyasaland (most of whom lived in Blantyre or Zomba) during the 1950s and 1960s was 9,300 (in 1960); the ratio of Africans to Europeans in Nyasaland in that year was 302:1. The penetration of "European culture" via mass media could not have been too deep; in 1968 less than 7 percent of rural Malawians (who made up 92 percent of the population) lived in a household with a radio.[41] Gear's claim is also less than convincing because it seems unlikely that appreciation for "European culture" would reach a zenith during the years of the Federation government. Though many Nyasaland Africans were converting to Christianity, prominent African Christian leaders of this era were more likely to foment distrust of government actions than they were to encourage acceptance of European culture.[42] In sum, the timing of the rise in attendance does not support the contention that it was a result of a newfound love of all things European.

The rise in attendances is in some part attributable to more accessible medical facilities. The number of rural dispensaries and "rural hospitals" (hospitals not staffed by a medical doctor) did increase, though not nearly as much as the postwar committee had originally proposed, growing only from 96 in 1946 to 112 in 1965. Though the Federal Ministry of Health proudly declared that the number of African hospitals in Nyasaland increased from 19 to 30 under its rule, most of these were smaller hospitals without doctors. As late as 1970 there was still only one "health unit" (a facility the size of a dispensary or larger) for every twenty thousand Malawians, one-half the ratio recommended by the World Health Organization at the time.[43] The rather slight increase in facilities is insufficient to explain a twelve-fold increase in outpatient attendance.

Changes in transportation, and in particular the spread of bicycle transport, did make medical facilities more accessible, but this can explain only a small part of the increase in attendance. Motor vehicle transport remained sparse throughout the colonial period. Nyasaland did experience a boom in bicycle ownership after the Second World War, increasing the range over which the sick could be transported (see figure 5.4).[44] But this change should not be overstated. In the late 1960s patients presenting to hospitals and dispensaries still came overwhelmingly from the immediate areas surrounding hospitals.[45]

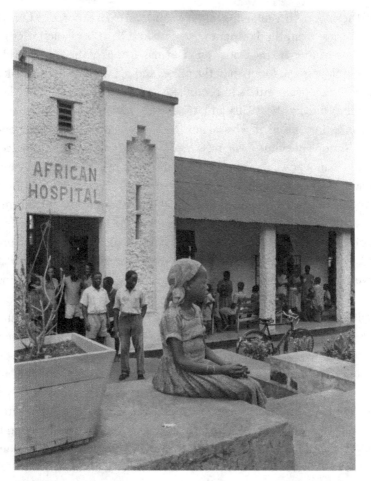

Figure 5.4 Outside Mlanje Hospital, February 1964. Note the bicycle on the bottom right.

Source: British Information Services, Central Office of Information, London. Reproduced with permission of UK National Archives.

Patients also came in larger numbers because the quality of the health facilities had improved. Roughly coincident with the rise in attendance at government facilities was a marked increase in recurrent expenditure on the government health sector. As shown in figure 5.5, recurrent expenditure on health care in 1965 was more than two times higher in inflation-adjusted terms than in 1955 and more than six times higher than in 1945. The rate of this rise in spending far outpaced population growth (see figure I.2 in the introduction). Most of the Federation-era increase in government health-care spending was devoted either to staff salaries or to paying for (increasingly

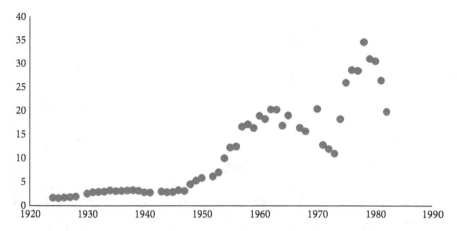

Figure 5.5 Recurrent government spending on Medical Department in Nyasaland/Malawi (UK pounds sterling, 2016 prices)

Sources: Annual reports of the Medical Department (pre-1964); Daniel Jack, *Economic Survey of Nyasaland, 1958–1959.* Ministry of Economic Affairs, Federation of Rhodesia and Nyasaland, 1959; Malawi, *A Conspectus including the Development Plan for 1965–69,* Blantyre: Malawi Ministry of Health, 1965.

expensive) drugs and supplies.[46] This rise in expenditures did not remedy many deficiencies in staffing and procurement. Even during years of budget cuts or acute staffing shortages, patients arrived in ever-increasing numbers.

The most important reason for the rise in attendance of Africans at government hospitals was the introduction of new drugs. The main event here is the revolution in antimicrobial therapeutics. In the United States, the first sulfonamide (sulfa) antibiotic reached the general public in the late 1930s. Penicillin was first mass marketed in 1945, followed in the coming years by bacitracin (1948) and chlortetracycline (1948). Effective therapy against pulmonary tuberculosis came with combination therapy including streptomycin (1948) and isoniazid (1952).[47] The antimalarial chloroquine reached consumers in the United States in 1946. Years—even decades—passed between the introduction of these drugs in Britain and their arrival in Nyasaland. Even after their introduction, these drugs were often strictly rationed. Still, they were powerful new tools. As demonstrated by figures 5.6a and 5.6b, the number of patients suffering from a number of common diseases who came to public-sector clinics rose precipitously in the aftermath of the introduction of novel therapeutics.

A rise in attendance figures for gonorrhea came after sulfa drugs became widely available in the 1940s. William Berry first used a sulfa drug called sulfanilamide (better known at the time by its trade name, M&B 693) at Mlanje

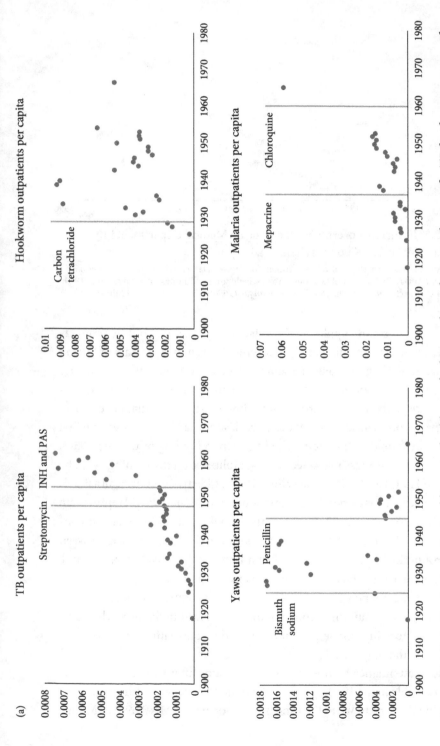

Figure 5.6a Outpatients per capita at public-sector health-care facilities and new drug introductions for TB, hookworm, yaws, and malaria

Sources: Annual reports of the Medical Department (pre-1964) and *Annual Report of the Work of the Nyasaland/Malawi Ministry of Health*. Zomba: Malawi Ministry of Health, 1965.

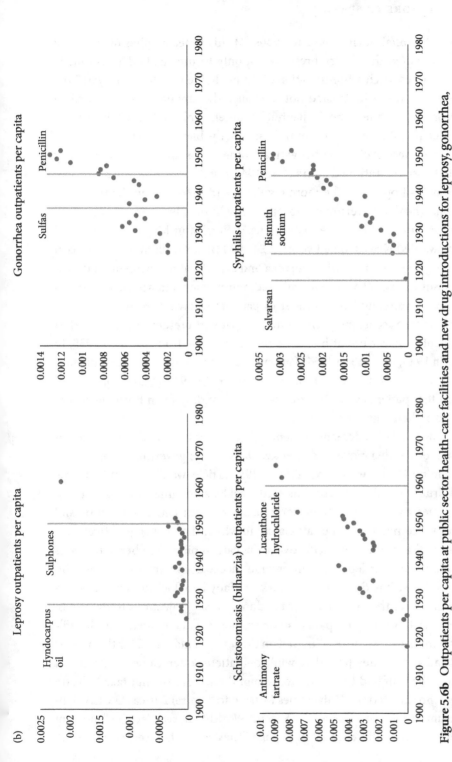

Figure 5.6b Outpatients per capita at public sector health-care facilities and new drug introductions for leprosy, gonorrhea, schistosomiasis, and syphilis

Sources: Annual reports of the Medical Department (pre-1964) and *Annual Report of the Work of the Nyasaland/Malawi Ministry of Health*. Zomba: Malawi Ministry of Health, 1965.

District Hospital during the late 1930s. At this time, supplies of this drug were so limited that Berry prescribed it only to inpatients. He also made sure to witness each administration of the medicine with his own eyes: "The dressers could not be trusted not to change the amount of the prescribed dose, or to substitute some similar but less potent tablet, retaining the surplus M&B for 'private practice,' or for their sale on the black market."[48]

Doctors were excited by the arrival of the new sulfa drugs, even if they had to be strictly rationed at first.[49] In 1941, the director of medical services wrote of his hope that "the more regular use of M&B 693 in the treatment of [gonorrhea] at government hospitals may in time bring infected persons in bigger numbers to those institutions."[50] Finally, in May 1945 the CDW Fund awarded Nyasaland a five-year, £42,000 (£1.68 million in 2016 prices) grant for free treatment of gonorrhea and syphilis at government and mission institutions.[51] This money allowed more patients to access sulfa drugs than ever before, and the number of patients receiving treatment for this condition rose accordingly. The number of patients presenting for gonorrhea treatment in government hospitals and clinics rose from 1,061 in 1935, to 2,089 in 1945, to 3,715 in 1951. Patients seemed to have growing confidence that treatment for this condition was effective. In 1944 medical officers reported that patients were less frequently absconding from hospitals before the end of their courses of treatment.[52]

During the 1950s demand for leprosy treatment increased after the introduction of another novel therapeutic. Dapsone, as government leprologist Dr. Gordon Currie would explain in a 1963 article, was "far from being the ideal drug." It had to be administered weekly, sometimes for years, and it sometimes caused permanent nerve damage.[53] But patients, doctors, and nurses welcomed the end of a long era in which the mainstay of treatment had been the infamously ineffective hydnocarpus oil. A number of missions had shuttered their leprosaria in previous decades, in part because, as John Iliffe explains, "the drugs did not work."[54] Many had flocked to mission-run leprosaria after the introduction of hydnocarpus oil injections in the 1920s. But by the 1940s neither patients nor providers had confidence in the efficacy of these drugs; those who lived on the settlements stayed for the meager food and shelter they provided, while outpatients often came for treatment because the staff had the power to exempt them from the hut tax.[55] Electra Dory, who directed the Universities Mission to Central Africa (UMCA) leprosarium in Likwenu during the Second World War, recalled the "apparent dejection and indifference" of the lepers: "They called themselves The Dead."

She remembered the futility of their regimens: "We rammed—I fear that is the only word that describes the treatment—we rammed in the oleaginous product of the *hydnocarpus wightiana*, causing in some cases more pain and destruction than the lepra bacilli."[56] Curative treatment was only possible after the arrival of dapsone therapy.[57]

This new efflorescence of public confidence was also seen in patients with other diseases. For tuberculosis, the rise in attendance followed the release of streptomycin and isoniazid at public hospitals in the mid-1950s. Penicillin, which began to arrive in small quantities at the end of the war, transformed therapy for syphilis.[58] Previous therapy for Africans diagnosed with syphilis was a series of sodium bismuth tartrate injections. These were painful and did not lead to a permanent cure.[59] By the late 1940s, physicians could rid bodies of syphilis and prevent its ravages with a single injection of penicillin. In the 1960s, attendance for schistosomiasis increased after the introduction of lucanthone hydrochloride. For malaria, the increase followed upon the dissemination of chloroquine.

More evidence that African patients generally evaluated the efficacy of therapeutics selectively is seen in the demand for injections. During the Second World War, medical officers lamented that many sick patients often demanded injections. William Berry ascribed this propensity to Africans' memories of yaws injections in the 1920s, which had brought dramatic cures.[60] Yet not all injections were equally popular. Medical officers complained that they could convince few patients to submit to antimony tartrate injections for schistosomiasis. This was, in general, an indolent infection; it could result in blood in the urine or eventually bladder cancer, but it was not as disfiguring as yaws, and the injection itself could precipitate serious malarial infections or abscesses.[61] African patients were, in Megan Vaughan's words, "discriminating" in their approach to injections.[62]

Some prominent contemporary commentators on colonial medicine interpreted the increasing numbers of patients presenting for treatment as evidence of rising incidence of disease.[63] But the rise in attendance was more likely a product of greater confidence in the efficacy of biomedicine. Such was the opinion of the medical officer in Mzimba, who reported in 1956 that "the increase in patients in hospital with Pulmonary Tuberculosis is not thought to represent an increase of the disease in the district. . . . All but one of the cases in hospital were chronic in nature, mostly with fibrosis and cavitation."[64] By 1956, routine curative treatment for tuberculosis in Nyasaland's district hospitals was two out of three drugs (streptomycin, isoniazid, and

PAS) "over a long period of time." This was not, by Malawian standards, inexpensive therapy, and shortages of these drugs were common. Still, they had become the standard of care.[65] Recent studies of AIDS treatment demonstrate that, in similarly impoverished settings, the introduction of effective chemotherapeutic agents correlates to a rise in reported cases, particularly when treatment is provided free at the point of care.[66] In midcentury Nyasaland as well, the availability of drugs was a major factor behind the increase in reported cases of many diseases presenting at government health facilities.

Medicine under Federation Rule

By the 1950s, then, Nyasaland's government finally had healing technologies that Africans patients wanted. But the rise in attendance at government facilities coincided with the coming of a government that Africans in Nyasaland most decidedly did not want. The increase in attendance occurred just in time for the era of the Federation of Rhodesia and Nyasaland, a decade-long and ultimately abortive political experiment at the close of the colonial era.

The Federation was the culmination of decades of effort. During the interwar years, white settlers in Southern and Northern Rhodesia began a campaign to join their two territories under a single government. In the mid-1930s, white settlers in Nyasaland argued that shared government would bring economic benefits to their territory as well. Settlers resumed advocacy for a shared regional government after the Second World War. Part of the urgency they felt stemmed from a growing fear that without a stronger union between their previously separate colonies, the seemingly inevitable move toward majority rule would sweep them from power. When Conservatives retook power in the 1951 UK elections, the Colonial Office's erstwhile objections to a federated government vanished. In 1953, the Central African Federation—including Southern Rhodesia, Northern Rhodesia, and Nyasaland, with a capital in Salisbury—was inaugurated.[67]

Both urban and rural Africans in Nyasaland objected to a political system that moved political authority from London to Salisbury. Many Africans in Nyasaland had spent time in Southern Rhodesia; they knew its racist policies. They did not trust Godfrey Huggins, prime minister of Southern Rhodesia (as well as a physician), when he promised the new federation would be a "partnership" between whites and blacks. Perhaps their concern derived from the fact that shortly after Huggins pledged to the Colonial Office that he would pursue "partnership," he reassured his fellow white settlers that it would be "the partnership between a rider and his horse."[68] On a tour of British Africa, Joan Wicken observed that Nyasaland's African population believed they "must do something now before [they] get into a position like that in Southern Rhodesia," where Africans were subjected to pass laws and had endured the alienation of huge portions of their land.[69] The inclusion of Nyasaland in the Federation was likely part of a deal in which British officials agreed to allow federation in exchange for the new government's assumption of Nyasaland's debts.[70] In a 1962 pamphlet, Federation officials claimed they had included Nyasaland "at the insistence of the British Government. . . . Britain had found the financial burden of the backward and impoverished Protectorate becoming increasingly onerous."[71] Thus in 1953 Nyasaland became the unwanted, impoverished, rebellious third member of a Federation dominated by white settlers.[72]

Under the new government's constitution, health was a federal, rather than a territorial, responsibility.[73] The Southern Rhodesian negotiators who helped shape the Federal Constitution had two reasons to favor the designation of health as a federal responsibility. The first was that a Federal health service could be a focus of propaganda for the new government. As early as 1939, Viscount Bledisloe—chair of a commission that favored a Central African federation—had argued before the UK House of Lords that Southern Rhodesian settlers were devoted to improving the health and education of Africans.[74] By taking control of health, a "big-spending" department with visible everyday functions, the Federal government could secure legitimacy, if not among black Africans, then at least among officials in Whitehall. Such legitimacy would help Federation supporters convince London to grant them a fully independent, white-led state.[75]

Another reason Southern Rhodesian negotiators pressed to make health a responsibility of the Federal government was that doing so promised to save their own territorial government a good deal of money. The Federation was in essence a vehicle to transfer financial resources from Northern Rhodesia's copper mines (nationalized since the early postwar years) to Southern Rhodesia and, to a lesser extent, Nyasaland. Between 1955 and 1961, Southern Rhodesia received roughly 64 percent of Federal expenditure, though it contributed only 50 percent of Federal revenue.[76] Southern Rhodesian officials were eager to use the plentiful Northern Rhodesian revenues to pay for their own Medical Department.

Federal control over health care took effect on July 1, 1954. Thereafter, health-care budgets for the three territories were decided by the Federal Parliament, a legislature designed to protect settler interests. The Parliament consisted of thirty-five members, twenty-six of whom were elected by settlers. Nyasaland, for its part, had only seven members: four elected by settlers, two Africans nominated by the governor, and one missionary selected by the governor to represent "African interests."

Promises about health care had featured prominently in pro-Federation arguments. In 1945, one such advocate, Roy Welensky, argued that health services for Africans would expand more rapidly under Federation rule than under the Colonial Office.[77] He was not incorrect. During the Federation era, spending on services in Nyasaland (including medical services) did rise markedly. Nyasaland received more funding than it contributed to the Federal budget, and officials in Salisbury took every opportunity to remind the world of this fact. In the very first month of Federal responsibility for health care, Manoah Chirwa, one of the two African members of parliament from Nyasaland, complained that African interests had been neglected in the Federation budget. Reverend Percy Ibbotson, a white missionary selected to represent Southern Rhodesia's "African interests," chided Chirwa and proceeded to list the projects related to African health and welfare slated for construction.[78]

Ibbotson's response to Chirwa indicates a desire to demonstrate beneficent motives, particularly as opposition mounted. From the outset, the Federation government was unpopular among Africans in Nyasaland. The Nyasaland-born, London-based physician Hastings Kamuzu Banda penned arguments against the Federation, beginning with a letter to the Bledisloe Commission in 1938. In 1949, Banda coauthored a pamphlet with Zambian activist Harry Nkumbula outlining a case against the Federation.[79] In April 1953, just before the Federation came into being, the Nyasaland African Congress (NAC) organized a nonviolent resistance campaign that included a strike by civil servants and farm laborers as well as boycotts of tax payments and purchases at European-owned stores.[80] This campaign coincided with growing resistance among smallholder farmers to other colonial policies. Chief Gomani of Ncheu told his subjects to disregard unpopular soil erosion regulations enacted by the Department of Agriculture. In May 1953 police deployed to Ncheu to apprehend Gomani, but a crowd fended off the policemen while the chief escaped.[81] Though the agricultural regulations predated the Federation, the NAC leadership linked opposition to the agricultural regulations to their anti-Federation campaign. In the Lower Shire Valley, women sang a song about the regulations in which they called for "death" to "Federation *capitãos*."[82]

None of these protests succeeded in preventing the advent of the Federation on August 1, 1953. But protests continued. That same month, African tenants on settler-owned tea and tobacco estates rebelled against increasing labor demands and shrinking land allocations. The tenants were particularly enraged by two stories, one about a plantation manager who had stripped naked a woman he found collecting firewood on his estate, and another a rumor of a planter who had killed two men who were stealing oranges. These stories confirmed the commonly held image of whites as *chifwamba* (cannibals), in search of African bodies. Tenants refused to work on European estates, and railway workers went on strike. Protestors blocked roads with trees, cut telephone wires, destroyed the homes of a half dozen chiefs, vandalized European-owned homes and businesses, and beat tax collectors. With Nyasaland's police overwhelmed, and the territory's troops fighting Chinese guerrillas in Malaya, Governor Geoffrey Colby had to request policemen from neighboring colonies to reassert control. They did so, but only after killing eleven Africans and injuring seventy-two more.[83]

While during the 1930s and 1940s most officials in London felt little urgency to spend more on health care in Nyasaland, even as they granted budget increases for health care in more restive corners of the West Indies and West Africa, the unrest of 1953 impelled Governor Colby and Federal prime minister Huggins to expand both policing and health services. In 1954 Nyasaland's police commissioner, Charles Apthorp, established a branch, called the Police Mobile Force, consisting of fourteen European officers and two hundred Africans. The force, designed for "use in disturbed areas," was quickly deployed to southern districts, where they beat villagers in house-to-house raids. In the years that followed, the Mobile Force continued to patrol the territory, enforcing agricultural rules and responding to civil unrest.[84]

Still, as Pierre Bourdieu observed, the carceral "right hand" of the state is often accompanied by a welfarist "left hand."[85] Health services in Nyasaland were not nearly so robust as in Bourdieu's France, but officials did publicize them in an effort to draw attention away from popular discontent. Medicine was the symbol of imperial virtue, often in lavish ceremony and florid language. Built at a cost of £702,000 (£15.8 million in 2016 prices), the Queen Elizabeth Central Hospital was dedicated at a ceremony attended by the Queen Mother in Blantyre in 1957.[86]

The Federation's early years saw increases in spending on health. Recurrent Medical Department expenditure in Nyasaland more than doubled, in inflation-adjusted terms, between 1951 and 1958 (see figure 5.5).[87] Recurrent medical expenditure as a percentage of total recurrent expenditure increased from 7.3 percent in 1952 to 9.9 percent in 1958.[88] Per capita recurrent Medical Department expenditure more than doubled between 1953 and 1958 (see figure I.2 in the introduction). New construction also accelerated; Nyasaland Medical Department's capital expenditures rose, in inflation-adjusted terms, more than sixfold between 1953 and 1959.[89]

During this expansion, critics of the Federation continued to point to inequitable policies. Even though Nyasaland was a net recipient, it received a much smaller share of Federation medical expenditure than Northern or Southern Rhodesia (all three territories had similar populations).[90] New drugs in high demand were more expensive than older therapies and, as the next sections detail, Federation officials frequently rebuffed Nyasaland physicians' requests.

To many Africans, the main problem with the Federation was not the Medical Department's budget. More fundamentally, they resented being ruled by avowed white supremacists in Southern Rhodesia. Rural Africans also opposed the continuation of *thangata* and the harsh enforcement of anti-erosion agricultural regulations. They protested the increase in poll tax rates, which rose from 17s/6d in 1954 to 30s in 1961.[91] Indirect tax increases and cuts to maize subsidies also disproportionately affected Africans.[92] Among Medical Department staff, discontent with Federation rule had significant effects, as African staff had their responsibilities downgraded and privileges stripped. Between 1953 and 1958, the number of employees in Nyasaland's Medical Department fell from 1,241 to fewer than 600.[93]

The widespread discontent found a voice in July 1958 when, after practicing as a physician in London and the Gold Coast for two decades, Hastings Kamuzu Banda returned to Nyasaland to a hero's welcome. Banda and other members of the recently formed Malawi Congress Party toured the nation, denouncing the "stupid Federation."[94] In March 1959, rumors circulated among settlers that MCP leadership was plotting a massacre. Nyasaland's governor declared a state of emergency, called up federal troops from Southern Rhodesia, and imposed martial law.[95] Hundreds of Africans (including Banda) were imprisoned and more than fifty killed.[96] Protests continued, as Africans called for Banda's release and an end to Federation rule.

In the midst of unrest, Federation officials redoubled their efforts to demonstrate legitimacy, to Whitehall as well as to Nyasaland's Africans, by increasing health spending. Recurrent expenditure on Nyasaland's Medical Department rose from £766,329 in 1959 (£16.4 million in 2016 prices) to £1,034,549 in 1962 (£20.3 in 2016 prices).[97] In inflation-adjusted terms, per capita recurrent government health spending was higher in 1962 than at any other point in Malawi's history between 1924 and 1982 (see figure I.2 in the introduction).

This spending favored European settlers and reflected the Federation's racist underpinnings. For instance, while Federation officials claimed that there was not enough money to replace many old and dilapidated African hospitals, funds were spent to ensure that even nominally multiracial hospitals had not only racially segregated wards but also segregated kitchen facilities.[98] And while more money was spent on health care in Nyasaland during the Federation than ever before, Northern and Southern Rhodesia, which each had larger white settler populations, continued to receive far greater shares of the Federal budget. In the fiscal year 1954–1955, Nyasaland received only 9.8 percent of total Federation Medical Services expenditures. This figure barely changed in succeeding years, rising only slightly, to 11.7 percent in 1958–1959.[99] Unrest could help impel increases in health spending, but it could not equalize budgets across racial and territorial lines.

Nevertheless, Federation propagandists made medicine central to official rhetoric during and after Nyasaland's state of emergency. On New Year's Day in 1960, the pro-Federation daily *Nyasaland Times* announced that the new ninety-bed Nkata Bay District Hospital was "virtually complete." It had been built, the article noted, "with funds provided by the Federal Government," and contained "a modern operating theatre and X-ray plant."[100] That same year, Federation consultant Harry Gear penned an essay in the pages of the *Lancet*, declaring: "Medicine's true teachers and disciples give more to Africa than medical care in a hospital or clinic. Their integrity and philosophy are a demonstration of the goodness to be found in their culture."[101] Citing *Proud Record*, an apologia written by Southern Rhodesian physician Michael Gelfand and published by the Government Printer in Salisbury, the *Nyasaland Times* announced in May 1960 that there was "twice as much for health" in 1958 as in the year before federation (1952).[102]

Recognizing that the fate of their regime would be decided in London, Federation officials launched a public relations campaign focused on British newspapers. The advertisements sought to show that the Federation had unburdened the British government of costly responsibilities. They assumed that the metropolitan public was tiring of quelling nationalist movements and attempting to make good on expensive promises of development.[103] One ad that appeared in the *Evening Standard* in late 1960 made health care a barometer of the regime's beneficence: "Only a rapidly expanding Federal economy can provide the educational and health facilities and employment needed by this rapidly growing population. . . . The health service has been greatly extended."[104] The advertisement was explicit in linking the health benefits of federation to the quest for continued legitimacy. In bold letters at the end of the ad, the copy read, "It would be a tragedy for all races in the Federation if this remarkable progress were stopped or reversed, if these great achievements were nullified, if economic and financial order were to break down and give way to chaos."[105]

Speaking to audiences in the United Kingdom, Federal prime minister Roy Welensky lost no opportunity to extol the benefits that his government had brought to Africans. In a 1961 speech at the University of Birmingham, Welensky claimed that Africans living in the Federation enjoyed "probably the finest health service on the continent."[106] During another speech that year, he spoke of the "diagnostic X-rays and simple laboratories and operating theatres" that had become "a *sine qua non* at all hospitals from the district level upward."[107] In a late plea to save his government, he noted "the time is now more than ripe for the Federation to take a completely fresh look at what the nation now has provided in capital works and all the recurrent expenditure that results therefrom in the provision and maintenance of the . . . services and facilities, staff to run the institutions, drugs, food for the patients and all the other items that contribute to the total cost of providing hospital services."[108] Health spending was, to Welensky, one of the best retorts to the unceasing calls to dissolve the Federation.

Welensky and his aides knew, by this point, that they were in a last-ditch struggle to save their regime. With a British public weary of colonial rebellions, particularly after Mau Mau in Kenya and the Malayan Emergency, UK prime minister Harold Macmillan signaled his preparedness to grant independence to many of the empire's remaining holdings. In January 1960, after a visit to Nyasaland, Macmillan admitted he had a dour opinion of "the cause of Federation." It was, he observed, "almost desperate because of the strength of African opinion against it."[109] In response to Macmillan's admission, in a speech the next month, that a "wind of change" was sweeping across Africa, the Ministry of Information in Salisbury published a pamphlet on the benefits of the Federation to Nyasaland. The introduction read like a plea and a threat: "In light of current developments . . . it now seems opportune to survey the tremendous benefits Nyasaland has received from Federation and what the cost would be should that Territory decide to break away."[110] The first chapter was a paean to the growth of the health sector, extolling "the human drama of the most undeveloped and backward part of the Federation being lifted in less than a decade to a parity in health services with its more highly industrialized and sophisticated neighbors."[111] Federation officials still hoped that spending on health would vindicate their larger project.

The Malawi Congress Party and Smallpox Vaccination

Far from being a force for pacification, medical and public health services became a locus of political conflict in late Federation-era Nyasaland. While the Malawi Congress Party gained popular support, officials in Salisbury and Zomba accused Banda and other MCP leaders of denying patients access to health-care facilities. In a session of Nyasaland's Legislative Council in July 1960, Michael Blackwood claimed MCP members were forcing sick African patients to vacate government and mission hospitals.[112] Kanyama Chiume, the MCP's publicity secretary, denied the accusations, calling them "a pack of fabrications . . . to try and discredit the Malawi Congress Party in the eyes of the world."[113]

Accusations against the MCP only grew more heated. In October 1960 the *Nyasaland Times* reported that a compulsory smallpox vaccination campaign had run into opposition in the Central Province. Young children ran away from vaccinators, a native authority told a vaccination team to leave, and another team was stoned by a crowd.[114] Initially this resistance was reported without any mention of the MCP. But by late November, the pro-Federation *Nyasaland Times* was blaming the opposition to smallpox vaccination on "intimidation" by "Malawi Congress Party followers."[115]

On December 6, the *Nyasaland Times* ran a front-page photo of an African infant with smallpox (see figure 5.7). Below the horrifically pock-marked body, a caption read:

Take a good look at this little pain-ridden child. He's barely six months old—and will be scarred for life if he does not die. This picture is not a "Federal" picture. It was taken by a man with no political axe to grind. Take another good look at smallpox and remember the handiwork of political agitators in the Central Province of Nyasaland.[116]

Public health reports and medical publications echoed the accusation of sabotage. As the *Annual Report on Public Health in the Federation for 1960* lamented, "Attempts to bring the outbreak under control were hampered by the political unrest and the incitement and intimidation of the people to evade and disrupt vaccination programs."[117] Writing in the pages of the *British Medical Journal* in July 1961, months after resistance to vaccination had ceased, J. Moat Sword, senior medical officer for the Central Province, attributed the smallpox "epidemic" to "political opposition to vaccination campaigns."[118]

A full-throated denunciation of MCP interference is found in a 1962 Federation pamphlet, which refers to health in Nyasaland during the Federation as a "Success—marred by politics." After recounting statistics on the increases in spending, patient attendance, and new facilities, the pamphlet lamented, "This happy picture was sadly marred some 18 months ago when a campaign of disturbance and intimidation was started against the Federal health services . . . leading officials of this political party who, while taking great care to obtain their own vaccinations, travelled around the country, urging villagers and schoolchildren to boycott the vaccinators. . . . Smallpox epidemics broke out among schoolchildren, and many of them died as a result."[119] The pamphlet also made explicit the use of health services as a symbol of legitimacy by accusing MCP leaders of seeking to sabotage them. The pamphlet argued, "The attitude of extremist politicians in Nyasaland is that if health services have to be Federal Government ones they would rather have no health services at all." But, the authors continued hopefully, "with the wonderful hospital facilities all over the country, and the experience of the deaths from smallpox of unvaccinated children . . . the people of Nyasaland . . . are becoming more and more aware of the anarchy in health matters which would arise once the Federal services were completely taken away."[120]

MCP leaders denied the accusations. In *Tsopano*, the party's newsletter, Chiume called the accusations "unfounded and false." Instead, he countered, "it was a man with UFP [Welensky's party] sympathies, perhaps employed as an *agent provocateur*, who went to persuade people not to accept vaccination as it would cause sterility." The entire "comic opera" was an attempt to slander Dr. Banda and the MCP.[121] Historian John McCracken and

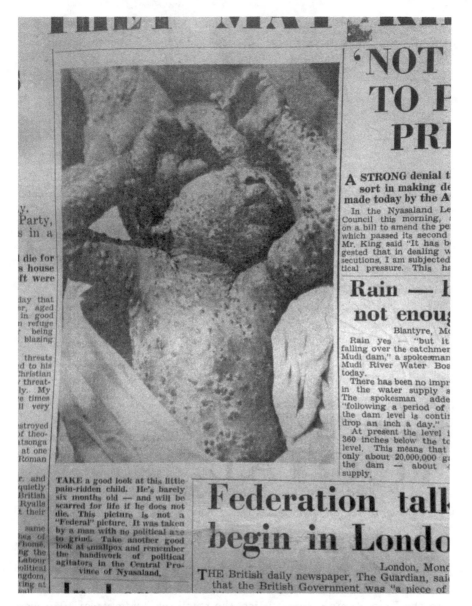

Figure 5.7 Infant with smallpox, Central Province, Nyasaland, 1960

Source: Nyasaland Times, December 6, 1960. Reproduced with permission of Malawi National Archives.

Banda biographer Philip Short also disputed the Federation's charge of MCP intimidation. Resistance to vaccination was, McCracken argued, "more an expression of popular mistrust than the result of political action."[122] Given the concomitant reactions against agricultural regulations and the imposition of federation, opposition to state-run compulsory vaccination was predictable.

The existing historiography has not, however, analyzed the technological shortcomings of the vaccine itself and the political economy of its distribution. Such an analysis would demonstrate that resistance to vaccination was also a function of the lack of efficacy of vaccination campaigns. Africans in Nyasaland had long experience with smallpox vaccination. Compulsory since 1908, smallpox was the only vaccine black Malawians routinely received before 1973.[123] The inability of government-run campaigns to prevent epidemics had become evident to many Africans as early as the first decade of the twentieth century. By the 1930s, official reports of "evasion" and refusal to submit to compulsory vaccination were commonplace.[124] An intensive campaign had been launched in the Central and Southern Provinces in 1948, but a new epidemic arose less than a decade later, in 1956. As vaccinators returning to affected villages in Kasungu that year observed, "The women and children run away and hide in the bush until the vaccinators have left."[125]

It is unsurprising then, that in the midst of protests and widespread distrust of government, rural Africans in some villages were unwilling to submit to a procedure of seemingly dubious merit administered by a widely reviled regime.[126] Compulsory vaccination (as well as burning the huts of smallpox cases) resembled other forms of coercive state action, such as tax collection, forcible labor recruitment, and door-to-door beatings by the Police Mobile Force. While voluntary curative medicine was becoming increasingly popular, compulsory vaccination was as distrusted as ever.

In any case, the 1960–1961 epidemic might be attributable less to political opposition than to problems with handling the vaccine. According to the Federation's own statistics, the smallpox epidemic of 1960 was no worse than other recent epidemics. During a smallpox outbreak in Northern Rhodesia that took many more lives than Nyasaland's 1960–1961 epidemic, officials did not blame political opponents, either in Nyasaland or Northern Rhodesia[127] In fact, medical authorities in both territories attributed the ferocity of the epidemic mainly to inefficacious vaccines. "Many cases showed signs of previous vaccination," reported the Medical Department, and few newly vaccinated children showed "takes" (the characteristic lesions at the injection site demonstrating a desired immune reaction).[128] By 1956, the Federation Ministry of Health had discontinued use of lanolinated lymph in favor of glycerinated lymph. This new lymph showed "noticeable improvement" in the rate of takes, but lost potency at high ambient temperatures. Because many of Nyasaland's facilities lacked refrigeration, the vaccine often lost potency by the time it was injected.[129] Anticipating this problem, Southern Rhodesian officials used more expensive freeze-dried vaccines, but only in parts of their own territory.[130] Despite these known deficiencies, when the 1960–1961 epidemic struck, Federation authorities blamed only the MCP; their reports contained no discussion of the rate of takes or of potential problems with the vaccine itself.

At the same time, Banda did not do as much as he could have to quell opposition to vaccination. In London in November 1960, just before negotiations over the future of the Federation, a reporter from the *Rhodesia Herald* asked Banda to instruct people to stop resisting vaccinators. The reporter claimed Banda demurred, insisting there was no smallpox epidemic in Nyasaland, only propaganda by the pro-Welensky press. He had come to London, he added, not as a physician, but as a politician.[131] Though the episode was recounted by an unsympathetic newspaper, Banda's response did indicate a disinclination to quell popular resistance, of any kind, if it could help destabilize the "stupid Federation."[132]

Banda's leadership in the fight for independence would win him the trust of many Malawians. Popular belief in the beneficence of Banda's new government helped break the cycle of self-reinforcing doubt, in which resistance to vaccination campaigns (by a distrusted colonial government) had helped spur repeated outbreaks, which in turn spurred more distrust of the vaccination campaigns.[133] Medical authorities in the Federation reported a "much readier acceptance of vaccinations" in Nyasaland in the year following the 1961 elections, which Banda's MCP won in a landslide.[134] Progress against smallpox accelerated after independence. With freeze-dried vaccine donated by UNICEF and without popular opposition, smallpox was eradicated from Malawi in 1971.[135] But a decade earlier this feat seemed a long way off, and smallpox control remained an arena for political conflict.

Medical Practice under the Federation: Rationing Drugs, Supplies, and Personnel

Beneath the slogans and propaganda that formed the discursive contests over medicine, what was the lived experience of medical practice in Nyasaland during the Federation years? In this section, the focus turns from political parties and pamphlets to correspondence between doctors, auxiliaries, and pharmacists. Given the centrality of new drugs to the rise in attendance at public-sector hospitals and dispensaries—and to Federation propaganda campaigns—health-care providers' near-constant frustration over rationing of essential medicines and supplies marked a jarring departure from official rhetoric. The administrators charged with managing central pharmacy stores and apportioning medical budgets denied hospitals and dispensaries the supplies necessary to treat the influx of patients. Yet medical practitioners— including British doctors with a firm belief in the superiority of European over African life—were loath to practice what they considered substandard medicine. The acrimony of these debates recalled the ardor of the disputes between the Colonial Office and directors of medical services calling for greater spending during the 1930s.

Limits on spending for new drugs meant that for the average patient in Nyasaland, new therapeutics for many diseases arrived much later than in America or Western Europe. In the treatment of malaria, one of the most common illnesses among Africans in Nyasaland, patients attending government facilities suffered even greater delays in access to new treatment. Mepacrine, an antimalarial known for its severe adverse neurological effects and prolonged treatment course, fell into disuse in the pharmacies of wealthier countries by the mid-1940s, as it was replaced by chloroquine. But for the next decade and a half, mepacrine remained the standard of care for the treatment of Africans in Nyasaland. The director of medical services noted the reason: in the mid 1950s, chloroquine was almost seven times the cost of mepacrine.[136] Only when the price of chloroquine fell below that of mepacrine did it become the treatment of choice in Nyasaland.[137]

Low levels of funding also resulted in shortages of new drugs to treat tuberculosis. While supplies of streptomycin had been limited in the United Kingdom in 1946, patients in Nyasaland still faced shortages of the drug almost a decade later. In 1954, streptomycin was distributed to Nyasaland's hospitals on a strict quota that was insufficient to treat all of the patients with active pulmonary tuberculosis infections. Isoniazid remained out of stock at the central pharmacy for months at a time.[138] "What do I do for pulmonary TB?" asked an exasperated medical officer at Mzimba in a letter to the director of medical services.[139] Two years later Dr. John Goodall, Nyasaland's medical specialist, complained to Director of Medical Services Howard Murcott that TB patients were again being denied treatment because the central pharmacy was without streptomycin. The Federal Ministry of Health had not dispatched the amount he had ordered. Goodall reported, "It is impossible to continue to treat tuberculosis patients in any satisfactory way."[140]

Treatment of tuberculosis with newer therapeutics was expensive, considering Nyasaland's meager health-care budget. In 1964, a year of therapy with isoniazid plus streptomycin cost thirty-five times the annual per capita Medical Department expenditure.[141] But Goodall was not satisfied with persistent shortages of necessary drugs. Like de Boer, he had first practiced colonial medicine in South Asia, where he had grown used to more amply funded medical services. His sympathies were definitely procolonial, and he blamed Hastings Kamuzu Banda for spoiling a formerly "happy and contented country."[142] Goodall did not see Africans and Europeans as equals, but he did expect that he would have the drugs and equipment necessary to maintain his own professional standards.

Perhaps the most colorful expressions of professional frustration concerned the poor quality of surgical supplies. In commenting on the director of medical services' decision to substitute his request for bone drills with "ordinary engineer's twist drills" supplied by a local firm,[143] one physician resorted to language that was—by the standards of this genre of correspondence—dripping with condescension:

> The drills fit. However, unless they are made from Vitallium or stainless steel there is a very real risk of bone porosis due to small pieces of the drill metal wearing off. . . . I imagine that is why the proper bone drills are more expensive—they are made for the job.[144]

Drugs and equipment were not the only essential components of a health-care system that were in short supply during the Federation era. Even as overall spending increased rapidly, the number of personnel in Nyasaland's Medical Department steadily decreased during the 1950s. In 1959, doctors, nurses, hospital assistants, and other medical personnel stationed in Nyasaland and working for the UK Colonial Medical Service had to decide whether they would transfer into the Federal Service or resign. Up until that point, they had been allowed to remain in the Colonial Service and work for the Federal Ministry of Health.

Many did not wish to make the transfer. African staff objected to rule by Southern Rhodesia. Some expatriate physicians had political and ideological objections to Southern Rhodesian racial policy, but for many the greater drawback to the transfer was the fact that they would have to relinquish the career prospects and benefits of the Colonial Service, including pensions. In the years leading up to this mandatory transfer, many medical personnel resigned. The Medical Department's staff numbered 1,241 in 1951, but by the end of June 1958 it had dropped to 599. In all, less than half of the African staff employed by Nyasaland's Medical Department at the start of the Federation transferred to the Federal Service.[145] So even as health-care spending increased, the numbers of African and expatriate medical staff fell during the Federation years.

Physician-anthropologist Paul Farmer has written about the process of "socialization for scarcity," wherein doctors, public health professionals, and patients in resource-poor settings become accustomed, after years of paltry budgets, to dismal standards of medical provision.[146] But in Nyasaland, the persistence of vocal dissatisfaction from medical officers indicates that many of them never became socialized for scarcity. In unceasing demands for sufficient stocks of essential medicines, better drugs, functional diagnostic equipment, and proper surgical supplies, the doctors objected to irksome delays, requisition denials, and substandard equipment. The tone of correspondence between medical officers and officials in the colonial capital often turned testy, as central administrators objected to cost overruns while medical officers rested their claims on inviolable professional standards.

In chapter 3 I argued that the prosopographical profiles of the colonial medical officers helped explain their expectations of colonial medicine. Nyasaland's doctors were not a racially progressive group. Joan Wicken observed during the mid-1950s that while the Gold Coast had integrated hospitals prior to independence, Nyasaland retained racially segregated facilities.[147] Nyasaland's European doctors rarely objected to this segregation, but they did resent drug shortages and broken equipment. Rather than resorting to notions of racial equality or the right to health care, medical officers most often invoked the dignity of their profession. Facing constant claims of scarcity, medical officers persisted in demanding recently released chemotherapeutics and specialized equipment.[148] They insisted that they could only faithfully discharge their duties if given the tools they had been trained to use.

The Dissolution of the Federation

Federal officials had worked assiduously to paint a picture of generosity in Nyasaland's medical provision, but once the Federation's fate was sealed, they cut budgets as deeply as they could. After years of accusing the MCP of sabotaging efforts to improve health, in 1963 Federal officials began tearing drugs and supplies from the shelves of Nyasaland's hospitals.[149]

In early 1962, officials in the Colonial Office concluded it was inevitable that the UK government would accede to MCP demands to dissolve the Federation. In an August 1961 election, the MCP won 99 percent of the African vote.[150] Hastings Kamuzu Banda transformed from imprisoned firebrand to prime minister of Nyasaland in little more than a year. In December 1962, Richard Austen ("Rab") Butler, head of the Colonial Office's Central African Office, announced to Parliament that Nyasaland would withdraw from the Federation. Butler and Banda had agreed, by that point, that Nyasaland would gain full independence from Britain by mid-1964.[151]

Even as anti-Federation forces prevailed in Nyasaland, the balance of power in Southern Rhodesia shifted in favor of more ardent white supremacists. In Southern Rhodesia's December 1962 election, Welensky's Federal Party lost power to the Rhodesian Front, which promised to declare Southern Rhodesia an independent state under white rule. This they would do in November 1965, but in the interim the Rhodesian Front dispensed with the pretense of "partnership."[152] Between July 1962 and July 1963, the Federal Ministry of Health organized the removal of £11,000 (£211,000 in 2016 prices) in medicines, equipment, and supplies from Nyasaland to Southern Rhodesia.[153] Sally Hubbard, a visiting British nurse working in Zomba's African Hospital, ruefully recalled "a frustrating morning with an official who could not believe that there just was not any more linen or other equipment lurking somewhere."[154]

The situation would continue to decline, as budget cuts and mass resignations followed the handover of health-care services to Nyasaland's government. The main impetus for the budget cuts was Banda's determination to keep a promise he had made to Butler in their 1962 negotiations on the transition to independence. Banda had pledged that within ten years, he would move the new country from an initial reliance on British aid to budgetary self-reliance.[155] Intent to keep this pledge, at the end of 1963 Banda's minister of finance Henry Phillips slashed spending on former Federal services—including health care—by 15 percent.[156] Meanwhile, most government physicians, fearing for their livelihoods after the dissolution of the Federation and independence, left the colony. In May 1964, Nyasaland had no radiologist, no psychiatrist, and no director for its Public Health Laboratory. The number of government medical officers fell from thirty in 1962 to twelve in 1964.[157] On the eve of the British departure, the Medical Department had descended into freefall.

Conclusion

During the Federation era, medicine was a political symbol put to creative use by both rulers and ruled, Europeans and Africans, practitioners and patients. Medicine proved so suddenly relevant because of a rapid change in the popularity of government medical facilities among Africans during the 1950s and 1960s. The lines outside government clinics each morning grew steadily during the Federation period, as more and more patients sought cures for their ills.

Given the white supremacist ideology dominant among Southern Rhodesian politicians, it seems counterintuitive that health-care spending rose to new heights during the Federation. But Federal officials were eager, during a time of political ferment, to evidence concern for African lives. Though the construction and renovation of health facilities, the hiring and training of health professionals, and the stocking of pharmacy shelves did not keep pace with the demand, all increased during the 1950s and 1960s. Federation propaganda made much of the government's work in health services and became only more self-laudatory during times of unrest and political uncertainty. Particularly during the two moments of the most profound unrest, in 1953 and in 1959–1960, as politicians in the United Kingdom and Southern Rhodesia debated the political future of Nyasaland, health care became a central point of political propaganda for both pro- and anti-Federation forces. The increase in expenditure on medical services during this era supports the school of thought that attributes social change to disruption.

But while public spending on medical services increased at unprecedented rates, to unprecedented heights, medical providers and African patients in Nyasaland agreed that public facilities left much to be desired. Overcrowded facilities were always low on drugs and short of personnel. These shortages would only grow worse as Malawi moved toward independence. But to the millions of Malawians who had endured colonial and Federation rule, medical care had become, by 1964, a popular service. So when, just after independence, a new government decreed that government health services would no longer be free at the point of care, the backlash was swift and fierce. Malawians would remind Banda, in ways he could not afford to ignore, that they had not struggled for freedom only to lose access to medical care.

6

A Freedom to Die For, 1964–1982

Prelude

Walking down the main dirt road of the Neno *boma* (district capital) one morning in January 2015, I saw men and women using bicycles to carry large bags filled with urea fertilizer. I asked one young man where he had obtained his bag. He pointed to a primary school about one hundred meters up the road. I asked him if he had purchased the fertilizer: *Munagula feteleyza?* He answered no, he had *received* it: *Ayi, ndinalandira feteleyza.* The distinction was an important one, as the price of imported fertilizer had skyrocketed with the recent devaluation of the Malawian kwacha.

Parked in front of the school was a large blue truck with an empty bed. The driver explained that he had driven from Blantyre that morning with 270 bags, which had been distributed that morning. This distribution, he explained, was a public works program, wherein heads of households identified as vulnerable by village headmen were employed in fixing roads. In return for labor, each household head received a fifty-kilogram bag of fertilizer as well as maize seed.

This was one among a number of public antipoverty interventions, including targeted cash transfers, cash-for-work programs, subvention of farm inputs, and free health care and primary education. For most Malawians, social support was crucial for survival, yet relatively little of it came in the form of government programs. One particularly common form of kinship-based social support was fosterage, wherein young children lived in the homes of relatives other than their birth parents. This was especially important for families with many young children; for parents in this stressful time of the life cycle of a family, there were many mouths to feed and few hands to help in the fields and around the home. A year earlier, Francis had sent his daughter Lucia to "visit" (*kucheza*) her maternal grandmother in Lilongwe for three months. For weeks while living with Francis I thought Monica was also Edith's and Francis's daughter because he called her "my child" (*mwana wanga*). But while inquiring about extended family, I finally

No More to Spend. Paul Farmer, Oxford University Press (2020). © Oxford University Press.
DOI: 10.1093/oso/9780190066192.001.0001

discovered that Monica was actually the daughter of Edith's brother, David. Edith and Francis were helping to care for Monica for a time while David and his wife—who were poorer than Francis and Edith—cared for their newborn baby.

In other households in Nyanza village, grandparents cared for grand-children. In some cases, the parents had died young, while in others they were away working in Lilongwe or South Africa. In a number of these households, the grandparents were barely able to provide for the children. An old woman with a marked limp said she had given birth to seven chil-dren, but only two survived. Two of her late daughters had each given birth to five children. Seven of those children now lived with her. The grandmother said she received some support from her other three grandchildren, who were older. One worked at the resort nearby, another worked in Blantyre, and the third lived in a nearby village. But she had the greatest hope for a particular grandson, currently in his penultimate year of secondary school. She showed me his report card, which listed him as third in his class. His teacher complimented his "seriousness." Beaming with pride, the grand-mother described her expectations for the boy: "He will take care of me" (*adzasamalira ine*). The care could not come a moment too soon. Only a few days earlier, while straining to carry a bag of fertilizer to her field, she had slipped and dropped the sack on her foot. Today it was swollen and painful, but she did not think she had broken any bones. She said she did not think it would do her any good to go to the clinic.

Many adults in Nyanza had to provide not only for young children, but also for their elderly parents. For the previous two years, Francis's mother Anna had found it difficult to complete her daily chores. She suffered from osteoarthritis so advanced that she could walk only slowly, and with discom-fort. Her husband Chisomo, Francis's stepfather (Francis's father had died twenty-five years earlier), was even more disabled. The medical assistants who saw him in rushed visits at the nearby Monkey Bay hospital had diag-nosed him with benign prostatic hyperplasia, a common condition among older men the world over, though he had never undergone a more exten-sive workup to rule out other conditions. He lived in such chronic pain that he rarely ever rose from his banana-leaf mat. The couple could do little to support themselves. Neither Anna nor Chisomo could complete the walk to the maize fields to help with planting or weeding, though they tended a tiny garden behind their home. It was left to Francis to do much of the work for his ailing mother and stepfather. He gave them a portion of each year's harvest. Edith often cooked extra food for them. "I have taken them into my hands," Francis explained, "so now it is as if I have two houses."

Even within his immediate family Francis had to cope with expensive needs. For the past two years, the eight-year-old Lucia had complained of intermittent dull pain in her chest and abdomen. This often kept her home from school, and her teacher reported that she lagged behind in some subjects. When Lucia first complained of this pain, Francis had taken her to the private clinic twelve kilometers away in Cape Maclear—a fee-charging clinic, but one that was widely thought to give more thorough exams than the public hospital in Monkey Bay. The doctor there could find nothing to explain the symptoms and transferred her to Mangochi District Hospital, where she remained as an inpatient for two weeks. After those physicians failed to explain her condition, Lucia and Francis went to Zomba Central Hospital. She received an X-ray there, but no diagnosis. Her sojourn continued to Kamuzu Central Hospital in Lilongwe, where she stayed for four days but without obtaining any answers or relief. She still complained about the pain, which could reduce her to tears for hours at a time. Whenever Lucia's pain came up in conversation, the expression on her parents' normally cheery faces quickly turned to distress.

Francis did not complain much about his responsibilities. But he did admit that they prevented him from building up savings. Though most of Lucia's care was at public clinics, weeks of food and long trips to hospitals proved expensive. In addition to providing food for his parents and a home for his niece, Monica, and his nephew, Samuel, Francis had also just finished paying for four years of secondary school fees for his late sister's son, William. These obligations had depleted his "capital" (here Francis used the English word). Francis and Edith rarely produced a harvest beyond their household's own subsistence needs, so they made very little money from crop sales. Francis felt he rarely had any savings to guard against a bad harvest or another family emergency, let alone save for a business investment. With his limited collateral he was unlikely to qualify for a small business loan from the bank in Monkey Bay. Even if he did, the annual interest rate charged for such a loan was nearly 30 percent.

Francis's experience showed the lengths to which Malawians had to go to support kin. While newspaper columnists denounced the "culture of dependency," rural Malawians I spoke to often said it was the government that was overly demanding.[1] As Francis explained in a conversation about taxation, "The government finds ways to get money from the poor." In the colonial era this took the form of the hut tax. Under Hastings Kamuzu Banda, who ruled from 1964 to 1993, every man, woman, and child had to buy an MCP card every year. In the "multiparty" era, since 1993, consumption taxes increased the prices of basic goods. People expected benefits from their government because they had been made to pay for them.

Introduction: The Historiography of Banda's Postindependence Health Policy

The historiography of medicine in postindependence Malawi is much thinner than that of its colonial precursor, Nyasaland. Probably the most widely read history of medicine in Malawi is Megan Vaughan's *Curing Their Ills*, but this book focuses on the period 1890–1950.[2] Markku Hokkanen's *Medicine, Mobility and the Empire* draws upon a wide array of sources but restricts its temporal purview to the precolonial and colonial eras.[3] John McCracken's magisterial *A History of Malawi* ends its narrative in 1966.[4] Colin Baker's article on the government medical service in Malawi, published in 1976, contains only two pages on the health sector since independence.[5] Malawi-born physician John Lwanda has published two books containing helpful discussions of postcolonial medicine, though he calls these works "preliminary" in recognition of the dearth of existing original research.[6] Public health and medical journals contain countless studies of the AIDS epidemic, and recent ethnographies are rich; still, the first two decades after 1964 are rarely mentioned in these literatures.[7]

Much of the history that is written of the postindependence period focuses on the neglect of government medical services during the long reign of Hastings Kamuzu Banda (1964–1993). In one of the few studies of post-independence medical services, Eric de Winter notes that between 1964 and 1971, the government completed only two new hospitals (at Rumphi and Kasungu).[8] Lwanda argued that "the colonial, Banda, and post-Banda regimes did not . . . prioritise the health sector."[9] Another Malawian physician, Austin Mkandawire, observed that as late as 1972, eight years after independence, the government retained the colonial-era system of segregated hospitals. In Zomba, the hospital for whites, commonly known as "Top Hospital" (ostensibly because of its location above the main city center), received better funding than "Bottom Hospital" (lower on the hill), attended by black Malawians.[10] In 1975 Kathryn Morton concluded that "there has been little expansion of government health facilities since independence."[11]

At first glance, these portraits of abject medical neglect are surprising, for Banda was a medical doctor. One might assume that a man who for so long claimed his aim in life was to return to Nyasaland to work as a doctor would have taken steps to rapidly improve the threadbare provision of health care for Africans once he came to power.[12] But, as the poet and political prisoner Jack Mapanje remarked, "Dr. Banda built more prisons than hospitals."[13]

Still, characterizations such as Mapanje's must be examined in light of other facts. Recurrent expenditure nearly doubled in the decade after independence.[14] In addition, aside from a brief three-month period in 1964, Malawi remained one of very few African countries to provide most government health care without fees at the point of service.[15]

How do we make sense of the fact that Banda guaranteed Malawians some modicum of free health services, especially given his well-documented lack of interest in health care? I argue that although Banda did not consider health care a priority, the popularity of biomedicine in Malawi, as well as expectations engendered by his own use of kinship obligations in political rhetoric, did not allow him to ignore the sector entirely. In order to understand the political significance of medicine in postindependence Malawi, it is helpful to turn to an ancient debate about the role of the state in private life. Scholars working in southern Africa have long recognized the *lack* of separation between what Aristotle termed the *oikos* (the home) and the *polis* (the public sphere). The logic of judgments about local moral worlds informs those judgments that citizens and subjects make about distant politicians and institutions.[16] They are not divided spheres with separate logics. In both, generosity and social solidarity have been central concerns.[17]

Such an admixture of public and private has long been a source of anxiety among social theorists in the global north. The German philosopher Jürgen Habermas argued that a citizenry beholden to the state for material security (formerly a concern only of the *oikos*) is no longer well-placed to engage in "rational-critical" debate about the proper limits of state action.[18] Though the western European bourgeois public sphere had once been primarily concerned with protecting negative rights, the rise of the welfare state decreased the potency of political discourse. Instead of being opposed by a critical public sphere, the state was being called upon by citizens to interfere in more and more areas of life. To the casual eye, this critique appears applicable to early postindependence Malawi. Banda sought to use social services to consolidate support. He actively fostered the connection between *oikos* and *polis* whenever he used the terminology of kinship to address crowds at openings of new government hospital wings. Habermas might interpret such acts as attempts to foreclose critical debate, and indeed, Banda was trying to foster political quiescence.

But the history of social protection in Malawi demands a more detailed analysis. *Oikos* and *polis* were intermingled long before independence, and both Banda and the Malawian public drew upon notions of wealth and obligation that were historically distinct from those of western Europe. Public benefits had long been a major focus of political debate, and with the rising popularity and capability of biomedicine Banda had to reckon with the state's role in its provision. This reckoning led to a complex fabric of rhetoric and policy, one not readily categorized along the familiar twentieth-century left-right political spectrum.

This chapter chronicles three moments in postindependence Malawi in which the rhetoric and practice of the state's obligation to its citizenry fashioned a variety of (often surprising) policies. The first section recounts an episode early in Malawi's history when Banda was compelled to reverse a decision to impose user fees at public-sector health facilities. The second section seeks to explain Banda's opposition to population control in part through his reliance on an ideology of "wealth-in-people," the notion (which he often repeated) that the source of his power was the number of people for whom he was responsible. Finally, the focus turns to diplomatic policy, to explore how Banda justified his alliances with controversial foreign regimes by explaining how they helped him improve health care. Pressing biosocial concerns—health, fertility, and even survival—were an inextricable part of political discourse and practice. The juxtaposition of the disinterested, "rational-critical" *polis*, wholly removed from concerns of the material concerns of *oikos*, proves too narrow an aperture through which to understand the political history of postindependence Malawi.

User Fees and the Struggle for Legitimacy

On Malawi's first day as an independent nation (July 6, 1964), outpatients attending government hospitals and rural health centers began to be charged a fee. Throughout the colonial era, Africans had been made to attend segregated and inferior facilities, but at these hospitals and dispensaries they were charged nothing.[19] At the dawn of the new nation, this changed. For decades, officials in British Africa had rebuffed suggestions from Whitehall to charge user fees, often with the argument that health care was one of the few tangible benefits that Africans had come to expect in return for taxation and subjugation.[20]

But the new policy did not come from thin air. A number of colonial administrators and commentators had long argued that the colonial and Federation-era systems of free care perpetuated atavistic laziness. Speaking to a branch of the British Medical Association in Northern Rhodesia in 1960, Prime Minister of the Federation of Rhodesia and Nyasaland Roy Welensky declared that it was time for an end to the days of "something for nothing."[21] Others, like Dr. Harry Gear, a consultant to the Federal Ministry of Health, considered free medical care an ominous precursor to socialism.[22] Thus, even as health-care fees represented a jolting change, they did not mark a complete rupture with the ideas of the past.

UK minister of home affairs R.A. 'Rab' Butler, who had been tasked by Prime Minister Harold Macmillan with Central African affairs, raised the issue of fees in negotiations with Banda over Nyasaland's secession from the Federation. In a December 1962 meeting, Butler told Banda he would have to decrease overall public spending and find new revenues to pay for health care.[23] During a visit to Nyasaland in late January 1963, Butler clarified further that at some point, Africans should be made to pay fees at government health facilities.[24] Years later Glyn Jones, Nyasaland's last colonial governor, would look back on the fees as a wise policy aimed at restraining expenditure. "I regarded [Banda] as being a very honorable man," he said, "in that he did his best to fulfill the conditions that the British Government tried to attach to the secession. . . . [Y]ou wouldn't have blamed him for playing for popularity—and my God, he didn't, he brought in those . . . charges for the health services."[25]

Banda would later claim no knowledge of the health-care fees, but his own history indicates he had little aversion to them. In November 1960, an official in the intelligence service in Salisbury had sought unflattering stories about Banda from his years as a physician in Ghana (prior to 1957, the British Gold Coast) during the 1950s. The officer reported that Banda had set up an unlicensed network of dispensaries in a rural region of north Ashanti. There, the story went, Banda told his attendants—trained in a "week-end course"—to charge patients 10 shillings and 6 pence (£13 in 2016 prices) per consultation. Banda, the official claimed, kept 90 percent of the revenues for himself even as he stocked the dispensaries with supplies and drugs purchased by the government. From this scheme, Banda reportedly made a profit of £1,000 per month (£25,000 in 2016 prices).[26]

Given that the provenance of this account was a Federation official seeking to sabotage Banda, it may be exaggerated or even fabricated. What is known is that Banda maintained a private practice in Kumasi, and that after independence, Ghana's Ministry of Health suspended Banda's medical license for six months.[27] No historian has yet definitely discovered the reason for this punishment.[28] Still, what is known of Banda's medical career suggests he was likely no stranger to, or opponent of, fees.

The first fees, introduced before independence, were aimed at pregnant women. In April 1963, seeking to save on expenditures at the close of the Federation and no longer worried about currying favor with the general African population, the Federal Ministry of Health took what the *Central African Journal of Medicine* hailed as "the first step towards charging Africans for medical services." The fee, of 1 pound and 10 shillings, would cover "antenatal attention, the confinement and any attendant medical or surgical care and also post-natal attention if necessary."[29] Sally Hubbard, a visiting British nurse, described the effects on the maternity ward in Zomba: "Where anyone thought the women would be able to get the money from was a mystery. The maternity ward emptied overnight and the fear spread to other wards where the patients thought they would also be charged."[30]

The notion that maternity patients should be the first to be charged fees would have been unthinkable to colonial medical administrators during the interwar years, when underpopulation and insufficient fertility were considered major problems and officials encouraged clinic-based births.[31] As early as the late 1940s, the pendulum had swung back; the dominant official concern became *over*population.[32] The discursive shift helped move health policy away from the earlier focus on maternal and child health.[33]

If the empty maternity wards were disquieting to Hubbard and others, the sight paled in comparison with the effects of outpatient charges that came in July 1964. These fees, imposed on Malawi's first day as a new nation, were not widely publicized. Their announcement came in a notice authored by Secretary for Health Dr. Robert Park and published in the first issue of Malawi's government gazette. Starting July 6, outpatients were to be charged three pence (3d), an amount known in much of British southern Africa as a "tickey."[34] Three pence was, at the time, a standard hourly wage for unskilled urban laborers.[35] But for rural Malawians, cash was rarely readily at hand,

and the fee would prove a significant deterrent. In June 1964, the last month before the fee was instituted, 308,381 outpatients attended government facilities. By August 1964, the first full month of the outpatient fee, attendance had fallen precipitously, to 122,996 (see figure 6.1).

In the weeks after the "tickey fee" was imposed, MPs heard complaints from their constituencies. MCP spokesman Kanyama Chiume, who had recently been appointed foreign secretary, recalled the popular reaction:

> Wherever we went, we were bombarded with questions as to whether this was the freedom we had told people to die for. One old man in Usisya, my home, showed me a wound caused by an axe which was becoming septic because he could not afford the new fees. "How do you expect us to be enthusiastic about self-help schemes?" he asked me, "when if we hurt ourselves in the process, you ask us to produce money to be treated in a country where you cannot give us jobs from which to earn our living?"[36]

This question invoked politically salient obligations: namely, to ensure employment and medical care in exchange for both labour and legitimacy from his people.

Cabinet members who opposed the fees would invoke these obligations ever more forcefully, as the fees became one among many issues that alienated Banda from his erstwhile allies. In September 1964, Chiume and other

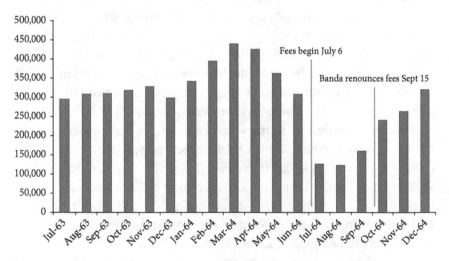

Figure 6.1 Outpatient attendances at government facilities, 1963–1964
Source: A Conspectus Including the Development Plan for 1965–69, Malawi Ministry of Health.

members of Banda's cabinet confronted the prime minister over the fees as well as a number of other issues, including low pay for civil servants; the slow pace of "Africanization" of government posts; and Banda's friendly relations with Mozambique, Southern Rhodesia, and South Africa. In much of the historiography of this episode, which came to be known as the Cabinet Crisis, the tickey fee plays a bit role in comparison with the ministers' other complaints.[37] But among the major issues, the fee was the only one with real significance in the daily lives of Malawi's largely rural and impoverished population.[38] Banda would paint his conciliatory relations with white-dominated governments in southern Africa as a boon for his people. Civil service salaries were of little concern to the majority of the populace, but Banda could ill afford to be seen as uncaring about health.

The ministers were also aware of the political significance of health care. Henry Chipembere, a young minister who had been among those who encouraged Banda to return to Nyasaland six years earlier, said the three-pence fee was "a heavy burden which prevented many people from taking their fever-stricken children to the dispensary." He lamented the government's attempt to limit expenditure using such charges, a tactic he called "economizing at the expense of the people's health."[39] Chipembere and other ministers eventually resigned from Banda's cabinet in protest. At a September 1964 rally near his home in Fort Johnston, Chipembere said the fees illustrated that "the present Malawi government is worse than Welensky's Federal government."[40]

For months, Banda's hold on power remained uncertain. Through late 1964 and early 1965, Chipembere and a few hundred followers hid in the Namizimu Forest north of Fort Johnston. Banda put a price on Chipembere's head, but out of either fear or loyalty, locals would not reveal his whereabouts.[41] After a failed attempt to invade Zomba, Chipembere fled to the United States in April 1965. Ironically, part of the reason for his departure was that he needed diabetes treatment not available to him in Malawi.[42] Banda's regime was saved, in part, by the government's ill-equipped health-care system.[43]

The Cabinet Crisis was the greatest threat to Banda's rule until he was finally forced from power in the early 1990s. He did not change his foreign policy or increase pay for civil servants, but he quickly distanced himself from the fee policy. A newspaper article reported that at a rally in Palombe a week after the parliamentary debate, Banda claimed his rebellious ministers "had bribed medical aides in the hospitals to refuse treatment to poor people so that there would be resentment." The article continued, "The Prime Minister promised the people that no one would be refused medical treatment because he had not got a 'tickee.' "[44] Though Malawi's *Government Gazette* does not document any official repeal of the fee, the Ministry of Health reported in 1965 that the outpatient fee simply "fell into desuetude."[45] Maternity fees, on the other hand, continued to be collected at most hospitals. In 1967 a midwife at a government dispensary in Monkey Bay told a touring official that average monthly deliveries had dropped from twenty-seven in the late Federation era to twelve because "people are not anxious to pay the fee."[46]

In addition to turning the blame for the fees back onto his rivals, Banda sought to reassert legitimacy through acts of generosity. Three days after his Palombe speech, Banda ordered that an earlier donation he had made to hospitals—a gift of more than 2,000 chickens and over 250,000 eggs—should be used "only to feed poor African patients."[47] The need to demonstrate concern for the poor after the battle over fees reflected his evolving understanding of the public's expectations of public provision.

A week later the nation's largest daily newspaper featured a photograph of Dr. Banda wearing a dark three-piece suit and tinted glasses, leaning over the bed of a female patient during a visit to the Queen Elizabeth Hospital, his gentle visage illuminated by sunlight streaming in through the window (see figure 6.2). This reminder of his career as a doctor was none too subtle. The article also noted that Banda had taken money out of his own pocket to give to individual patients.[48] In the midst of the greatest threat to his political career to date, Banda focused his publicity on shows of solicitude for the sick.

Banda still considered his hold on power precarious. In early 1965 his public speeches were entirely occupied with the hunt for Chipembere.[49] After Chipembere fled, Banda remained concerned about other ex-ministers in exile, particularly Yatuta Chisiza, his own former bodyguard.[50] Chisiza was killed in a failed invasion of Malawi from Tanzania in October 1967. Then another threat arose in the form of a rumor. Between November 1968 and March 1970, at least thirty-three people died in a series of murders in the Blantyre suburb of Chilobwe. One of the most popular explanations for the spate of killings was that the government was allowing white South Africans to steal Malawians' blood as repayment for loans Banda had taken out to build the new capital at Lilongwe.[51] Banda's health-care policy can only be understood in the context of this unrest and distrust. In an uncertain political environment, Banda would not risk such an unpopular decision as the reimposition of user fees.[52]

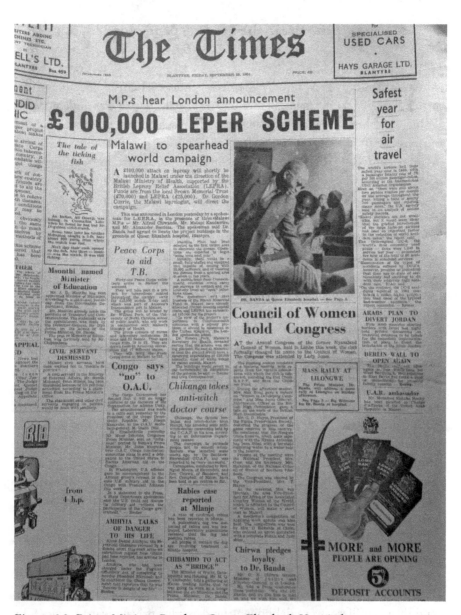

Figure 6.2 Prime Minister Banda at Queen Elizabeth Hospital

Source: Nyasaland Times, September 25, 1964. Reproduced with permission of Malawi National Archives.

Scarce Health Care in the Postindependence Economic Boom, 1965–1975

Malawi's economy grew rapidly after independence, buoyed by rising prices for cash crops on international markets. The health sector was not a priority. While neighboring Zambia opened a medical school and nearly tripled the number of urban clinics in the first decade after independence, Malawi's Ministry of Health did comparatively little to improve access to health services.[53] Scarcely more than 1 percent of the government's development budget went toward health services, compared to more than 2 percent in Tanzania,[54] despite the fact that in 1970 there was still only one "health unit" (a facility the size of a dispensary or larger) for every twenty thousand Malawians, roughly one-half the recommended World Health Organization minimum at the time.[55]

Under Banda, the government's response to requests from local leaders for new facilities was to instruct localities to rely on voluntary labor. A 1974 government publication declared "a remarkable spirit of self-help has achieved magnificent results."[56] Views on the ground were less rosy. Local administrators found it exceedingly difficult to convince poor farmers to contribute time and funds (in addition to taxes) to poorly coordinated construction projects. In 1968, for instance, the government of Malawi secured funding from the Beit Trust Fund to replace a rural dispensary in Fort Johnston district (today, Mangochi district). The funds were exhausted after the construction of the dispensary, so officials decreed that the staff housing had to be constructed using self-help labor. Two years later there was still no staff housing because, in the words of the secretary for health, "the spirit of self-help was not coming forth."[57]

Not everyone was asked to make such sacrifices. The Ministry of Health operated private wards in government hospitals, which promised prompt attention and experienced providers to paying patients. But Ministry of Health accountants complained that many "VIPs"—MPs, cabinet ministers, and their families—were delinquent on debts for private-ward services. In March 1973, prominent political figures with long-standing debts included President Banda's private secretary Cecilia Kadzamira, Minister of Finance Aleke K. Banda, and Reserve Bank of Malawi governor John Z. Tembo.[58] While delinquents debtors could face legal action, a Ministry of Health accountant was warned by his superior that "accounts relating to prominent figures are not to be referred to the State Counsel without the prior authority of the Principal Secretary."[59] Responsibility and self-help were lessons meant only for the poor.

For health-care providers in Malawi's public sector, independence did not bring an end to the struggle to provide decent care. After the brief dip during the three months of the tickey fee, outpatient attendance at public facilities began to rise again, climbing from 8.7 million in 1965 to 11.1 million in 1969.[60] Aging and poorly equipped facilities struggled to keep up with the influx of sick bodies.[61] The small but vocal cadre of physicians in district hospitals proved unwilling to accustom themselves to the practice of medicine without medicines. A Dutch doctor working at Nkhata Bay in the late 1960s bitterly recalled the futility of his pleading letters to the Central Medical Stores, which often ran out of such basic items as "tetracycline, ferrous sulphate, chloroquine, penicillin, Lysol, acetyl salicylate and dressings."[62] Often he could not intubate his patients "because the proper tubes were not obtainable for a long time."[63]

While doctors and nurses in the central hospitals complained of deficiencies at their facilities, the auxiliaries in rural areas toiled in far worse conditions. In the late 1960s, while serving on a Rockefeller Foundation commission, US physician John Bryant visited a hospital in the town of Port Herald. He observed,

> There is not a single doctor, not a single nurse. . . . The outpatient service is jammed with a pressing, murmuring throng. . . . Two medical assistants are surrounded at their desks. . . . Diagnoses are made on the basis of the first words uttered by the patient and are at the simplest possible level. Each takes one or two minutes. . . . The medical assistants see about three hundred patients during the morning. A baby has "warmth of the body." The blood is examined for malaria: positive. The treatment: chloroquine. Everyone with fever is assumed to have malaria. . . . The next has abdominal pain. What do you do about abdominal pain in two minutes?[64]

Bryant described this scene to illustrate a conundrum facing contemporary international health experts about the value of unsupervised medical auxiliaries in rural Africa. Was their care worse than none at all? Bryant did not put himself on either side of the debate, nor did he condemn the auxiliaries or the Ministry of Health for the low standards. But Malawi's public sector was in no one's eyes a model of medical provision.

Fertility Control versus Mortality Control

The obstacles to a decent heath system were not all domestic. During Malawi's first few years of independence, the nation's new leaders often found themselves rebuffed when they asked for international funding for health projects. At the October 1969 annual meeting of the World Bank in Washington, Minister of Finance Aleke Banda met with Abdel El-Emary, director of the Bank's Africa Department. Late in the meeting, the minister of finance mentioned that Malawi was planning to ask for assistance in financing health care. El-Emary demurred, saying he "could not make any positive statement on Bank interest or involvement in the area of health."[65]

A few months earlier, World Bank official John Adelman had written a report on Malawi that explained the bank's position, which relied heavily on claims of scarcity. In the absence of family planning, Adelman argued, combatting disease was a waste of money: "It is difficult to press for a large scale general attack on these problems, both because of financial limitations and also because one is reluctant to encourage a major mortality control campaign prior to seeing some official receptivity to a fertility control campaign."[66] Adelman had shared these thoughts with Malawian officials prior to his departure, prompting a critical response from President Banda. A letter addressed to World Bank president Robert McNamara included the following passage:

> One of the officials of the Bank who was here recently . . . mentioned the question of population explosion in this country. He said that our annual birth rate was too high and that we should do something about it. I disagreed with him. . . . Population explosion is not a problem in Malawi for the next fifty years, if not a hundred years. The problem is development for which we need finance.[67]

Banda could hardly have written a passage more offensive to McNamara. An adamant proponent of population control, McNamara believed decreasing the fertility rate should be a major priority in poor countries. He said as much when he responded to Banda less than a week after receiving the letter:

> The concern I have expressed on a number of occasions is with a situation in which the rate of population increase is outstripping . . . the rate

of economic growth, with the result that economic development does not result in human development. . . . [I] firmly believe that family planning is important for all developing countries which have excessively high rates of population increase.[68]

This disagreement would sour personal relationships between Banda and many leading officials in international development institutions.

The idea that per capita economic growth in poor countries was being hindered by rapid population increase garnered more support during the early 1960s. Private and public sources of international aid propounded the virtues of population control. At its June 1962 board of directors meeting, the Ford Foundation approved $10.7 million for population control; much of this funding went toward intrauterine device insertion campaigns.[69] Beginning in 1966, the US Agency for International Development devoted ever-larger sums to similar efforts, particularly in India.[70] Robert McNamara, who had previously served as US defense secretary, became a vigorous proponent of population control soon after assuming the position of World Bank president in 1968. Like Adelman, McNamara did not favor financial support for health care in borrower nations that had not yet achieved declines in fertility rates. As he explained during a 1969 meeting of the World Bank President's Council, "usually health facilities contributed to the decline of the death rate, and thereby to the population explosion."[71]

World Bank reports on Malawi during the late 1960s and early 1970s made the nation's rising population a more central concern than its dearth of health care. In a report of a 1971 mission to Malawi, the only mention of medicine or public health came in the section devoted to "population pressure," which nearly made a virtue of the country's absence of health services: "The structure of population and the high fertility ratios, in addition to the pressure of population on land, could create a serious demographic problem, particularly if there is some improvement in health services."[72] The report noted per capita recurrent public expenditure on health was only 85 (US) cents per year while annual per capita development expenditure on health was 3 cents. The authors worried that this situation was politically untenable: "Sooner or later, there is bound to be increased pressure for an improvement in health."[73] But they did not look forward to this eventuality, as it would bring forth "a marked reduction in infant mortality" and a consequent rise in population. To the authors of this World Bank report, astronomical rates of infant mortality were a rather useful check on overpopulation.

While the World Bank and USAID called for IUDs and sterilization, Banda lent no public support to birth control measures in Malawi. He banned books on birth control and deported a Dutch missionary who had delivered lectures on the subject.[74] In early 1965, a medical officer's request for the oral contraceptive Anovular from Malawi's Medical Stores was canceled on the grounds that "contraceptives are not supplied from Government Hospitals."[75] Historians of Malawi, and Banda himself, have offered varied reasons for his opposition to birth control. As he explained in his letter to McNamara, Banda saw population growth as desirable. He often declared Malawi was blessed with vast expanses of fertile soil, which could support millions more.[76] To some observers, Banda's position could be explained by his puritanical beliefs. Banda did not drink or smoke, promulgated laws against drunkenness. and banned Malawian women from wearing minidresses or even trousers.[77]

If in some ways Banda's cultural views fitted well with the contemporary western backlash against the sexual revolution, his stance on population also drew on ideas that cultural conservatives in the United Kingdom would have considered scandalous. In 1947, while working as a physician in London, Banda and the Scottish missionary Cullen Young coauthored a preface to *Our African Way of Life*, a volume of essays written by African students in Nyasaland. In the preface, Banda and Young defended a male initiation ceremony, known as *vinyau*, practiced by Banda's people, the Chewa:

> For some sixty years we have frowned upon and, indeed, opposed what we— Government and Mission—took to be a more or less licentious "harvest" or "fertility" orgy local to the Chewa and Chipeta areas. Actually . . . it is a central part of the educational technique, fundamental to the preparation of the male for adult life within the community and maintaining at the heart of the community itself a continuing reverence for the social ideal as Africa sees it.[78]

The logical consistency in Banda's sexual politics lay not in its adherence to cultural conservatism along the lines of some Christian churches, but in what anthropologists and historians of Africa have called "wealth-in-people." This is the idea that people—rather than money or other material resources—were primary in understanding wealth in land-rich, labor-scarce African societies. Since the 1970s this idea has been used to make sense of the rapid assimilation of the conquered and the destitute into new social groupings, and of inclusive definitions of kinship.[79] Even if Banda did not use this term, his politics appeared designed to demonstrate wealth-in-people. Metaphors of abundance and of vastly extended kinship relations were central to his rule.

The centrality of wealth-in-people—and specifically, wealth in women—to Banda's political symbolism was explicit in *Malawi News*, the mouthpiece of the MCP. In a January 1961 article entitled "Kamuzu Speaks to His Amazon Army," the reporter referred to the women at Banda's speech as "his women."[80] This attribution of all women to Banda persisted well into his reign. Wherever Banda delivered a public address, organizers made sure he was greeted not only by cheering thousands, but also by enthusiastic and well-rehearsed groups of praise-singing local women. Banda called these women his *mbumba*, which among the matrilineal Chewa refers to a group of sisters and their daughters living under the protection of a maternal uncle or elder brother known as an *nkhoswe*. If the analogy was not clear enough, Banda made it explicit by constantly referring to himself as "*nkhoswe* number 1."[81] By assuming the role of *nkhoswe* to women throughout Malawi, Banda indicated he was responsible for their flourishing, and he would in turn be made ever more wealthy and powerful by the fruits of their wombs.[82]

At the opening of Dedza District Hospital in 1975, *mbumba* sang songs during pauses in Banda's speech. The link between the acclaim of mothers and Banda's legitimacy as ruler was explicit in the opening verse:

If ndife amayi (We are mothers/women)
Ochokera ku Dedza (From Dedza)
Tangomvani mawu a Ngwazi (Hear the words of our Hero)
Chitukuko m'Malawi (On the development of Malawi)[83]

Banda thanked them for their "gratitude." The women made clear, if they had not already, that they credited Banda personally for the new hospital:

Ife ndife amayi (We are mothers/women)
Tinyadira chipatala (We are proud of the hospital)
Tangoona a Ngwazi amangitsa chipatala. (See that our Hero has built a hospital)

The presence of so many women singing Banda's praises was evidence of his greatest source of wealth—his wealth-in-people.

The importance of wealth-in-people was also evident in Banda's "donations" of food to hospital inpatients. These "personal donations" were a simulacrum,

for Banda had generated his wealth through a series of elitist and confisca-
tory state policies. The government marketing board (ADMARC) paid maize
producers far less than prevailing global prices. Banda then funneled the marketing board's profits into aid and credit for large agricultural, industrial, and
retail concerns, many of which he controlled and owned through a holding
company called Press Ltd.[84] Regardless of the provenance of his wealth,
though, the parallel between caregiving by kin and Banda's "gifts" to the sick
was striking. Among friends and kin, the gift of food, particularly the *ndiwo*
(relish, or side dish) that accompanies the staple maize meal, is a particularly
potent demonstration of generosity. Louis Joseph Chimango, who became
Banda's minister of health in 1978, used one of Banda's donations to purchase
"poultry products, bread, fruit, green maize and fresh fish." While the government budget covered the cost of *nsima*, the basic maize staple, Banda himself contributed the *ndiwo*. As if the parallel between caregiving by kin and
Banda's role as *nkhoswe* were not clear enough, Banda's officials arranged to
have this food distributed by the League of Malawi Women.[85]

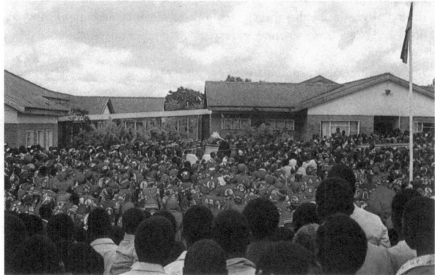

The Official opening of Gogo Chatinkha Maternity wing was accompanied with pomp and colour. Above, the Life President mobbed by his "Mbumba" on arrival for the opening ceremony, 25 December 1980.

Figure 6.3 President Hastings Kamuzu Banda, surrounded by his *mbumba*,
opening the Gogo Chatinkha Maternity wing at Queen Elizabeth Central
Hospital, Blantyre, December 25, 1980

Source: *Malawi: Fruits of Independence, 1966–1986* (Blantyre, Malawi: Department of Information,
1986). Reproduced with permission of Malawi National Archives.

The political potency of women as symbols of Banda's wealth was on full display on Christmas Day, 1980, when Banda went to the Queen Elizabeth Central Hospital to open a new maternity wing. The opening of the wing—which, as the Ministry of Information touted, had been built using personal funds donated by the president himself—was a joyous celebration of this abundance, with Banda surrounded by his *mbumba* clad in blue and red *zitenje* (cloths) bearing likenesses of his face (see figure 6.3). While such episodes demonstrated Banda's wealth-in-people, a source of symbolic potency and political strength, they also exposed a potential vulnerability. As the self-proclaimed protector of Malawi's people—and specifically the fecundity of its women—the president could ill afford to appear to neglect their health. This created an opening for an elite reformer willing to complain, since negative publicity about government health facilities would challenge Banda's status as "*nkhoswe* number 1." Indeed, Banda's decision to build a new maternity wing at Queen Elizabeth Central Hospital, opened with such fanfare, came in response to a complaint made at great personal risk by a Malawian physician.

The challenge was delivered by forty-two-year-old Dr. John David Chiphangwi, one of the nation's few black Malawian doctors. The son of a tea-estate clerk and a primary schoolteacher, he had received his medical education in Scotland and Uganda before returning to Malawi in the early 1970s. He quickly earned a reputation for dedication to his patients at Queen Elizabeth Central Hospital, where he served as head of the Department of Obstetrics and Gynecology. In 1978, during one of Banda's annual Christmas pilgrimages, Chiphangwi was tasked with showing him around the maternity ward. It was well known to all the doctors that Banda wanted the tour to present him in the best possible light, so it was standard practice to hide patients who slept on the floors. Chiphangwi was frustrated by his dingy, dilapidated, overcrowded ward and was unwilling to hide the realities of everyday practice. On Christmas Day, he accompanied a stone-faced, obviously embarrassed Banda through the congested ward. Chiphangwi's colleagues fled and feared they might never see him again.[86] But the gambit worked. Shortly after the visit, Banda announced plans to build the Gogo Chatinkha Maternity Wing (named after his sister), where Chiphangwi would treat patients for another quarter of a century.[87] Without this deft protest, the maternity wing might never have been built. Wealth-in-people was therefore a double-edged sword for Banda, as it provided an opportunity for an elite reformist to challenge him.

Health in a Political Economy of Exploitation

By the early 1970s, the unrest of Malawi's 1960s had abated. The cabinet ministers who had rebelled against Banda were exiled, dead, or forgotten. The World Bank and bilateral donors thought Banda's economic policies were masterful.[88] Furthermore, without the armed rebellions that had so preoccupied him during the 1960s, Banda faced, from a cynical political perspective, less of an imperative to use spending on health care as a political palliative.

Banda relished this quietude and used the opportunity to centralize power.[89] He extolled "obedience" and "unity" as two of the cardinal virtues for citizens of the new nation. Malawians quickly learned that the consequence of disobedience could be imprisonment, disappearance, or death.[90] In 1971, the MCP named him Life President. The following year, Banda declared "everything is my business. . . . When people think of the government in the village, to them it's Kamuzu."[91] Indeed, everything *was* his business. By the mid-1970s, Banda came to own many of the nation's grandest agricultural estates. He purchased much of the nation's industrial sector and used state funds to build ornate homes for himself around the country.[92] British officials, who oversaw substantial infusions of aid to Malawi during its early years of independence, criticized these "palaces" as unseemly uses of public funds, but Banda argued that his people expected him to live in such residences.[93] Banda never portrayed himself as a common man.[94] He amassed great wealth, and he reminded his people that he was "not poor."[95] But he insisted he used his wealth to help people. In a 1975 speech, he explained why he had drawn from his own account to construct student housing at the College of Nursing: "To me, money is of importance only for what I can do with it."[96]

Banda also realized he could claim credit for international aid. Much of his time was spent traveling the world asking foreign leaders for development assistance. Though he sought to wean Malawi quickly from British grants-in-aid, Banda was keen to secure funds from other countries and international bodies. The search for aid was, for Banda, a demonstration of both personal skill and national sovereignty. By securing support from a variety of sources, Banda could claim he had not surrendered the nation's independence to any single outside power.[97] Banda made a show of this search. Addressing a crowd in Neno in 1968, Banda declared, "I, your Kamuzu, have to find money somewhere to build more roads, more bridges, more schools, more hospitals everywhere in the country."[98]

In his requests for aid, health care was not Banda's first priority. For years he remained focused on grand infrastructure projects, chief among them a plan to move the capital from Zomba to Lilongwe.[99] Nonetheless, Banda recognized the political significance of access to biomedicine. Between 1966 and 1974, outpatient attendance at government facilities increased by 26 percent.[100] His speeches stressed his success in improving access to health care. In his 1966 inaugural address, Banda drew attention to his recruitment of staff from Israel and other countries. He also touted the new National School of Nursing, opened in 1965 with instructors sent by the United Kingdom and Canada, and hailed a four-hundred-bed hospital to be built in Zomba with a loan from West Germany.[101]

As the leader of an impoverished nation with few mineral resources, Banda had little to offer foreign governments. Malawi did, however, have a seat in the UN General Assembly, and embattled governments saw value in allying with Malawi, a black-led African nation.[102] By publicly supporting foreign governments with less-than-sterling reputations in black Africa, Banda was able to secure grants, concessional loans, and in-kind assistance.

One example of Banda's manipulation of contingent political circumstance occurred during the mid-1970s, when the Gulbenkian Foundation, a private organization based in Portugal, funded the construction of the new district hospital in Dedza. At the hospital's official opening, Banda told the crowd that he had secured the funds by proposing a quid pro quo with Portugal, a colonial power then facing armed resistance in Mozambique:

> I happened to have known this foundation called Gulbenkian. . . . I said, "Tell your chairman I know your government says it wants friendship with us here, particularly with me. If your government wants to be friendly with me, it must help me build a new hospital at Dedza. If it refuses then I will not believe it if it says it is my friend.". . . Within two or three weeks I got a letter to say, "O, we can at least let you have K144,000."[103]

Ten years earlier, in the midst of the Cabinet Crisis, Banda's rebellious ministers had denounced his willingness to ally Malawi with odious colonialists like the Portuguese. In this address and in others, Banda defended his policies by trying to demonstrate how they provided tangible benefits.[104]

Beyond southern Africa, Banda sought assistance from other nations eager for allies. In 1964, Israel contributed five medical officers and two senior physicians to the Ministry of Health, which was still reeling from a spate of departures. In the first months of Malawi's independence, these Israeli doctors would run some of the nation's largest hospitals.[105] The majority of Malawian nurses who trained between 1964 and 1972 received their training in Israel.[106] During these years, Israel was not yet the pariah it later became among majority-ruled nations in Africa. Yet even after the 1973 Arab-Israeli War led most Black African states to suspend diplomatic relations with Israel, Malawi was one of only four to maintain them.[107]

Even when dealing with states that were not so controversial, Banda ensured that partisanship paid dividends. In general he took the side of the Western bloc in the Cold War and sought to garner financial benefits from close relations with the United States and western Europe.[108] In 1965 Banda told the UN General Assembly that "history, logic, justice and fair play leave Malawi with no choice but to recognize the government in Bonn as the legal government of Germany." Shortly thereafter, the West German government expressed its appreciation by offering a £1 million loan (£18.2 million in 2016 prices) to replace Zomba's General Hospital.[109]

At least ten foreign governments, including Japan, the United Kingdom, and the United States, provided support for health-care projects during the 1970s.[110] With the benefit of this funding, recurrent health-care expenditure increased, in inflation-adjusted terms, more than threefold between 1973 and 1978 (see figure 5.5 in chapter 5). Still, expenditures on health care remained paltry. Between fiscal years 1976/1977 and 1980/1981, the Ministry of Health claimed an average of only 6.8 percent of the Malawi government's recurrent budget and 1.8 percent of the development budget.[111]

International advisers did not object. Even after the World Bank began to provide financing for health care in the mid-1970s, bank officials remained dismissive of the possibility of any sustained effort to build the health sector. Theorists of "modernization" like Arthur Lewis and Walt Rostow (both were read avidly by Malawian nationalist leaders and early postcolonial economic policymakers) argued that health-care spending constituted unproductive "consumption," which poor countries like Malawi could ill afford.[112] This discourse, too, was part of the social construction of scarcity, for it rendered health-care spending as profligacy. In internal memos at the World Bank's East Africa Department, officials argued that Malawi's low level of health-care spending was evidence not of "neglect," but only of "the paucity of funds available" to fill "bottomless pits" of need.[113]

Conclusion

In *The Ideas in Barotse Jurisprudence*, social anthropologist Max Gluckman argued that relations resembling kinship could be established through acts of material generosity. This materiality of obligation was especially true in relations between ruler and subject. A maxim of the Barotse people of southern Africa held that "the good subject is the one who is generous as a child is to a parent; the good lord is the one who is generous as a parent is to a child."[114] The anthropologist Meyer Fortes derived a similar lesson from his time among the Tallensi in West Africa: "A kinsman of any degree is a person whose welfare one is interested in and whom one is under a moral obligation to help in difficulties, if possible."[115]

This understanding of popular expectations of kin, and those who would claim to be kin, can help explain the politics of medicine in Malawi at the dawn of independence. Since the arrival of effective new drugs after the Second World War, government hospitals and dispensaries had grown more popular among the general population. Medicine's newfound capacity to protect the sick from suffering and premature death carried with it a new set of political obligations.

Banda learned the potency of this obligation soon after independence, when he sought to quell the popular reaction to the imposition of user fees. Though he did not invest heavily in medicine in the early postindependence years, he did abandon the fees and then made grand displays of any new government developments in the health sector. His "personal donations" to hospitals were public demonstrations of solicitude for the destitute sick. Banda had spent much of his life outside southern Africa. In his manner and historical sensibility, he identified more with the London bourgeoisie among whom he had lived for so long. But as leader of Malawi, there were social facts that he could not afford to ignore. The obligation to provide for the sick, or to at least appear to do so, was one such fact.

Throughout the first two decades of Banda's iron rule, medicine was not a central priority, but it was not entirely forgotten. After independence, Banda used government medical services much as he used his ubiquitous ceremonial flywhisk (a symbol of his *kukhwima* [skill in magic]) to ward off the bad omens threatening his own regime.[116] Yet in the midst of Banda's grand displays of concern, Malawians continued to suffer for want of decent curative and preventive health-care services. Measles vaccination, for instance, was nearly universal for children in the United States by the mid-1950s. But in 1979, measles remained the leading cause of inpatient pediatric deaths in Malawi's government hospitals.[117] The other two leading causes of pediatric inpatient deaths, pneumonia and malaria, were readily treatable conditions.[118] Banda's rhetoric about health care may have helped to secure his regime, but the lack of attention to health care in his budgets helped Malawi maintain its position toward the bottom of international health indices.

Banda was the physician-president who constantly portrayed himself as the benevolent *nkhoswe* of his people. There is, of course, a profound contradiction here. On the one hand, Banda relied on the symbolism of female fertility to legitimate his rule. On the other hand, the ban on birth control and the persistence of fees for hospital deliveries show a disregard for maternal health. But even if budget figures and health policies did not demonstrate a focus on health outcomes, health, and in particular fertility, were central to the symbolism of Banda's long rule. This symbolism, specifically Banda's reliance on the rhetoric of wealth-in-people, left him open to the charge of hypocrisy and forced him, at times, to spend at least some of the state's resources on health care.

7

"Vaccines or Latrines?" 1983–2016

Prelude

"If you could leave this place, you would," said an elderly man waiting in line to see a nurse at a mobile clinic in a camp for people fleeing rising waters. In early January 2015 large swaths of Malawi and Mozambique suffered the region's worst flood in at least a half century. The United Nations estimated 170,000 people were displaced, while at least 150 people died. Crops were washed away and livestock drowned. Thousands sought shelter in hastily constructed camps. Alongside doctors from a Malawian nongovernmental organization (NGO), I visited some of them. Red Cross nurses reported seeing scabies, diarrhea, and malaria. Scores of women complained of generalized body pain, which one doctor called a somatic manifestation of stress.

The annual rains were usually a welcome sight, and initially their arrival was a relief. After applying fertilizer and planting their crops in November 2014, farmers waited anxiously for the rains, which usually begin by mid-November but did not start that year until mid-December. Once they began, though, they would not relent. By the second week of January, the Shire River had flooded its banks and began to fill the surrounding valley. Refugees in Nchalo described waters that rose to the necks of full-grown men. Livestock were washed away. Malawians described the disaster with a refrain repeated so often that it seemed everyone was quoting Coleridge: "Water, water everywhere."

By February 2015, a shifting cast of NGOs provided ad hoc relief at one camp. Tents from UNICEF, the Red Cross, and the Malawi Army had been cobbled together, but many leaked in the heavy rains. The World Food Programme and World Vision distributed soy, beans, and cooking oil. Médecins Sans Frontières built latrines and staffed a mobile clinic. Illovo, a sugar company with a plantation nearby, parked a tank of potable water at the side of the road. One afternoon, without any notice, a local Muslim charitable society unloaded a truck full of groceries in front of the camp. Hungry men

No More to Spend. Paul Farmer, Oxford University Press (2020). © Oxford University Press.
DOI: 10.1093/oso/9780190066192.001.0001

and women jostled for the sudden windfall. Government officials conducted head counts of camp residents.

But there was little coordination. The camp was crowded, its location miserable. Placed in the middle of a barren, unshaded field, the tents became ovens in the midday sun. There was relative comfort nearby. A half mile away, a lodge offered ample shade and breakfast to NGO administrators with per diems and SUVs.

While the destruction of housing was a disaster, the most fearful sights came when the waters subsided. By late January, the valley was usually lush with maize, cotton, and rice. But this time when they looked around, people saw only a thick layer of sand suffocating their crops. Though the region's semisubsistence farmers were accustomed to a precarious existence and seasonal hunger, this was an unbearable shock. Most families had already run out of food stored up from the May 2014 harvest. Even without these floods, the months from January to April were commonly known in Malawi as *nyengo njala* (the hungry season). During that time, as families exhausted the previous harvest and waited for the next, dedicated malnutrition wards in hospitals filled with children with crispy orange hair, distended bellies, swollen feet, and twig-like arms. In most years, impoverished men and women sought out *ganyu* (piecework labor) in the fields of wealthier farmers. But after the floods, even this work had disappeared.

Most flood victims I interviewed were quick to list exactly what they needed. They called for emergency food relief and expanded public works programs to keep families fed. They asked for seed and fertilizer to allow them to make one last-ditch attempt to replant their crops before the rains stopped for the year. Most of the displaced dreaded the prospect of sitting idle in sweltering camps, on church floors, or in repurposed schoolrooms, subject to the whims of whatever NGO decided to visit. But for most, help did not come. Two months later, as the window for replanting crops closed, many Malawians had nothing left to their names but ruined fields and collapsed homes.

Parts of the country spared the torrential rains were struck by drought. Francis's village was one such place. One morning in February, after a night of rainfall, Francis looked relieved. His nascent maize crop was about to enter a crucial phase. Without sufficient moisture in the soil, the silken tassels that signaled a healthy crop would not emerge on time. "I was worried," Francis admitted. He hoped the rains would continue. But his hopes were dashed. Over the coming weeks, unrelenting sunshine parched the soil and scorched the stalks. Tassels, those harbingers of full stomachs, sprouted late or not at all.

The joyful spirits that accompanied strong harvests came to few Malawians in 2015. Malawians' reliance on high-risk, high-reward maize—a crop that can yield bounteous harvests but is susceptible to drought—did not pay off that year. After a record 2014 harvest of 3.9 million tons, the floods and droughts of 2015 depressed that year's harvest to only 2.9 million tons. By December 2015, shortages had pushed maize prices to record highs.[1]

These disasters revealed the nature of wealth in rural Malawi. People measured prosperity not by the ability to conspicuously consume luxuries (few had any), but rather by the number of misfortunes (sickness, flood, drought, changes in government programs) they could withstand before tumbling into penury. When Francis's nephew William could no longer afford school fees after the deaths of his parents, he could turn to Francis to pay them. Wealth entailed networks of support that allowed individuals to deal with tragedy and disaster. Francis and his family had the means to shield themselves against the coming onslaught of hunger, but without public action to ensure access to food, many other Malawians did not.

Introduction

This chapter chronicles, in brief, the history of Malawi's health sector from the early 1980s until the mid-2010s. While conducting research, I did not have access to government records covering this period, due in part to the thirty-year moratorium on files at Malawi's National Archives. There exists, however, a wealth of secondary literature on health services and governance during this era. The literatures produced by anthropologists, physicians, public health researchers, economists, demographers, and political scientists who study the more recent past make it possible to delineate continuities and discontinuities in Malawi's government medical services.

Scarcity has been an especially potent social construct during Malawi's age of AIDS. Arising shortly after the imposition of "structural adjustment," a set of austerity-based policy prescriptions favored by the World Bank and IMF for struggling nations like Malawi, the burgeoning new pandemic was more deadly because of the nation's already-depleted public health and medical care systems. Among those who engaged in arguments about the inescapability of scarcity were educators and students at Malawi's new medical school and policymakers discussing user fees. But in the battle over AIDS treatment, elite reformists challenging the construction of scarcity were finally successful. These efforts, more than any others, belied the century-long claim that there was simply no more to spend. Yet even as international funding and local efforts have saved hundreds of thousands of lives, Malawians continue to complain, with justification, that their health-care system provides far less than it should.

Debt and Structural Adjustment

Before the 1980s, Malawi's development trajectory appeared, to many outside observers, commendable. Under Banda, Malawi's economy grew rapidly. Between 1970 and 1979, Malawi's real GDP grew at an average rate of 6.3 percent per annum, and real GDP per capita at a rate of 3.9 percent per annum. By controlling powerful parastatal corporations with interlocking directorates, borrowing heavily using government guarantees, and paying smallholder growers far less than the market value for their products at the government marketing boards, the life president funneled the state's resources into tobacco estates and nascent industrial concerns. With strong international prices for the nation's major cash crops—tobacco and tea—the estate sector remained profitable for the few who controlled it. A USAID mission summarized the situation: "Malawi's private sector is alive, doing well, and owned by the government."[2]

But the economic crises that affected much of the rest of the world during the 1970s did not long spare Malawi, which remained one of the world's poorest countries. Drought struck much of the nation during 1979 and 1980. At the same time, the auction price of flue-cured tobacco, Malawi's major export, tumbled by 36 percent.[3] A cascade of setbacks ensued. Increasing fuel costs after the 1979 Iranian Revolution drove up the cost of importing fertilizer and depleted Malawi's reserves of foreign exchange. A dramatic increase in international interest rates led to a rise in the share of Malawi's government budget that had to be devoted to servicing foreign debts. This figure rose from 7 percent in 1977 to 19 percent in 1980. After a bloody civil war in Mozambique led to the closure of the heavily trafficked road to the port in Beira, imports and exports were diverted to much more expensive routes. Malawi's GDP fell by 5.2 percent in 1981 and would not regain its former levels of growth for decades.[4] Inflation rose from 9 percent in 1978–1979 to

33 percent in 1988–1989. Meanwhile, over a million refugees fleeing the war in Mozambique placed further demands for food and medical assistance on the government.[5]

Despite these challenges, Banda remained resolute about completing his favored projects. He continued to direct government revenues toward the construction of an international airport and buildings in the new capital city of Lilongwe as well as toward his own palaces. In aggregate terms, however, Banda was no spendthrift. He and his Ministry of Finance had long made the achievement of annual recurrent budget surpluses a priority. Even when such surpluses were no longer possible, Banda sought to limit expenditures on any budget items he did not consider priorities. One area that was not central to his vision for Malawi's development was health care, which would suffer in the austerity imposed in the aftermath of the economic downturn. The share of Malawi's recurrent budget devoted to health care, already low during the 1970s, declined still further, falling from 7.4 percent in 1978 to 5.2 percent in 1982.[6] During his last full year as president (1993), Banda directed more state resources toward government residences than toward medicines and vaccines.[7]

Such stringency had real consequences for public health. Malawi had launched its Expanded Program on Immunization in 1979, with the goal of immunizing all children under twelve months of age against six preventable diseases: measles, tuberculosis, whooping cough, diphtheria, poliomyelitis, and tetanus. But with the cuts to funding, vaccination rates actually deteriorated. By 1985 only 35 percent of children were fully immunized at twelve months.[8]

In the midst of multiple crises at the close of the 1970s, Banda turned to the IMF and World Bank for assistance. In exchange for short-term loans, these international financial institutions demanded a number of conditions designed to ensure prompt repayment to international creditors.[9] Seeking relief from its shortage of foreign currency and mounting debts, Malawi accepted a loan from the IMF in 1979. In exchange, the government promised to halt increases in government expenditure and to raise taxes. When this aid proved insufficient to weather the onslaught of economic shocks, Malawi submitted to three successive "structural adjustment programs"— more loans in exchange for promises of austerity, economic liberalization, and privatization—in 1981, 1982, and 1985.[10]

Malawi's debts, the consequence of Banda's focus on agricultural estates, palaces, and personal vanity projects such as a new capital city, were as misbegotten as the TZR railway debt of the 1920s. And as in that era, debt payments crowded out spending on basic social services. Structural adjustment programs were, in the main, designed to ensure that foreign creditors were repaid, and indeed external debt servicing came to occupy a large proportion of government spending, rising to 25.8 percent of recurrent expenditure in 1981–1982, and to 38.3 percent by 1986–1987.[11] Though the World Bank initially encouraged Malawi to maintain levels of recurrent expenditure on agriculture, health, and education, by the mid-1980s its overriding objective for Malawi's budget was a decrease in total recurrent expenditure.[12]

From the start of negotiations over the terms of its loans, World Bank officials tried to convince Banda to impose user fees on government medical services.[13] Many other nations that submitted to structural adjustment loans did introduce such fees. Zambia began charging point-of-care fees at government medical facilities in 1991, and Uganda followed suit in 1993.[14] But Malawi did not join them. In fact, by the year 2000 Malawi, Tanzania, and South Africa were the only nations in sub-Saharan Africa where public-sector medical services remained free at the point of delivery.[15] Though Banda said little publicly about the motivations behind his refusal to institute fees, the memory of the tickey-fee debacle may well have made him wary of renewed demands for user fees by foreign creditors.

Even if access to the underfunded health system remained unhindered by user fees, other programs valued by Malawi's poor did suffer cuts as a result of structural adjustment. In Nyanza village, one woman remembered that during the 1980s she received two bags of fertilizer every year from the government, free of charge. But as a condition of its second structural adjustment loan, Malawi agreed to abolish its fertilizer subvention program.[16] Such disinvestment in smallholder production contributed to a rise in malnutrition; the percentage of children under five who were underweight rose from 19 percent in 1975 to 30 percent in 1998.[17] By the end of the Banda era, all semblance of social protection was disintegrating, while even more terrible calamities loomed.

The Multiparty Era and the AIDS Epidemic

The earliest evidence of HIV in Malawi comes from a retrospective examination of blood samples collected in 1982 in Karonga. The virus appears to have been introduced by migrants returning home from the mining towns of

Katanga in Zaire and the Zambian Copperbelt.[18] In January 1983, Malawi's *Medical Quarterly* published a case report of a fifteen-year-old boy with skin nodules and a mass in his chest. He was found to have a then-rare form of cancer known as Kaposi's sarcoma.[19] There was no mention of HIV, for the virus itself was not discovered until the following year.

Over the next decade, AIDS transformed from a mysterious illness into a social conflagration. Because of the long delay between initial infection and symptoms, few people appeared ill even as the virus spread. But spread it did; among women attending antenatal clinics in Blantyre, HIV prevalence rose from 2.6 percent in 1986 to over 30 percent in 1998. Infection rates were lower outside major cities, but by 2002 the infection rate was 11 percent in rural areas.[20] In 1988, the Employment Bureau of Africa stopped recruiting Malawians to work as migrant laborers in South Africa's mines, citing high rates of HIV.[21] Malawians already in South Africa were taunted by coworkers, who called them "dying people."[22] Back in Malawi, AIDS ravaged communities. In the 1990s, people came to expect that every weekend would involve at least one funeral.[23] The epidemic precipitated a steep decline in life expectancy, from forty-five years in 1989 to thirty-seven years in 2003.[24]

Life-saving combination antiretroviral therapy (ART) became available in wealthy nations in 1996, but almost no Malawians had access to these drugs before the mid-2000s. Hospitals seemed to observers to be little more than inhumane warehouses for the dying. In 1998, a journalist bore witness to the carnage:

> The patients lie two to a bed and on the floor, waiting to be sent home to die. Tattered blankets brought by relatives drape their shrunken bodies, because Lilongwe Central Hospital doesn't have any linen. . . . Public offices grind to a halt because so many workers are away at funerals.[25]

Medical facilities were so underfunded, underequipped, and understaffed that the few remaining doctors felt unable to handle much of anything. Not since the Great War had medical staff in Malawi expressed such frustration and helplessness. A British expatriate physician working at a hospital in northern Malawi reported that his facility had for months been stocked out of bare basics such as cotrimoxazile (an antibiotic to prevent opportunistic infections in people with HIV), acetaminophen, and chloroquine, and it had even run out of antiseptic alcohol.[26]

The sense of futility and the widespread belief in the inevitability of continued scarcity led some in the medical community to offer previously unthinkable proposals. In 2003 Michael King, an expatriate surgeon at Queen Elizabeth Central Hospital and a longtime proponent of population control, wrote a letter—entitled "AIDS: Are We Really Serious?"—to the editor of the *Malawi Medical Journal*. In it, King proposed "strategies for combating AIDS" that "have not been given adequate consideration." Among these strategies was a policy in which anyone planning to begin a job, university, or training program should be made to submit to an HIV test. Omitting such testing was "beyond reason," King suggested, as "Malawi, with its scarcity of money, has to make sure its public funding is used to the best advantage for the people of the nation."[27] King was suggesting, without saying so explicitly, that those who tested positive for HIV should be denied access to jobs, training, and schooling. The letter prompted a critical response from Vicky Lavy, another expatriate physician working in Queen Elizabeth Central Hospital. She retorted, "Excluding positive people from employment would considerably reduce the potential workforce, as well as making life even more difficult for those living with HIV."[28] While these physicians argued over the propriety of such measures, the possibility that international funding might be used to purchase AIDS drugs seemed so far outside the realm of possibility as to merit no mention.

Among the physicians who persevered despite the carnage were Malawian doctors. Banda's government finally approved plans for a medical school in 1986.[29] John Chiphangwi, the obstetrician who had successfully challenged Banda to improve maternity services at Queen Elizabeth Central Hospital during the late 1970s, was the founder and moral leader of Malawi's new medical school. As the physician-anthropologist Claire Wendland chronicled in an ethnography of the medical school, Chiphangwi's example suffused the ethos of the school. Medical student Evelyn Kazembe seemed to exemplify this sentiment, which Wendland found in so many of her classmates: "I just had this heart for the people. To serve."[30]

Still, without access to life-saving antiretroviral therapeutics, Malawi's new doctors could do little to help their patients with AIDS. By 2002, over 70 percent of bed occupancy in Malawi's hospitals was attributable to AIDS-related illnesses.[31] By 2004, 74,000 Malawians died of AIDS-related causes each year.[32] An estimated 960,000 of Malawi's 12.7 million Malawians were living with HIV.[33] For every ten new nurses who graduated from Malawi's training institutions, four died from AIDS.[34] Only nine facilities in the public sector offered ART. Together they provided treatment to only 3,000 patients.[35]

The confluence of falling commodity process, structural adjustment–linked declines in social service spending, and the rise of AIDS fed distrust of Malawi's political system. In March 1992, Malawi's Catholic bishops wrote a pastoral letter that was read before congregations around the country. Among other injustices, the letter called attention to unequal access to education and health. The bishops refused to accept facile claims of scarcity: "One cannot claim to uphold the principle of the sanctity of life if provision has not been made for even minimal health care for every person. . . . [I]f this problem is to be tackled, it will demand allocation of more resources from the state."[36]

The pastoral letter opened the floodgates of protest and unrest. Workers went on strike and marched in the streets of Blantyre.[37] In October 1992, major international donors froze all aid to Banda's regime except for emergency food aid and refugee relief.[38] In 1993, Banda still felt secure enough in his hold on the populace to call for a referendum. To his surprise, when voters were given the choice between continued single-party rule and multiparty democracy, 64 percent chose the latter. The next year, in the first multiparty election since independence, Banda lost to Bakili Muluzi, a former secretary-general of the MCP.

Shortly after taking office, Muluzi took steps to consolidate support among the rural poor, among whom Banda had been seen as a protector of material subsistence. Muluzi promised not only new civil and political rights, but also improved health care and education. In his most popular move, Muluzi abolished user fees for government primary schools; enrollment increased from 1.7 million in 1993 to 3.9 million in 1994.[39] He also refused to follow recommendations by the World Bank to institute user fees at health clinics. Whereas Banda had privately told World Bank officials he would institute the fees without ever doing so, Muluzi spoke publicly about his disagreement with World Bank recommendations. When its officials encouraged Muluzi to follow through on Banda's unfulfilled commitment to institute user fees, he rebuffed them, publicly declaring that he would not be responsible for "excluding the poorest members of our communities from access to health services."[40]

But despite Malawians' new freedoms and Muluzi's promises about social services, the "multiparty" era soon came to be associated in the popular imagination with famine. After a weak maize harvest in 1998 led the government to seek advice from the Rockefeller Foundation, it began a popular "starter pack" program, in which every household received a small packet of food and fertilizer. But facing pressure from donor governments, Muluzi drastically scaled back the program in 2001. In the next year, smallholder maize production fell by more than 25 percent.[41]

Under Banda the government had often made up for such shortfalls by selling from a "strategic grain reserve" at affordable prices. In 1979 Malawi had constructed massive concrete silos at Kanengo, which housed grain bought from farmers in good harvest years to be resold at reasonable prices in bad ones. In 1999, in fulfillment of a condition for a World Bank loan, Muluzi privatized the grain reserve. By June 2000 the grain had all been sold off, mostly to private speculators. When the next year's harvest proved weak, the government had no stores, and speculators charged exorbitant prices. After a half century without widespread famine, the scourge returned.[42] The president was late to declare a state of emergency, and international relief proved insufficient. One elected official in Malawi's south remembered 2002 as the year "nobody came to help."[43]

The AIDS Response Reaches Malawi

Amid AIDS and famine and immiserating policies, continued scarcity seemed so inevitable that some health-care workers curtailed their ambitions to the barest interventions. In 2003, instructors at the College of Medicine reported on a recent learning module that they had conducted for first-year students. In the session, students were made to debate the following proposition: "The recent trend of increasing investment in health care in low-income countries at the expense of environmental health measures will be detrimental to health outcomes overall." This debate might have become a common rehearsal of a centuries-old debate in public health, over the relative merits of curative medicine or sanitary measures, if not for the instructors' title for the debate: "Vaccines or latrines?" The authors showed little awareness that readers might be shocked at the idea that both interventions could not be pursued at once. The lowered expectations inherent in the debate showed just how far socialization for scarcity had advanced among some prominent members of Malawi's health sector.

Yet in their debate, students did not simply accept the premise that spending on vaccines must, of necessity, come from spending on latrines. One student, assigned to argue in favor of the proposition, contended not that medical expenditures should be cut, but that the focus of health policy should be "broadened" to include both biomedical and sanitary interventions. Another student, assigned to argue against the proposition, insisted that any true effort to prevent childhood deaths demanded not only new sanitation infrastructure but also oral rehydration therapy, antibiotics, antimalarial drugs, and vaccines.[44] If the professors were socialized for extreme scarcity, at least some of the students were not.

Many trained clinicians were just as dissatisfied with the state of affairs. In 2005, Tarek Meguid and Elled Mwenyekonde, a physician and clinical officer, respectively, in the department of Obstetrics and Gynecology at Bottom Hospital in Lilongwe, wrote a scathing "situational analysis." They deplored the overcrowded wards, the lack of public toilets, and the operating theater so shoddily designed and ill-equipped that "sterility becomes a myth."[45] They lamented the laboratory, which was so chronically short of equipment that "most of the time it is not possible to get even a full blood count."[46] Their despair drips off the page. They wrote, they explained, out of a "duty to continue to cry for help."[47]

Into this lifeworld of incredibly constrained possibilities a sudden injection of donor funds finally appeared in the mid-2000s. Activists, humanitarians, and politicians of vastly different ideologies from the Global North and South sparked the passage of legislation and the appropriation of funding for debt relief and increased international aid for health care. As a result, development assistance for health rose dramatically, from $9.8 billion in 1999 to $21.8 billion in 2007.[48] The role of transnational grassroots activism in helping to drive this increase has been well-documented and need not be retold here.[49] Less recognized is the key role of elite reformists, individuals who used fame and positions of authority to convince politically powerful decision-makers to increase spending on health care in nations like Malawi.

Elite reformists' main tool in this advocacy was not social disruption, or even monetary power, but rather what the philosopher Richard Rorty called "sentimental education." For instance, arch-conservative US senator Jesse Helms, long an opponent of both domestic AIDS funding and foreign aid, became a major supporter of international AIDS treatment programs shortly after speaking with Franklin Graham, the eldest son of the evangelist Billy Graham. Franklin Graham led a Christian relief organization called Samaritan's Purse. According to Helms's memoirs, during the year 2000 Graham convinced him that AIDS was taking a toll not only on homosexuals and promiscuous adults, groups that Helms considered immoral, but also children.[50] Helms claimed Graham was the first to explain to him the toll AIDS took on "innocent victims of this sexually transmitted disease," the millions of children who had either contracted the infection from their mothers or been orphaned by the death of a parent. No longer simply a punishment for the shameful, AIDS became in his eyes a scourge upon the blameless. With this revised understanding Helms, during the last two years of his long Senate tenure, was a major proponent of AIDS funding.[51]

Sentimental education was also central to the conversion of another key political leader, US president George W. Bush. Because of the association between the disease and immorality in conservative politics, a health adviser told an advocate in the 1990s that "the one thing Bush is really uncomfortable dealing with is AIDS."[52] This began to change when Franklin Graham, who had given the convocation at Bush's first inaugural in 2001, began speaking with Bush about the international AIDS pandemic during the first year of his presidency.[53] Graham often drew a link between Jesus's mercy and the modern AIDS crisis. Once Bush began expressing concern about AIDS, he also framed his response as a "mission of mercy."[54]

Shortly before he announced a new $15 billion AIDS initiative, Bush met with physicians such as Peter Mugenyi of Uganda and Paul Farmer, who worked in Haiti. Both told uplifting stories and showed dramatic before-and-after photographs of patients brought back from death's doorstep by ART.[55] Later in his presidency, Bush spoke often of this "Lazarus effect" and marveled at "dying communities being brought back to life, thanks to the compassion of the American people."[56] Emotionally laden appeals were therefore central to the push for the funding that helped Malawi and other poor countries deliver life-saving AIDS treatments to their people.

The success of advocates such as Franklin Graham was also a product of the particular social and political configurations that coincided with the global AIDS movement at the start of the twenty-first century. During the early 2000s, AIDS was a very visible global pandemic, with increasing coverage in the international media. The toll of AIDS on communities in the United States and Europe during the 1980s and 1990s had created sizable political constituencies concerned with the spread of the disease elsewhere. Most important, ART had transformed AIDS from an inevitably fatal disease into a manageable chronic condition. And although the high price of these medicines seemed, initially, to put them entirely beyond the reach of poor patients in poor countries, a steep decline in cost once generic manufacturers began mass production transformed the contours of the possible.[57] The combination of moral claims directed at elites and contingent political configurations helped spur a rapid rise in financial resources for health interventions in poor countries. Between 2002 and 2008, donor countries' contributions to global AIDS programs increased sixfold. These funds saved millions of lives.

In Malawi, the rise in foreign assistance for health occurred alongside increasing domestic government expenditures. No longer pressured by the World Bank and IMF to limit health-care expenditures after the institutions abandoned structural adjustment in the early 2000s, President Bakili Muluzi increased public expenditure on health from 2.9 percent of GDP in 2002 to 5.7 percent in 2004. As a percentage of annual government expenditures, health-care outlays rarely exceeded 9 percent during the 1990s, but by 2005 the share had reached almost 20 percent.[58] After winning Malawi's 2004 presidential election, Bingu wa Mutharika maintained this level of health-care spending as a percentage of GDP even as Malawi entered a period of rapid economic growth.[59]

The burgeoning levels of international and domestic funding made it possible for health officials to expand access to AIDS treatment while improving staffing in clinics and hospitals around the country.[60] In 2005, using funding from the Global Fund for AIDS, Tuberculosis, and Malaria, Malawi began providing free ART to adult patients.[61] A grant from UNITAID, an international airfare tax devoted to global health, allowed Malawi to provide ART to pediatric patients free of charge.[62] By March 2011, 433 clinics in Malawi treated more than 264,000 patients with ART.[63] Given the overwhelming toll that AIDS had taken on the nation's populace, the increasing access to ART had significant and salutary effects on overall mortality rates. A study in Karonga District found that all-cause adult mortality decreased by 32 percent between 2002 and 2008.[64]

Malawi also received assistance to address its shortage of health-care workers. Low pay and desperate working conditions had compelled many to leave the public sector. In response, in 2005 the Global Fund and the UK Department for International Development funded the six-year, $272 million Emergency Human Resources Programme (EHRP). This program provided a 52 percent salary increase for all health-care workers, expanded preservice training, and recruited expatriate doctors and nurses. Analyses found that the EHRP's salary "top-ups" helped stem the flow of health-care workers out of the public sector. In addition, the number of health professionals trained in Malawi each year increased from four hundred in 2004 to over one thousand by 2008.[65]

Medicine in Malawi since the 2008 Financial Crisis

After almost a decade of rapidly rising public-sector health-care spending in Malawi, the 2008 financial crisis brought a stark end to the trend.[66] The increase in international development assistance halted at a level far below the target of 0.7 percent of GDP agreed to by the leaders of developed nations in 2002.[67] The situation did not much improve after Western economies emerged from the recession that followed the crisis. Total global development assistance increased, on average, 11.2 percent per year from 2000 to 2010. But between 2010 and 2017, the increase slowed to 1 percent per year.[68] Peter Mugyenyi, whose work had helped convince President Bush to increase global health-care funding almost a decade earlier, wrote in 2010 that lower-than-promised donor funding had "forced many facilities to turn away new HIV-positive patients seeking ART."[69]

Politicians and their advisers in rich nations once again justified the persistently low levels of aid by invoking familiar claims of scarcity. During his 2008 campaign for the US presidency, Barack Obama had promised to increase funding to the President's Emergency Plan for AIDS Relief (PEPFAR) by $1 billion per year, but in his first budget request in 2009 he asked only for a $165 million increase. Obama himself expressed incredulity that AIDS activists were not satisfied with the size of his request. In a handwritten response to a May 2009 memo on global health funding, Obama remarked of AIDS activists, "How can they complain when we are increasing funding?"[70] Ezekiel Emanuel, an adviser in Obama's White House, remarked during a 2010 trip to Ethiopia that universal treatment for multi-drug-resistant tuberculosis might not be possible because "we absolutely have scarce resources to treat TB."[71]

These claims of scarcity were rarely accompanied by admissions of other realities. For instance, wealthy nations did little to stem the illicit financial flows leaving poor nations. By some credible estimates, the amount of money leaving Africa through illicit channels was equal to the amount entering through aid.[72] Nevertheless, the idea that scarcity was inescapable led to the resuscitation of old policy ideas. Malawi's Ministry of Health began considering the imposition of user fees at government clinics. The ministry justified these proposals with the claim that the government could no longer afford to treat patients for free at the point of care.[73]

Malawi's health-care workers were quick to note that even with the progress of the previous decade, much had been left undone. In a July 2011 interview Dorothy Ngoma, executive director of Malawi's National Organization of Nurses and Midwives, despaired over the state of the health sector:

> Don't let anyone convince you that [past efforts] have relieved the emergency. While we can see improvements in pockets, we are still in a crisis. Without money on the table, we can't make progress. . . . Where are our partners? . . . Why are there so many people dying for want of basic needs?[74]

By noting all the deficiencies in health care, Ngoma was attempting to challenge the dominant discourse of scarcity.

The inadequacy of medicine in Malawi finally came to the fore of civic debate in April 2012, when seventy-eight-year-old President Bingu wa Mutharika was rushed to Kamuzu Central Hospital in cardiac arrest after a massive heart attack. Doctors tried to resuscitate him, but without success. In the days that followed, a popular rumor began to spread: when the president arrived, the doctors at Kamuzu Hospital had not given him epinephrine, the main drug used in the cardiac resuscitation protocol, because the hospital was stocked out of the drug.[75] The government would not confirm the rumor, but Mutharika's purported death-by-stock-out came as little surprise to most Malawians, who had their own bitter experiences with a health-care system so poorly funded and managed that it could not save even the president.

The embarrassment of this episode and the priorities of Mutharika's successor, Joyce Banda, made health care central to the nation's political agenda, if only briefly. Joyce Banda (no relation to Hastings Kamuzu Banda), Malawi's vice president when Mutharika died, had been an advocate for women's health since surviving post-partum hemorrhage decades earlier. During her tenure as president, which lasted only two years, she oversaw the construction and staffing of new clinics with expanded obstetrics capabilities, and she encouraged village chiefs to refer pregnant women to the clinics. Her presidency was also marred by an embarrassing scandal when civil servants were found with cash pilfered from the public purse.[76] Though the president herself was never directly implicated, the scandal became the major story heading into the 2014 general election. In that vote, she was defeated by her predecessor's brother, Peter wa Mutharika. The younger Mutharika made health care less of a focus than either Bingu or Joyce Banda. During fiscal year 2016–2017, the Ministry of Health accounted for just 8 percent of public expenditure, down from 12.4 percent during 2009–2010.[77] By late 2016, local newspapers reported widespread drug shortages in hospitals and clinics.[78]

Conclusion

During a drive home from an outreach cervical-cancer-screening clinic in the rural Neno District in 2015, a veteran nurse remembered, "There were many medicines in the time of Kamuzu Banda," and "fewer stock-outs." But as Francis's wife Edith lamented, during the era of multiparty democracy, *mankhwala kulibe* ("There are no medicines"). Nearby government facilities, she said, were frequently stocked out of antibiotics like chloramphenicol, and even cheap analgesics like acetaminophen or aspirin. The staff at the hospital, she said, had a common piece of advice for patients: *Mugule!* ("Buy them yourself!"). Even if services at government health facilities remained nominally free at the point of care, costs such as the required "health passbook," the booklet that patients had to buy and carry with them in order for health-care workers to record diagnoses and treatments, might prevent them from coming at all.[79]

Though the funding increase halted after 2008, the injection of domestic and international resources into the health sector had allowed Malawi to make progress on a number of health indices. The death rate attributable to HIV/AIDS fell by 64 percent between 1990 and 2012. Over the same period, the death rate due to malaria decreased by 63 percent. Between 1990 and 2013, maternal mortality rates fell by 54 percent, and under-five mortality rates fell by 72 percent. These trends are hopeful but are not any better than other countries in the region. Aside from HIV/AIDS, where Malawi's treatment program has been hailed as a model, most of Malawi's other health indices mirror the averages for the World Health Organization's sub-Saharan African region.[80]

Since 1980, Malawians have endured a number of crises, including famines and structural adjustment and political upheavals. No disaster was so terrible as AIDS, which tore through families and communities, clinics and hospitals, exposing fatal vulnerabilities in social support and medical provision. Only a sudden and unexpected burst of global health funding, spurred in large part by leaders in rich nations who were never socialized for scarcity, proved capable of slowing the unrelenting slaughter.

Conclusion: Breaking the Spell of Scarcity

I should have died after my heart stopped. In August 2000 I was fourteen years old, playing in a baseball game in a tony suburb of Boston. As I led off of third base, my teammate at bat hit the ball right at me. Before I could get out of the way, the ball struck me in the chest and knocked me to the ground. Felled by a rare and almost always fatal event called *commotio cordis*, the impact of the ball sent my heart into arrhythmia and—soon thereafter—arrest. But on that day, a cardiac nurse was in the stands, and my coach was a trained emergency medical technician. Their prompt use of CPR brought back my pulse and then my consciousness.

Five years later in Kigali, Rwanda, I sat next to a hospital bed where a six-year-old girl, whom I will call Mary, lay dying. Her breaths were labored, her limbs emaciated. Her cough produced sputum tinged with blood. Mary suffered from multi-drug-resistant tuberculosis. In the United States, her prospects for survival would have been far better than mine were after my near-death experience. In Rwanda, though, Mary's doctors did not have the equipment that could rapidly determine the drug susceptibilities of her particular infection. Even after reaching a hospital bed in Rwanda's best tertiary care facility, Mary was doomed to perish because her doctors did not know which drugs to administer. Eventually, Mary's sputum was shipped to Boston for drug susceptibility testing, but by the time the results returned she was already dead.

I should have died, yet I lived. The presence of trained medical professionals at my game was my salvation. Mary should have lived, yet she died. How, I wondered, could we bring to an end such untimely death and avoidable suffering? When, as an undergraduate at Harvard University, I turned to the public health literature, the answers on offer were often disappointing. Policymakers and experts insisted campaigns to remedy gross disparities in access to health care were counterproductive. To them, the major task of public health was to apportion the existing pot of meager resources for poor countries, and to do so using utilitarian theory rather than lived experience as a guide.

Take, for instance, former World Bank chief economist William Easterly, who in 2006 declared, "Spending AIDS money on treatment rather than on

No More to Spend. Paul Farmer, Oxford University Press (2020). © Oxford University Press.
DOI: 10.1093/oso/9780190066192.001.0001

prevention makes the AIDS crisis *worse*, not better."[1] Easterly buttressed his assertion with a 2002 study, published in *The Lancet*, that concluded— without any high-quality evidence—that AIDS prevention was far more cost-effective than AIDS treatment.[2] Easterly did not call for more money, only a shift of existing resources. The ethicist Ezekiel Emanuel and his col- league Colleen Denny made their assumption about scarcity even more ex- plicit in the *New England Journal of Medicine* in 2008: "International aid is inherently limited," they argued. "Consequently, it is extremely important to consider how this finite aid is distributed." At one level this statement is a truism; any material or financial resource is, in the extreme, "inherently lim- ited." But what Emanuel and Denny meant was that international aid was limited *to its current levels*. In the next few paragraphs, the authors unabash- edly decided who should live and who should die. Aid spending, they con- cluded, should immunize children against pertussis rather than treat adults with AIDS.[3]

I was often assigned papers of this sort during an undergraduate sem- inar at Harvard. Seated around an ornate hardwood table in high-backed leather chairs, my classmates and I, the sons and daughters of financiers and physicians, were taught how to reason through "hard choices" about which basic health interventions the poorest people on the planet should receive, and which they should not. These decisions were to be made, we were taught, with distance and dispassion. Unschooled as we were in the acceptable limits of public health discourse, these exercises made us angry. The assumption that the size of the budget for global health was inevitably limited (presum- ably, to its current level) seemed too facile. To many of us, it also appeared a convenient construct for the complacent. Attempts in the literature to foreclose broader questions of political economy, to proceed relentlessly to deliberations over the division of existing resources, avoided a conversation that the wealthy—people like us—might find even more difficult. For, in a truly open and honest discussion, historically deep, geographically broad, and (for many) politically uncomfortable questions about distribution be- come unavoidable.[4] Only if we accept the allocation of resources as inevitable is expanded AIDS treatment the enemy of higher immunization rates.

These intellectual constraints appeared to elide the fact that there was a fundamental choice that preceded the divvying up of paltry resources among the world's poorest peoples. Indeed, some ethicists have acknowledged that exercises such as Easterly's and Emanuel's dealt with "second-order" questions while ignoring "first-order" questions about why allocations of financial resources for the health of the poor were so pathetic to begin with.[5] To be sure, the world is full of unavoidable scarcities, but in the twenty-first century, why did lecturers think it useful to ask budding medical students, as Malawi's College of Medicine did, to debate whether the Ministry of Health should focus on "vaccines or latrines"? Reducing public health to technical considerations of cost-effectiveness ignored the far more troubling questions about how the world's destitute sick had come to be seen as expendable. These are unavoidably historical questions.

These questions returned, again and again, during my time in Malawian villages. My original aim was to understand which medical interventions people had come to use at different points in Malawian history. My interlocutors were willing to try to answer my questions, though most elderly Malawians could not really remember the specific medicines they had been given as children. The more persistent and unavoidable topics of conversation concerned battles with subsistence. Their daily lives were filled with "second-order" questions about how to divide impossibly limited resources. Should I buy fertilizer or send my child to school? Should I keep my stored grain for the hungry season or sell some to pay for a bicycle ride to the clinic? Impoverished Malawians were experts in tragic choices.

At the same time, though, my interlocutors were aware that some of their scarcities were constructed. They knew the benefits of immunization, better housing, and more adequate food. They desperately sought each of these for themselves and their families. But they did not generally believe that decreasing budgets for drugs and staff at hospitals was the preferable way to increase spending on these other priorities. When asked where additional funds for such programs might come from, many pointed to public officials who stole from government coffers, or wealthy Malawians in the cities, or foreign governments with historic ties to Malawi. Looking far and wide, they could see that there was plenty of money available; it just was not available to them.

Impoverished Malawians never begrudged their neighbors' use of public-sector health resources. In the lakeshore village of Nyanza, I frequently had my clothes repaired by a paraplegic man who had survived polio. He used a hand-powered sewing machine; his young nephew aided him by turning the wheel. About a kilometer away lived a blind man who had lost his sight in the late 1970s to measles. Neither of these men blamed their debilities on Bamusa, a man in their village who had regained his sight following free cataract surgery in Zomba's Central Hospital. The cataract surgery was more expensive than a polio or measles vaccine, but none of the men saw a necessary trade-off between immunization and ophthalmologic surgery. They did not believe resources were so inescapably scarce as to demand such a choice. More could be spent to allow for both. The social construction of scarcity may have had a hold on the moral imaginary of elite academics—the effects of this thrall were found in my undergraduate public health seminar rooms and in the everyday lives of the poor—but my Malawian friends did not believe, as public health experts did, that access to health care was a zero-sum game they had to play with the lives of kin and countrymen.

Even in Malawi, which remains as of this writing one of the world's poorest countries, scarcity is a construction that obscures unequal wealth and exploitative extraction, and by so obscuring it aims to free the powerful from social obligations. During the First World War, colonial police conducted night raids to kidnap villagers and force them into the carrier service.[6] At the same time, colonial officials claimed to lack the resources to provide better care for the thousands of Africans who died as beasts of burden. In the 1920s, the UK Treasury demanded repayment for a misbegotten railway loan while refusing to improve African hospitals. Two decades later, the Labour Party deployed the myth of comprehensive "traditional social security" to place geographical bounds on its plans for social protection. Shortly thereafter, the Federation government in Salisbury painted its own health-care spending for Nyasaland's Africans as exorbitant, even as it spent far more per capita on health services for Europeans than for Africans. Throughout the 1960s and 1970s, Life President Banda and World Bank administrators constantly claimed Malawi's dismal health services were actually quite impressive in light of "funds available," even as Banda built personal palaces with state funds. By the late 1990s and early 2000s, as Malawians died in the hundreds of thousands from AIDS, international bodies and public health experts argued that bringing antiretroviral therapy to the African poor was ethically unsound, fiscally unrealistic, and logistically impossible. This history shows changing justifications for scarcity, but it also reveals a continuity that was not broken by independence or the advent of multiparty democracy.

The construction of scarcity had mortal consequences. The absence of nearby health-care facilities doomed many to needless suffering and premature death. For patients who did manage to make it to hospitals and health centers, broken X-ray machines and laboratory equipment left medical providers unable to render accurate diagnoses. Without enough adequately trained medical providers, women perished from treatable complications of labor and delivery. Stringent rationing and frequent shortages of antibiotics left thousands to die of treatable infections. Ineffective vaccines allowed smallpox to spread and bred distrust of public health campaigns. While Malawians paid taxes and submitted to forced labor under both colonial and postcolonial governments, little of the wealth extracted from their toil came back to them. The portrayal of existing standards of public health and medical provision as inescapable has long helped to keep them low.

But this history also reveals something else about the construction of scarcity: it is not always accepted. Two groups in particular were less convinced about the inevitability of extremely limited resources for the poor. The first were the poor themselves. Particularly after the therapeutic advances of the 1940s and 1950s, curative medical interventions became increasingly popular. The shifts in Africans' demands for health care are comprehensible as empirical responses to the changes in biomedical efficacy. Just as resistance to some preventive interventions can be better understood by examining the technologies (e.g., smallpox vaccines that were not heat stable), so too can the growing demand for curative medical interventions be understood as a rational response to the rise in biomedical efficacy. Once they found relief from their ills in biomedicine, Malawians proved resistant to efforts to keep them away from the clinics.

In periods of unrest such as the Federation era, threatened elites sometimes allowed slightly more resources for health care. Not every kind of unrest was capable of opening the purse. Labor strikes, for instance were more frightening to officials and holders of capital than millenarian religious movements, and so the former generally led to more health-care spending as a political palliative. But in most instances the poor had little power to garner such resources. Under the thumb of colonial rule, or authoritarian one-party government, or the constraints of structural adjustment, they had few democratic institutions through which they could demand anything.

The second group that has been obstinate in its refusal to accept the construction of scarcity are those elites who were personally involved in the care of the poor. In particular, physicians and low-level officials resented having to make second-order choices every day when they knew more was available. Facing frequent drug shortages, decrepit facilities, and understaffed clinics, they agonized daily over which patients should receive severely constrained resources. They realized that this was not inevitable, but rather the result of first-order choices about appropriations to the colonial Medical Department and (later) to Malawi's Ministry of Health. In trying circumstances, these elite reformists called for better drugs, supplies, and facilities.

This historical fact raises something of a problem because some, though certainly not all, of these elite reformists worked for and vocally supported an exploitative British colonial regime. It may seem regressive to look to colonial-era European doctors and nurses as role models, and indeed many of them held ideas about racial politics that would today rightly be considered reactionary. But there remain things worth emulating in their example. Global health practitioners and policymakers should be at least as skeptical about claims of scarcity in our time as Shircore and de Boer were in theirs. Just as de Boer suggested that tax revenues from mining might be used to benefit Nyasaland, advocates in the present should insist on greater creativity in securing the finances necessary to improve the health of poor people in poor countries. Nurses like Sally Hubbard saw the toll that user fees took on the health of pregnant women during the late Federation era. Modern-day elite reformists should be at least as attuned to the consequences for the poor of such barriers to care. And political activists and political officials should be at least as creative in devising funding streams for health-care systems of poor countries as MPs such as Percy and Davies were in their revision of the 1929 CDA.

In the postcolonial era, additional challenges to scarcity were leveled by health-care providers and other reformists. John David Chiphangwi faced down Hastings Kamuzu Banda on Christmas Day 1978, forcing the president to see the squalor and overcrowding of the Queen Elizabeth Central Hospital's obstetrics ward. Later, Peter Mugyenyi and Paul Farmer showed that effective AIDS treatment in poor countries was, in fact, possible. Alongside other advocates, these doctors advocated successfully for far greater health-care spending from rich countries than they had ever before received.

The construction of scarcity, though, is a resilient thing, and it cannot be overcome by doctors and nurses alone. Claims of scarcity survived the end of colonialism and dictatorship. They have delayed—and continue to delay—access to medicine and public health for billions of people. The construct persists, for the most part, because we continue to live in a world where nationality, language, class, race, gender, and proximity hold great influence over our willingness to care about the lives of other human beings. A world awash in wealth allows avoidable suffering not for want of new ideas or inventions, but because we still do not feel deeply enough for one another.

This history of indifference to human suffering, of the rationalizations devised to deflect responsibility, reveals that our sentimental education remains incomplete.

Yet as much as history gives reasons to despair, it also demonstrates that caring is not inevitably futile, that cynicism is not always vindicated. Anyone who interrogates claims of scarcity will inevitably face demands to be *reasonable*, to settle on some comforting boundary between the possible and the impossible. I have avoided doing so in this book, as the history told herein demonstrates that it is often a fool's errand. Writing in the late 1990s, for instance, most would have considered universal access to AIDS treatment in Malawi a fanciful wish, quite outside the realm of possibility. Within a few years, increased international aid made such access a reality, despite unceasing criticism that such provision was irresponsible given "inherently limited" funding. It is difficult, and probably foolhardy, to define a "reasonable" amount of spending, especially when the average American benefits from more public sector health expenditure in two days than the average Malawian does in an entire year.[7]

Perhaps historians of health could look to the geographer Mike Davis, who called on fellow scholars of climate change to seriously consider so-called "impossible solutions" so as not to "become complicit in the *de facto* triage of humanity."[8] The rhetoric of scarce financial resources has been used to render tractable problems intractable for so long that it now threatens the future of humanity. We need not condemn ourselves to perpetually impoverished ambitions, not while there is still so much to do, so much lost ground to make up.

Notes

Foreword

1. Thomas Winterbottom, *An Account of the Native Africans in the Neighbourhood of Sierra Leone* (London: C. Whittingham, 1803), 2:29–32. His description was detailed enough that infectious disease specialists still refer to glandular tumors on the nape of the neck as "Winterbottom's sign," calling into question subsequent assertions that trypanosomiasis was new to Sierra Leone. The same process of discovery and forgetting would later mark virgin-soil claims about Ebola in Upper West Africa.
2. See Captain A. C. H. Gray, "Reports on the Sleeping Sickness Camps, Uganda, and on the Medical Treatment of Sleeping Sickness Patients at the Segregation Camps, from December, 1906, to January, 1908," in *Reports of the Sleeping Sickness Commission of the Royal Society*, No. IX (London: Darling & Son, 1908), pp. 62–96.
3. See William A. Murray, "History of the Introduction and Spread of Human Trypanosomiasis (Sleeping Sickness) in British Nyasaland in 1908 and Following Years," *Transactions of the Royal Society of Tropical Medicine and Hygiene* 15, no. 4 (1921): pp. 121–128.
4. Inge Heiberg, quoted in Maryinez Lyons, "From 'Death Camps' to Cordon Sanitaire: The Development of Sleeping Sickness Policy in the Uele District of the Belgian Congo, 1903–1914," *Journal of African History* 26, no. 1 (1985): 81.

Introduction

1. Philip Mullenix, Scott Steele, and Charles Andersen, "Limb Salvage and Outcomes among Patients with Traumatic Popliteal Vascular Injury: An Analysis of the National Trauma Data Bank," *Journal of Vascular Surgery* 44, no. 1 (2006): 94–99.
2. Eric Frykberg, "Popliteal Vascular Injuries," *Surgical Clinics of North America* 82, no. 1 (2002): 67–89.
3. Personal communication with Dr. Luckson Dullie, February 2015.
4. For AIDS, see William Easterly, "Human Rights Are the Wrong Basis for Health Care," *Financial Times*, October 12, 2009; Andrew Creese et al., "Cost-Effectiveness of HIV/AIDS Interventions in Africa: A Systematic Review of the Evidence," *Lancet* 359, no. 9318 (2002): 1635–42; and Elliot Marseille, Paul B. Hofmann, and James G. Kahn, "HIV Prevention before HAART in Sub-Saharan Africa," *Lancet* 359, no. 9320 (2002): 1851–56. For multi-drug-resistant tuberculosis, see John Donnelly, "Emanuel on TB: 'The Challenge Is Enormous,'" *Science Speaks: Global ID News*, October 28, 2010. For cancer, see I. Magrath and J. Litvak, "Cancer in Developing Countries: Opportunity and Challenge," *Journal of the National Cancer Institute* 85, no. 11 (1993): 863; and T. A. Ngoma, "World Health Organization Cancer Priorities in Developing Countries," *Annals of Oncology* 17, no. 8 (2006): S9–S14.

5. Colleen C. Denny and Ezekiel J. Emanuel, "US Health Aid Beyond PEPFAR: The Mother and Child Campaign," *Journal of the American Medical Association* 300, no. 17 (2008): 2048–51.

6. Randall M. Packard, *A History of Global Health: Interventions into the Lives of Other Peoples* (Baltimore, MD: Johns Hopkins University Press, 2016).

7. Jim Yong Kim, quoted in Adriana Petryna and Arthur Kleinman, "The Pharmaceutical Nexus," in *Global Pharmaceuticals: Ethics, Markets, Practices*, ed. Adriana Petryna, Arthur Lakoff, and Arthur Kleinman (Durham, NC: Duke University Press, 2006), 1–32.

8. Joan E. Wicken, "African Contrasts," Alice Horsman Travelling Fellow, 1956–1957 (paper submitted to Somerville College, Oxford, January 1958), MSS.Afr.s.1726, BLOU, 7.

9. Ibid., 6.

10. Leigh Gardner, *Taxing Colonial Africa: The Political Economy of British Imperialism* (Oxford: Oxford University Press, 2012), 155–56.

11. Hansjörg Dilger, "Targeting the Empowered Individual: Transnational Policy Making, the Global Economy of Aid, and the Limitations of Biopower in Tanzania," in *Medicine, Mobility, and Power in Global Africa: Transnational Health and Healing*, ed. Hansjörg Dilger, Aboulaye Kane, and Stacey Langwick, 60–91 (Bloomington: Indiana University Press, 2012), 64. A cross-country analysis of eighty nations between 1973 and 1990 concluded that inflation was spurred most often by *military* expenditures rather than social spending (Song Han and Casey B. Mulligan, "Inflation and the Size of Government," *Federal Reserve Bank of St. Louis Review*, June 2, 2008, 245–68).

12. This assumption of inevitable scarcity is left unexplored in many other works. For instance, in his history of Malawi's medical services, John Lwanda contends that Malawi's early postcolonial government "did not have enough resources to run universal medical services." This statement is not further explored (John Lloyd Chipembere Lwanda, *Colour, Class and Culture: A Preliminary Communication into the Creation of Doctors in Malawi* [Glasgow: Dudu Nsomba, 2008], 38). John Iliffe blames the denial by Nyasaland's financial secretary of a native council's 1949 proposal to set aside a portion of the hut tax to assist orphans and disabled adults on "governmental poverty joined with official ideology." Iliffe does not analyze the reasons for "governmental poverty" or the balance of responsibility attributable to "poverty" and "ideology," respectively (John Iliffe, "The Poor in the Modern History of Malawi," in *Malawi: An Alternative Pattern of Development: Proceedings of a Seminar Held in the Centre of African Studies, University of Edinburgh 24 and 25 May, 1984* [University of Edinburgh Centre of African Studies: Edinburgh, 1985], 267).

13. Wicken, "African Contrasts," 70, 83.

14. Gardner, *Taxing Colonial Africa*, 238.

15. Malawi's nominal GDP per capita is, according to the IMF, USD$295. See International Monetary Fund, *World Economic Outlook Database—April 2017*.

16. "Free Heart Surgery Scheme for the Poor," *Hindu*, December 25, 2012.

17. See Paul Farmer, Matthew Basilico, and Luke Messac, "After McKeown: The Changing Roles of Biomedicine, Public Health and Economic Growth in Mortality Declines," in

Therapeutic Revolutions: Pharmaceuticals and Social Change in the Twentieth Century, ed. Jeremy Greene, Flurin Condrau, and Elizabeth Watkins (Chicago: University of Chicago Press, 2016), 186–217.

18. John McCracken, *A History of Malawi, 1859–1966* (Woodbridge, UK: James Currey, 2012), 57–65.

19. As an anonymous reviewer once contended, "It is important to remember that Nyasaland was a Protectorate, it was not intended to be a 'little England' with a government and institutions that would eventually be the same as in the UK."

20. P. J. Cain and A. G. Hopkins, *British Imperialism, 1688–2000*, 2nd ed. (London: Longman, 2001), 385–86. Also see Gardner, *Taxing Colonial Africa*, 3–4.

21. Michael Havinden and David Meredith, *Colonialism and Development: Britain and Its Tropical Colonies, 1850–1960* (London: Routledge, 1996).

22. Ewout Frankema, "Colonial Taxation and Government Spending in British Africa, 1880–1940: Maximizing Revenue or Minimizing Effort?," *Explorations in Economic History* 48, no. 1 (2011): 136–49.

23. Steven Feierman, "Struggles for Control: The Social Roots of Health and Healing in Modern Africa," *African Studies Review* 28, nos. 2/3 (1985): 73–147. Also see Rita Hinden, *Plan for Africa: A Report Prepared for the Colonial Bureau of the Fabian Society* (London: George Allen & Unwin Ltd., 1941).

24. In their seminal study on the profitability (or, by their account, the unprofitability) of the colonies for the British metropole (1865–1914), Lance Davis and Robert Huttenback admit that while "the British as a whole certainly did not benefit economically from the Empire . . . individual investors did." See Lance Davis and Robert Huttenback, *Mammon and the Pursuit of Empire: The Political Economy of British Imperialism, 1860–1912* (Cambridge, UK: Cambridge University Press, 1986), 306.

25. Frankema, "Colonial Taxation and Government Spending in British Africa," Appendix 1. Britain was not the only colonial power that was loath to open the metropolitan treasury for colonial development. Elise Huillery has calculated that between 1907 and 1957 the French metropolis provided only 2 percent of French West Africa's public revenue, while salaries for colonial executives and district administrators claimed more than 13 percent of local public expenditures. See Elise Huillery, "The Black Man's Burden—The Cost of Colonization of French West Africa," *Journal of Economic History* 74, no. 1 (2013): 6.

26. Shashi Tharoor, *Inglorious Empire: What the British Did to India* (London: Hurst Publishers, 2017).

27. Amartya Sen, *Poverty and Famines: An Essay on Entitlement and Deprivation* (Oxford: Oxford University Press, 1983).

28. Sen places great faith in the ability of democratic discourse to prevent famines, going so far as to claim "there has never been a famine in a functioning multiparty democracy" (Amartya Sen, *Development as Freedom* [New York: Anchor, 2000], 178).

29. "Appendix: Institute of Development Studies Conference Statement on Scarcity, June 2005," in *The Limits to Scarcity: Contesting the Politics of Allocation*, ed. Lyla Mehta (London: Routledge, 2010), 257–58.

30. Ted Schrecker, "Interrogating Scarcity: How to Think about 'Resource-Scarce Settings,'" *Health Policy and Planning* 28 (2013): 400–409.

31. For disease-specific histories, see Maryinez Lyons, *The Colonial Disease: A Social History of Sleeping Sickness in Northern Zaire, 1900–1940* (New York: Cambridge University Press, 1992); John Farley, *Bilharzia: A History of Imperial Tropical Medicine* (New York: Cambridge University Press, 1991); and Randall Packard, *The Making of a Tropical Disease: A Short History of Malaria* (Baltimore, MD: Johns Hopkins University Press, 2011). For histories of mission hospitals, see Markku Hokkanen, *Medicine and Scottish Missionaries in the Northern Malawi Region 1875–1930: Quests for Health in a Colonial Society* (Lewiston, NY: Edwin Mellen Press, 2007); Michael Jennings, "'Healing of Bodies, Salvation of Souls': Missionary Medicine in Colonial Tanganyika, 1870s–1939," *Journal of Religion in Africa* 38, no. 1 (2008): 27–56; Terence O. Ranger, "Godly Medicine: The Ambiguities of Medical Mission in Southeastern Tanzania, 1900–1945," in *The Social Basis of Health and Healing in Africa*, ed. Steven Feierman and John Janzen (Berkeley: University of California Press, 1992), 256–84; Charles Good, *The Steamer Parish: The Rise and Fall of Missionary Medicine on an African Frontier* (Chicago: University of Chicago Press, 2004); and Nancy Rose Hunt, *A Colonial Lexicon of Birth Ritual, Medicalization, and Mobility in the Congo* (Durham, NC: Duke University Press, 1999). For histories of government health services, see Ralph Schram, *A History of the Nigerian Health Services* (Ibadan: Ibadan University Press, 1971); Michael Gelfand, *Proud Record: An Account of the Health Services Provided for Africans in the Federation of Rhodesia and Nyasaland* (Salisbury, Southern Rhodesia: Government Printer for the Federal Information Department, 1960); Michael Gelfand, *A Service to the Sick: A History of the Health Services for Africans in Southern Rhodesia, 1890–1953* (Gwelo, Southern Rhodesia: Mambo Press, 1976); Ann Beck, *A History of the British Medical Administration of East Africa, 1900–1950* (Cambridge, MA: Harvard University Press, 1970); Ann Beck, *Medicine, Tradition, and Development in Kenya and Tanzania, 1920–1970* (Waltham, MA: African Studies Assn, 1981); R. T. Mossop, *History of Western Medicine in Zimbabwe* (Lewiston, NY: Edwin Mellen Press, 1997); and Colin Baker, "The Government Medical Service in Malawi: An Administrative History, 1891–1974," *Medical History* 20, no. 3 (1976): 296–311.

32. See, for instance, Maynard W. Swanson, "The Sanitation Syndrome: Bubonic Plague and Urban Native Policy in the Cape Colony, 1900–1909," *Journal of African History* 18, no. 3 (1977): 387–410; and Philip Curtin, "Medical Knowledge and Urban Planning in Tropical Africa," *American Historical Review* 90, no. 3 (1985): 594–613. There are, of course, a number of exceptions. One historian who explores both the exploitative nature of colonialism and the realities of medical care in the life of everyday Africans is Nancy Rose Hunt. See Hunt, *A Colonial Lexicon*.

33. For a sample of celebratory narratives, see Gelfand, *A Service to the Sick* and *Proud Record*. For a sample of the critical narratives, see Wolfgang U. Eckart, "The Colony as Laboratory: German Sleeping Sickness Campaigns in German East Africa and in Togo, 1900–1914," *History and Philosophy of the Life Sciences* 24, no. 1 (2002): 69–89; and Paul S. Landau, "Explaining Surgical Evangelism in Colonial Southern Africa: Teeth, Pain and Faith," *Journal of African History* 37, no. 2 (1996): 261–81.

34. Michael Worboys draws a particularly explicit link between budgetary neglect and innovation when discussing cuts to colonial medical spending during the 1930s. See Michael Worboys, "Colonial Medicine," in *Companion to Medicine in the Twentieth Century*, ed. Roger Cooter and John V. Pickston (London: Routledge, 2002), 67–80.

35. Julie Livingston, *Improvising Medicine: An African Oncology Ward in an Emerging Cancer Epidemic* (Durham, NC: Duke University Press, 2012); Nancy Rose Hunt, *A Colonial Lexicon*; Claire L. Wendland, *A Heart for the Work: Journeys through an African Medical School* (London: University of Chicago Press, 2010); and Stacey A. Langwick, "Articulate(d) Bodies: Traditional Medicine in a Tanzanian Hospital," *American Ethnologist* 35, no. 3 (2008): 428–39.

36. Shula Marks, "What Is Colonial about Colonial Medicine? And What Has Happened to Imperialism and Health?," *Society for the Social History of Medicine* 10, no. 2 (1997): 215.

37. The most careful historical investigation of the effects of health care on health outcomes in Africa may be Shane Doyle's study of three districts in Tanzania and Uganda: *Before HIV: Sexuality, Fertility and Mortality in East Africa, 1900–1980* (Oxford: Oxford University Press, 2013).

38. For more on statistics (and their absence) in Africa, see Morton Jerven, *Poor Numbers: Why We Are Misled by African Development Statistics and What to Do About It* (Ithaca, NY: Cornell University Press, 2013).

39. Vito Tanzi and Ludger Schuknecht, *Public Spending in the 20th Century: A Global Perspective* (Cambridge, UK: Cambridge University Press, 2000), 38. Also see World Health Organization, *The Abuja Declaration: Ten Years On*, 2011, http://www.who.int/healthsystems/publications/Abuja10.pdf.

40. World Bank Data Catalog, Health Expenditure Per Capita, https://data.worldbank.org/indicator/SH.XPD.PCAP

41. James C. Scott, *Two Cheers for Anarchism: Six Easy Pieces on Autonomy, Dignity, and Meaningful Work and Play* (Princeton, NJ: Princeton University Press, 2012), 16–17.

42. Philip A. Klinker and Rogers M. Smith, *The Unsteady March: The Rise and Decline of Racial Equality in America* (Chicago: University of Chicago Press, 1999).

43. Jim Paul, "Medicine and Imperialism in Morocco," *Middle East Research and Information Project Reports* 60 (1977): 3–12. Also see "Cote d'Ivoire: Free Health Care, for Now," *IRINnews*, http://www.irinnews.org/report/92701/cote-d-ivoire-free-health-care-for-now (accessed January 29, 2016).

44. Richard Rorty, "Human Rights, Rationality, and Sentimentality," in *Truth and Progress: Philosophical Papers*, vol. 3 (Cambridge, MA: Harvard University Press, 1998), 181. Rorty explains that the most convincing and politically efficacious answer to the question "Why should I care about a stranger, a person who is no kin to me?" is not "Because kinship and custom are morally irrelevant, to the obligations imposed by the recognition of membership in the same species," but rather "the sort of long, sad, sentimental story that begins . . . 'Because her mother would grieve for her.' Such stories, repeated and varied over the centuries, have induced us, the rich, safe, powerful people to tolerate and even to cherish powerless people."

45. The idea that the wealthy could discover greater sentimental concern for the poor was particularly prominent in the postwar scholarship of British social researcher Richard Titmuss. See, for instance, Titmuss, *Problems of Social Policy* (London: His Majesty's Stationery Office, 1950). Also see T. H. Marshall, *Citizenship and Social Class: And Other Essays* (Cambridge, UK: Cambridge University Press, 1950). For a discussion of moral commitments to welfare in southern Africa, see James Ferguson, *Give a Man a Fish: Reflections on the New Politics of Distribution* (Durham, NC: Duke University Press, 2015).

46. Peter Baldwin, *The Politics of Social Solidarity: Class Bases of the European Welfare State, 1875–1975* (Cambridge, MA: Cambridge University Press, 1990), 49.

47. Ibid., 53.

48. Paul Farmer, "Who Lives and Who Dies," *London Review of Books*, February 5, 2015.

49. Paul Farmer, "Global AIDS: New Challenges for Health and Human Rights," *Perspectives in Biology and Medicine* 48, no. 1 (2005): 10–16.

50. Peter Berger and Thomas Luckmann, *The Social Construction of Reality: A Treatise in the Sociology of Knowledge* (New York: Penguin, 1966), 78–79.

51. Ibid., 78–79.

52. Marc Bloch, *The Historian's Craft: Reflections on the Nature and Uses of History and the Techniques and Methods of the Men Who Write It*, trans. Peter Putnam (New York: Vintage, 1953), 39.

53. Northern Rhodesia's copper industry is a stark example of revenues lost to a foreign-owned extractive industry. In fiscal year 1937–1938, the expatriated profits of the territory's three major copper companies amounted to more than seventy times the Northern Rhodesian government's health-care budget. See Rita Hinden, *Plan for Africa*, 53–54, 102.

54. Baker, "Government Medical Service in Malawi," 296–311. Also see Harry S. Gear, "Some Problems of the Medical Services of the Federation of Rhodesia and Nyasaland," *BMJ* 2, no. 5197 (1960): 525–31; P. J. Freund, "Health Care in a Declining Economy: The Case of Zambia," *Social Science & Medicine* 23, no. 9 (1986): 875–88. For a more recent history that attributes a particular prominence to missions in Malawi, see Catherine Valentine, "Settler Visions of Health: Health Care Provision in the Central African Federation, 1953–1963" (master's thesis, Portland State University, 2017).

55. Michael King and Elspeth King, *The Story of Medicine and Disease in Malawi: The 150 Years Since Livingstone* (Blantyre, Malawi: Arco Books, 1992); and Austin C. Mkandawire, *Living My Destiny: A Medical and Historical Narrative* (Limbe, Malawi: Popular Publications, 1998). These mission-trained medical providers staffed clinics not only in Nyasaland but also in neighboring colonies such as Northern Rhodesia and Tanganyika. Patrick Malloy, " 'Holding [Tanganyika] by the Sindano': Networks of Medicine in Colonial Tanganyika" (PhD diss., University of California Los Angeles, 2003), 204.

56. Harry Gear, quoted in Baker, "Government Medical Service in Malawi," 296–311. Writing in 1925, Hans Coudenhove, who had lived in Nyasaland for decades, made the same point. Coudenhove, *My African Neighbors: Man, Bird, and Beast in Nyasaland* (Boston: Little, Brown, 1925), 8–9.

57. See, for instance, Good, *Steamer Parish*; James William Jack, *Daybreak in Livingstonia: The Story of the Livingstonia-Mission, British Central Africa* (London: Forgotten Books, 2012); Landeg White, *Magomero: Portrait of an African Village* (Cambridge, UK: Cambridge University Press, 1989); W. P. Livingstone, *Laws of Livingstonia: A Narrative of Missionary Adventure and Achievement* (London: Hodder and Stoughton, 1921); James Tengatenga, *The UMCA in Malawi: A History of the Anglican Church, 1861–2010* (Zomba, Malawi: Kachere Series, 2010); Mary McCulloch, *A Time to Remember: The Story of the Diocese of Nyasaland* (London: Charles Birchall and Sons, 1959); and Michael Gelfand, *Lakeside Pioneers: Socio-Medical Study of Nyasaland, 1875–1920* (Oxford: Basil Blackwell, 1964).

58. In 1962, Nyasaland had fewer mission hospitals (sixty-one) than either Southern Rhodesia (sixty-five) or Northern Rhodesia (eighty), even though Nyasaland had an estimated African population (2.93 million) higher than Northern Rhodesia's (2.46 million) and only somewhat lower than Southern Rhodesia's (3.64 million). See *Annual Report on the Public Health of the Federation of Rhodesia and Nyasaland for the Year 1962*, CSD 607, BL.

59. See, for instance, Joseph Hodge, *Triumph of the Expert: Agrarian Doctrines of Development and the Legacies of British Colonialism* (Athens: Ohio University Press, 2007); Packard, *A History of Global Health*; and Helen Tilley, *Africa as a Living Laboratory: Empire, Development and the Problem of Scientific Knowledge, 1870–1950* (Chicago: University of Chicago Press, 2010).

60. Johannes Fabian, *Time and the Other: How Anthropology Makes Its Object* (New York: Columbia University Press, 1983), 31.

61. For a history of the political economy of medical provision in South Africa, see Randall Packard, *White Plague, Black Labor: Tuberculosis and the Political Economy of Health and Disease in South Africa* (Berkeley: University of California Press, 1989).

62. John Iliffe, *The African AIDS Epidemic: A History* (London: James Currey, 2006), 102.

63. Steven Feierman, "Change in African Therapeutic Systems," *Social Science & Medicine* 13B (1979): 277–84. Also see Walter Bruchhausen, "Medical Pluralism as a Historical Phenomenon: A Regional and Multi-Level Approach to Health Care in German, British and Independent East Africa," in *Crossing Colonial Historiographies*, ed. Anne Digby, Waltraud Ernst, and Projit B. Mukharji (Newcastle, UK: Cambridge Scholars Publishing, 2010), 99–113.

64. For examples of hagiographic accounts by colonial apologists, see such works as Gelfand, *Proud Record* and *Service to the Sick*. For a canonical and wholesale critique of colonialism, see Walter Rodney, *How Europe Underdeveloped Africa* (London: Bogle-L'Ouverture Publications, 1972).

65. Kenan Malik, "The Great British Empire Debate," *New York Review of Books*, January 26, 2018.

66. Ferguson, *Give a Man a Fish*, 33.

67. Jeremy Greene, "Colonial Medicine and Its Legacies," in *Reimagining Global Health: An Introduction*, ed. Jim Yong Kim, Paul Farmer, Arthur Kleinman, and Matthew Basilico (Berkeley: University of California Press, 2013), 33–73.

Chapter 1

1. The suffix -*ni* in Chichewa, the most commonly spoken language in Malawi, is used to denote a command.
2. George Shepperson and Thomas Price, *Independent African: John Chilembwe and the Origins, Setting and Significance of the Nyasaland Native Rising of 1915* (Edinburgh: Edinburgh University Press, 1969), 179; John McCracken, *A History of Malawi: 1859–1966* (Woodbridge, UK: James Currey, 2012), 80.
3. Interview with Francis in Nyanza Village, Mangochi District, Malawi, March 20, 2015.
4. See, for instance, W. T. C. Berry, *Before the Wind of Change* (Suffolk, UK: Halesworth Press, 1984), 17.
5. Lewis Mataka Bandawe, *Memoirs of a Malawian: The Life and Reminiscences of Lewis Mataka Bandawe* (Blantyre, Malawi: Claim, 1971). Also see Edward Paice, *Tip and Run: The Untold Tragedy of the Great War in Africa* (London: Weidenfeld & Nicolson, 2007), 162–63.
6. Bandawe, *Memoirs of a Malawian*, 70–73; and Paice, *Tip and Run*, 162.
7. Interview with Francis in Nyanza Village.
8. King and King, *Story of Medicine and Disease in Malawi*; and Mkandawire, *Living My Destiny: A Medical and Historical Narrative* (Limbe, Malawi: Popular Publications, 1998).
9. Steven Heyneman, "The Evaluation of Human Capital in Malawi," World Bank Staff Working Papers, no. 420, xii.
10. David Livingstone, *Missionary Travels and Researches in South Africa: Including a Sketch of Sixteen Years' Residence in the Interior of Africa* (London: John Murray, 1857).
11. David Livingstone, *David Livingstone's Shire Journal, 1861–1864*, ed. G. W. Clendennen (Aberdeen: Scottish Cultural Press, 1993).
12. Livingstone, *Missionary Travels*.
13. Livingstone, *Laws of Livingstonia*, 92.
14. McCracken, *A History of Malawi*, 116.
15. Good, *Steamer Parish*.
16. Agnes Rennick, "Church and Medicine: The Role of Medical Missionaries in Malawi, 1875–1914" (PhD diss., University of Sterling, UK, 2003), 205.
17. McCracken, *History of Malawi*, 118–19.
18. For a more heroic narrative, see Michael Gelfand, *Lakeside Pioneers: Socio-Medical Study of Nyasaland, 1875–1920* (Oxford: Basil Blackwell, 1964). For missions as propagators of racialized ideas of medical difference, see Megan Vaughan, *Curing Their Ills: Colonial Power and African Illness* (Redwood City, CA: Stanford University Press, 1991).
19. *Annual Medical and Sanitary Report for the Year Ending 31st December 1940* (Zomba, Nyasaland: Government Printer, 1941). Also see Advisory Commission on the Review of the Constitution of the Federation of Rhodesia and Nyasaland, *Survey of Developments Since 1953: Cmmd. 1149* (London: Her Majesty's Stationery Office, 1960), 140–41; and G. van Etten, "Toward Research on Health Development in Tanzania," *Social Science & Medicine* 6, no. 3 (1972): 343.

20. John Reader, *Africa: A Biography of the Continent* (New York: Vintage, 1999), 579.

21. Griffith Bevan Jones, *Britain and Nyasaland* (London: Allen & Unwin, 1964), 53.

22. Michael Worboys, "Manson, Ross and Colonial Medical Policy: Tropical Medicine in London and Liverpool, 1899–1914," in *Disease, Medicine and Empire: Perspectives on Western Medicine and the Experience of European Expansion*, ed. Milton Lewis and Roy Macleod (London: Routledge, 1988), 21–38.

23. Vaughan, *Curing Their Ills*, 30–32.

24. W. H. Mercer, "The Colonial Office List for 1913: Comprising Historical and Statistical Information Respecting the Colonial Dependencies of Great Britain" (London: Waterlow & Sons Ltd., 1913), 274.

25. John Lwanda, *Colour, Class and Culture: A Preliminary Communication into the Creation of Doctors in Malawi* (Glasgow: Dudu Nsomba, 2008), 47; and Rennick, "Church and Medicine," 125.

26. Markku Hokkanen, "Towards a Cultural History of Medicine(s) in Colonial Central Africa," in *Crossing Colonial Historiographies: Histories of Colonial and Indigenous Medicines in Transnational Perspective*, ed. Anne Digby, Waltraud Ernst, and Projit Mukharji (Newcastle, UK: Cambridge Scholars Publishing, 2010), 147.

27. John M. Janzen, *The Quest for Therapy in Lower Zaire* (Berkeley: University of California Press, 1978), 221.

28. Rennick, "Church and Medicine," 301. Also see D. Maier, "Nineteenth Century Asante Medical Practices," *Comparative Studies in Society and History* 21, no. 1 (1979): 63–81.

29. Daniel R. Headrick, "Sleeping Sickness Epidemics and Colonial Responses in East and Central Africa, 1900–1940," *PLoS Neglected Tropical Diseases* 8, no. 4 (2014): 1–8. Also see Jan Vansina, *Paths in the Rainforest: Toward a History of Political Tradition in Equatorial Africa* (Madison: University of Wisconsin Press, 1990).

30. Steven Feierman, "Struggles for Control: The Social Roots of Health and Healing in Modern Africa," *African Studies Review* 28, no. 2/3 (1985): 73–147. Also see Elias Coutinho Mandala, *The End of Chidyerano: A History of Food and Everyday Life in Malawi, 1860–2004* (Portsmouth, NH: Heinemann, 2005).

31. Markku Hokkanen, "The Government Medical Service and British Missions in Colonial Malawi, c. 1891–1940: Crucial Collaboration, Hidden Conflicts," in *Beyond the State: The Colonial Medical Service in British Africa*, ed. Anna Greenwood (Manchester, UK: Manchester University Press, 2016), 47–48. Also see Charles J. Griffin and Walter E. Demuth, "No. 4 of 1903, Epidemic and Contagious Diseases, Rules, 117/1911, 21st July 1903, Sleeping Sickness," in *Proclamations, Rules and Notices Relating to the Nyasaland Protectorate in Force on the 31st December, 1914* (Zomba, Nyasaland: Government Printer, 1915), 40–43.

32. Rennick, "Church and Medicine," 299.

33. Rennick, "Church and Medicine," 301. Also see Megan Vaughan, "Health and Hegemony: Representation of Disease and the Creation of the Colonial Subject in Nyasaland," in *Contesting Colonial Hegemony: State and Society in Africa and India*, ed. Dagmar Engels and Shula Marks (London: British Academic Press, 1994), 173–201.

34. Markku Hokkanen, *Medicine and Scottish Missionaries in the Northern Malawi Region 1875–1930: Quests for Health in a Colonial Society* (Lewiston, NY: Edwin Mellen Press, 2007), 146, 298.

35. Rennick, "Church and Medicine," 300.

36. Ibid., 301.

37. Ibid., 305.

38. Ibid., 304.

39. For more on the role of trust in public acceptance of public health interventions such as vaccines, see H. Birungi, "Injections and Self-Help: Risk and Trust in Ugandan Health Care," *Social Science and Medicine* 47, no. 10 (1998): 1455–67. Also see Robert Aronowitz, *Risky Medicine: Our Quest to Cure Fear and Uncertainty* (Chicago: University of Chicago Press, 2015), 214; and Julie Livingston, Keith Wailoo, and Barbara M. Cooper, "Vaccination as Governance: HPV Skepticism in the United States and Africa, and the North-South Divide," in *Three Shots at Prevention: The HPV Vaccine and the Politics of Medicine's Simple Solutions*, ed. Keith Wailoo, Julie Livingston, Steven Epstein, et al. (Baltimore, MD: Johns Hopkins University Press, 2010), 231–53.

40. Vaughan, "Health and Hegemony," 185–86.

41. For a brief account of the wars of conquest led by Harry Johnston between 1891 and 1894 while in the employ of both the British government and the BSAC, see McCracken, *History of Malawi*, 57–67.

42. McCracken, *History of Malawi*, 85.

43. Randall Packard, "The Invention of the 'Tropical Worker': Medical Research and the Quest for Central African Labor on the South African Gold Mines, 1903–36," *Journal of African History* 34, no. 2 (1993): 271–92.

44. Berry, foreword to *Before the Wind of Change*.

45. McCracken, *A History of Malawi*, 148.

46. Paice, *Tip and Run*, 13–15.

47. Shepperson and Price, *Independent African*.

48. Ibid.

49. R. W. Lyall Grant, A. M. D. Turnbull, J. C. Casson, et al., "Report of the Commission appointed by his Excellency the Governor to Inquire into Various Matters and Questions concerned with the Native Rising within the Nyasaland Protectorate," January 14, 1916, in *Voices from the Chilembwe Rising*, ed. John McCracken (Oxford: Oxford University Press, 2015), 586–96.

50. McCracken, *History of Malawi*, 143–44, 159–60.

51. Paice, *Tip and Run*, 265.

52. Headrick, "Sleeping Sickness Epidemics and Colonial Responses." Also see Paice, *Tip and Run*.

53. McCracken, *History of Malawi*, 149.

54. Melvin E. Page, *The Chiwaya War: Malawians in the First World War* (Boulder, CO: Westview Press, 2000), 46–47.

55. Ibid., 45–46. Also see Jan-Bart Gewald, *Forged in the Great War: People, Transport and Labour; The Establishment of Colonial Rule in Zambia, 1890–1920* (Leiden: African Studies Centre, 2015), 16.

56. Gewald, *Forged in the Great War*, 43.
57. Elias Mandala, "Feeding and Fleecing the Native: How the Nyasaland Transport System Distorted a New Food Market, 1890s–1920s," *Journal of Southern African Studies* 32, no. 3 (2006): 505–24.
58. Baker, "Government Medical Service in Malawi," 296–311.
59. Page, *Chiwaya War*, 110–11.
60. Gewald, *Forged in the Great War*, 44, 94.
61. Gewald, *Forged in the Great War*, 112–13.
62. Francis Baily, *Twenty-Nine Years' Hard Labour* (London: Hutchinson & Co., 1934), 95–96.
63. Page, *Chiwaya War*, 113–14.
64. Paice, *Tip and Run*, 395. Rough estimates of the number of deaths from the 1918–1919 Spanish influenza pandemic in sub-Saharan Africa place the total at 1.5 to 2 million.
65. Hector Duff to Secretary of State for the Colonies, April 14, 1919, CO 525/82, No. 135, UKNA.
66. *Official History of the War: Medical Services General History*, vol. IV (London: H. M. Stationery Office, 1924), 477–78.
67. Ibid., 492.
68. Ibid., 490.
69. Page, *Chiwaya War*, 113.
70. Quotation from Henry Hearsey, *Annual Medical Report on the Health and Sanitary Condition of the Nyasaland Protectorate for the Year Ended 31st December, 1918* (Zomba, Nyasaland: Government Printer, 1919). Also see King and King, *The Story of Medicine and Disease in Malawi*, 106.
71. Baker, "Government Medical Service in Malawi," 301.
72. Henry Hearsey, "Medical Treatment of Natives. Rural Dispensaries, by Office of the Principal Medical Officer," August 25, 1921, S40/1/3/2, MNA.
73. "Chief Secretary, Zomba to District Residents," September 6, 1921, S40/1/3/2, MNA.
74. Principal Medical Officer H. Hearsey to Chief Secretary, Zomba, May 1, 1921, S40/1/3/2, MNA.
75. Richard Rankine to Secretary of State for the Colonies Winston Churchill, December 12, 1921, T161/156, UKNA. Also see Acting Chief Secretary to Principal Medical Officer H. Hearsey, December 3, 1921, S40/1/3/2, MNA.
76. "EA Estimates 1010: Acting Governor to Secretary of State," January 5, 1922, T 161/156, UKNA.
77. Undersecretary of State Gilbert Grindle to Chancellor of the Exchequer Robert Home, February 8, 1922, T 161/156, UKNA.
78. Untitled Treasury Department analysis, February 21, 1922, T 151/156, UKNA.
79. G. L. Barstow to Undersecretary of State for the Colonies Gilbert Grindle, March 9, 1922, T 161/156, UKNA.
80. Richard Rankine to Principal Medical Officer H. Hearsey, April 12, 1922, S40/1/3/2, MNA.
81. Principal Medical Officer Henry Hearsey to Acting Chief Secretary, April 18, 1922, S40/1/3/2, MNA.

82. Colin Baker, "Tax Collection in Malawi: An Administrative History, 1891–1972," *International Journal of African Historical Studies* 8, no. 1 (1975): 40–62.
83. Principal Medical Officer H. Hearsey to Chief Secretary, Zomba, May 1, 1921.
84. Robert I. Rotberg, *The Rise of Nationalism in Central Africa: The Making of Malawi and Zambia, 1873–1964* (Cambridge, MA: Harvard University Press, 1965). Also see Baker, "Government Medical Service in Malawi."
85. Joseph M. Hodge, *Triumph of the Expert: Agrarian Doctrines of Development and the Legacies of British Colonialism* (Athens: Ohio University Press, 2007), 118–21.
86. Lord Frederick J. D. Lugard, *The Dual Mandate in British Tropical Africa* (London: Routledge, 2013), 92–93
87. Ann Beck, *Medicine, Tradition, and Development in Kenya and Tanzania: 1920–1970* (Waltham, MA: African Studies Association, 1981), 15–16.
88. John Iliffe, *East African Doctors: A History of the Modern Profession* (London: Cambridge University Press, 1998), 60–61.
89. Van Etten, "Toward Research on Health Development in Tanzania," 338. Also see Oswald Masebo, "Society, State and Infant Welfare: Negotiating Medical Interventions in Colonial Tanzania, 1920–1950" (PhD diss, University of Minnesota, 2010), 186.
90. Hodge, *Triumph of the Expert*, 123; and Patrick Malloy, "'Holding [Tanganyika] by the Sindano': Networks of Medicine in Colonial Tanganyika" (PhD diss., University of California Los Angeles, 2003), 206.
91. Raymond Busy, "Blantyre Government Hospitals and Dispensary General Report 1921," 1922, S1/1728/27, MNA, 3.
92. "AG Eldred, Senior Medical Officer, Blantyre to Acting Principal Medical Officer Raymond Busy," July 10, 1924, S1/1728/27, MNA.
93. F. E. Whitehead, *Annual Medical Report on the Health and Sanitary Condition of the Nyasaland Protectorate for the Year Ended 31st December, 1925* (Zomba, Nyasaland: Government Printer, June 11, 1926), 13.
94. F. E. Whitehead, *Annual Medical Report on the Health and Sanitary Condition of the Nyasaland Protectorate for the Year Ending the 31st December, 1928* (Zomba, Nyasaland: Government Printer, July 10, 1929), 6.
95. Hokkanen, "Government Medical Service," 53.
96. Malloy, "'Holding [Tanganyika] by the Sindano,'" 210–15.
97. Whitehead, *Annual Medical Report on the Health and Sanitary Condition of the Nyasaland Protectorate for the Year Ending the 31st December, 1928*, 66.
98. F. E. Whitehead, *Annual Medical Report for the Year Ended 31st December, 1927* (Zomba, Nyasaland: Government Printer, June 16, 1928).
99. Whitehead, *Annual Medical Report on the Health and Sanitary Condition of the Nyasaland Protectorate for the Year Ended 31st December, 1925*, 13–14.
100. Lwanda, *Colour, Class and Culture*, 30.
101. The causative agent in yaws is *Treponema pertinue*, whereas the causative agent in venereal syphilis is *Treponema pallidum*. There is evidence of cross-protective immunity between yaws and venereal syphilis. See T. Guthe, "Clinical, Serological and Epidemiological Features of Frambosia Tropica (Yaws) and Its Control in Rural Communities," *Acta Derm-Venereol* 49 (1969): 343–68.

102. For more on Castellani's mixture, see "Internal Treatment of Yaws, Condensed by The Journal of Tropical Medicine and Hygiene," *Journal of the American Medical Association* (April 17, 1915): 1363.

103. Whitehead, *Annual Medical Report on the Health and Sanitary Condition of the Nyasaland Protectorate for the Year Ended 31st December, 1928*, 11, 43.

104. H. G. FitzMaurice, "Appendix IV: Notes on the Treatment of Yaws with Novarsenobillon and with Sodium Bismuth Tartrate," in *Annual Medical Report on the Health and Sanitary Condition of the Nyasaland Protectorate for the Year Ended 31st December 1928*, 43.

105. H. B. Follit, "Some Notes on the Treatment of Yaws in Nyasaland," in *Annual Medical Report on the Health and Sanitary Condition of the Nyasaland Protectorate for the Year Ended 31st December 1925* (Zomba, Nyasaland: Government Printer, 1926).

106. Klaus Strebhardt and Axel Ullrich, "Paul Ehrlich's Magic Bullet Concept: 100 Years of Progress," *Nature Reviews Cancer* 8 (2008): 473–80.

107. See J. O. Shircore, "Yaws and Syphilis in Tropical Africa: Mass Treatment with Bismuth-Arsenic Compounds," letter to the editor, *Lancet* 208, no. 5366 (1926): 43–44.

108. Terence O. Ranger, "Godly Medicine: The Ambiguities of Medical Mission in Southeastern Tanzania, 1900–1945," in *The Social Basis of Health and Healing in Africa*, ed. Steven Feierman and John Janzen (Berkeley: University of California Press, 1992), 266.

109. Shircore, "Yaws and Syphilis in Tropical Africa."

110. FitzMaurice, "Appendix IV."

111. Ranger, "Godly Medicine," 265, 268.

112. Guthe, "Clinical, Serological and Epidemiological Features of Yaws," 345–47.

113. John B. Christopherson, "The UMCA and Medical Work at Magila," *Central Africa* 39 (1921), 91. Also see Ranger, "Godly Medicine."

114. Whitehead, *Annual Medical Report on the Health and Sanitary Condition of the Nyasaland Protectorate for the Year Ended 31st December, 1928*.

115. Christopherson, "UMCA and Medical Work at Magila," 86–91; and Ranger, "Godly Medicine."

116. Baker, "Tax Collection in Malawi," 48.

117. Berry, *Before the Wind of Change*, 17.

118. Mandala, *End of Chidyerano*, 49–51.

Chapter 2

1. Joan E. Wicken, "African Contrasts," Alice Horsman Travelling Fellow, 1956–1957 (paper submitted to Somerville College, Oxford, January 1958), MSS.Afr.s.1726, BLOU, 23–24.

2. Medical assistants and clinical officers are the two major "mid-level" or "auxiliary" health cadres in Malawi. Medical assistants (and hospital assistants) have been trained at missionary schools in Malawi (by various names, with varied requirements), since the nineteenth century, and at government institutions beginning in the mid-1930s. Since 2000, the required training to become a medical

assistant (by obtaining a certificate in clinical medicine) is two years of postsecondary, preservice didactic training. Since independence, medical assistants have mostly been tasked with outpatient care. Clinical officers were introduced in Malawi in 1980. To become a clinical officer (by obtaining a diploma in clinical medicine), one must complete three years of postsecondary, preservice didactic training and one year of internship. Clinical officers are expected to care for hospitalized patients and outpatients as well and to perform some surgical procedures, including Caesarean sections. While most of the country's few physicians (260 for a population of 13 million) work in urban areas, medical assistants and clinical officers are often tasked with providing care in rural dispensaries and district hospitals. Government and missionary training institutions offer a number of nursing degrees, which require between one and three years of preservice and in-service training. See Adamson S. Muula, "Case for Clinical Officers and Medical Assistants in Malawi," *Croatian Medical Journal* 50, no. 1 (2009): 77–78. Also see *Nurse/Midwife Training Operational Plan: Field Assessments, Analysis and Scale-up Plans for Nurse Training Institutions* (Lilongwe, Malawi: Ministry of Health, 2011).

3. In order of number of filled posts in 2010, the cadres of health workers in Malawi's public health sector were nurses (including midwives), then medical assistants, then clinical officers, then environmental health officers (who are tasked with community public health work), and finally physicians. See Annex 2, *Malawi Health Sector Strategic Plan, 2011–2016* (Lilongwe, Malawi: Ministry of Health, 2010).

4. Health Compass, "'Moyo ndi Mpamba, Usamalireni!' Inspiring Behavior Change in Malawi" (accessed March 6, 2018) https://www.thecompassforsbc.org/sbcc-spotlights/moyo-ndi-mpamba-usamalireni-inspiring-behavior-change-malawi.

5. L. J. L. Nthenda, "H.M. Treasury and the Nyasaland Administration, 1919–40" (PhD diss., Oxford University, 1972); D. J. Morgan, *The Origins of British Aid Policy, 1924–1945* (London: Brill, 1980); and E. A. Brett, *Colonialism and Underdevelopment in East Africa: The Politics of Economic Change, 1919–1939* (London: Heinemann, 1973).

6. From the south bank of the Zambesi, goods would be transported across the river, then loaded onto an existing rail line connecting Beira to Port Herald (now Nsanje).

7. Leroy Vail, "The Making of an Imperial Slum: Nyasaland and Its Railways, 1895–1935," *Journal of African History* 16, no. 1 (1975): 100.

8. Landeg White, *Bridging the Zambesi: A Colonial Folly* (London: Macmillan, 1993), 42–44, 57–59.

9. Ibid., 43.

10. White, *Bridging the Zambesi*. Oury made Sharpe a director of the Mozambique Company, the Zambesia Mining and Development Company, and Beira Works Ltd. See Robert B. Boeder, *Alfred Sharpe of Nyasaland, Builder of Empire* (Blantyre, Malawi: SoMA, 1981).

11. Cynthia Ann Crosby, "A History of the Nyasaland Railway, 1895–1935: A Study in Colonial Economic Development" (PhD diss., Syracuse University, 1974), 145–48.

12. Vail, "Making of an Imperial Slum," 102.

13. G. H. Pirie, "The Decivilizing Rails: Railways and Underdevelopment in Southern Africa," *Journal of Economic and Social Geography* 73, no. 4 (1982): 221–28.

14. F. Skevington, "Memorandum re: Estimates of the Nyasaland Protectorate for the year 1921–22," February 9, 1921, T 161/91, UKNA.

15. Nthenda, "H.M. Treasury and the Nyasaland Administration," 256.

16. Ibid., 258.

17. Glyn Jones, H. Norman-Walker, Henry Phillips, et al., "Colloquium on Nyasaland Finance," April 23, 1980, Mss.Afr.s.1742, Box 1, File 27, BLOU.

18. Nthenda, "H.M. Treasury and the Nyasaland Administration," 260.

19. David John Morgan, *The Official History of Colonial Development: The Origins of British Aid Policy, 1924–1945* (London: Humanities Press, 1980), 39–40.

20. Rudolf von Albertini, *Decolonization: The Administration and Future of the Colonies, 1919–1960* (New York: Holmes & Meier Publications, 1982), 103.

21. Paul Denman and Paul McDonald, "Unemployment Statistics from 1881 to the Present Day," *Labour Market Trends* 4, no. 1 (1996): 5–18.

22. Philip Williamson, "'Safety First': Baldwin, the Conservative Party, and the 1929 General Election," *Historical Journal* 25, no. 2 (June 1982): 397.

23. Ian M. Drummond, "More on British Colonial Aid Policy in the Nineteen-Thirties," *Canadian Journal of History* 6 (1971): 189–95. For Milner's proposal of an "Imperial Development Fund," see Viscount Milner, *Questions of the Hour* (London: Hodder and Stoughton, 1923), 155.

24. Vail, "Making of an Imperial Slum," 108.

25. For more on the history of Treasury control over the colonies, see Richard M Kesner, *Economic Control and Colonial Development: Crown Colony Financial Management in the Age of Joseph Chamberlain* (Westport, CT: Greenwood Press, 1981).

26. Stephen Constantine, *The Making of British Colonial Development Policy, 1914–1940* (Totowa, NJ: F. Cass, 1984), 143.

27. Williamson, "Safety First"; also see Philip Williamson, *Stanley Baldwin: Conservative Leadership and National Values* (Cambridge, UK: Cambridge University Press, 1999), 37.

28. "Stanley Baldwin Speech to Open Conservative General Election Campaign," *Times (of London)*, April 19, 1929, The Times Digital Archive.

29. "The Colonial Empire: Lines of Future Development," *Times (of London)*, May 1, 1929, The Times Digital Archive.

30. John Gallagher, *The Decline, Revival and Fall of the British Empire: The Ford Lectures and Other Essays*, ed. Anil Seal (Cambridge, UK: Cambridge University Press, 1982), 116.

31. "Schemes of Work: Mr. Thomas on His Plans," *Times (of London)*, July 4, 1929, The Times Digital Archive.

32. "Colonial Development; Help from Annual £1,000,000 Fund," *Times (of London)*, July 11, 1929, The Times Digital Archive; "Parliament: The Colonies and Unemployment; Development Loans," *Times (of London)*, July 13, 1929, The Times Digital Archive; "Memorandum Explaining the Financial Resolution of the Colonial Development Act," Command Paper (UK Treasury Department, 1929).

33. Morgan, *Official History of Colonial Development*, 41–43.
34. William Lunn, Colonial Development Bill, 1929, *Hansard*, vol. 230, c474, House of Commons Debate, July 17, 1929.
35. Philip Williamson, "Percy, Eustace Sutherland Campbell, Baron Percy of Newcastle (1887–1958), Politician and Educationist," in *Oxford Dictionary of National Biography* (Oxford: Oxford University Press, 2004).
36. Ibid.
37. "Obituary: Arthur Vernon Davies, OBE, MB, ChB," *BMJ* 2, no. 4261 (1942): 297.
38. Morgan, *Official History of Colonial Development*, 53.
39. This bridge would connect the TZR with another, older railroad that ran between the northern side of the Zambesi and the southern Nyasaland city of Port Herald. The bridge would obviate the need for ferry transport across the river.
40. From Morgan, *Origins of British Aid Policy*, 53 (emphasis added).
41. Nthenda, "H.M. Treasury and the Nyasaland Administration," 272.
42. Leo S Amery, *Colonial Office*, *Hansard*, vol. 235, c 1963 House of Commons Debates, February 24, 1930.
43. Morgan, *Origins of British Aid Policy*, 55–56.
44. R. D. Bell, "Report of the Commission Appointed to Enquire into the Financial Position and Further Development of Nyasaland," Colonial Office No. 352 (London: His Majesty's Stationery Office, 1938), Box 3, No. 20, SoMA. 174.
45. Nthenda, "H.M. Treasury and the Nyasaland Administration," 263.
46. Morgan, *Official History of Colonial Development*, 55.
47. Jeremy Wormell, "Blackett, Sir Basil Phillott (1882–1935), Civil Servant," in *Oxford Dictionary of National Biography* (Oxford: Oxford University Press, 2004).
48. Neal R Malmsten, "British Government Policy toward Colonial Development, 1919–1939," *Journal of Modern History* 49, no. 2 (1977): D1249–87.
49. Thomas Drummond Shiels, *Colonial Office*, *Hansard*, vol. 240, c1498 House of Commons Debates, June 26, 1930.
50. Morgan, *Official History of Colonial Development*, 55.
51. Ibid.
52. Ibid., 47–48. Also see Shiels, *Colonial Office*, June 26, 1930.
53. "Obituary: John Owen Shircore, C.M.G., M.B.Edin., M.R.C.P.E.," *Lancet* 262, no. 6676 (1953): 94. Patrick Malloy, "'Holding [Tanganyika] by the Sindano': Networks of Medicine in Colonial Tanganyika." (PhD diss., University of California Los Angeles, 2003), 208.
54. J. O. Shircore, "Yaws and Syphilis in Tropical Africa: Mass Treatment with Bismuth-Arsenic Compounds," *Lancet* 208, no. 5366 (1926): 43–44.
55. Ibid.
56. John Owen Shircore, *Report on the Nyasaland Medical Service with Special Reference to a Grant Under the Colonial Development Fund* (Zomba, Nyasaland: Government Printer, 1930), Box 15, No. 2, SoMA, 3.
57. *Annual Medical Report on the Health and Sanitary Condition of the Nyasaland Protectorate for the Year Ending the 31st December, 1930* (Zomba, Nyasaland: Government Printer, 1931), Box 15, 24, SoMA.
58. Shircore, *Report on the Nyasaland Medical Service*, 5.

59. Shircore, *Report on the Nyasaland Medical Service*, 4.

60. See ibid., 18; and see *Annual Medical Report on the Health and Sanitary Condition of the Nyasaland Protectorate for the Year Ending the 31st December, 1931* (Zomba, Nyasaland: Government Printer, 1932), UMMC, 4.

61. *Annual Medical Report on the Health and Sanitary Condition of the Nyasaland Protectorate for the Year Ending the 31st December, 1931.*

62. "Table A: Recommended and Approved Grants to Be Met from the Fund for the Five-Year Period Ending 31 December 1935, in Provision of Medical Facilities," CO 525/177/1/18, Colonial Office Records, UKNA, 74.

63. Morgan, *Origins of British Aid Policy*, 51, 59.

64. Ibid., 114–15.

65. Austin C. Mkandawire, *Living My Destiny: A Medical and Historical Narrative* (Limbe, Malawi: Popular Publications, 1998), 87. Also see A. D. J. B. Williams, *Annual Medical & Sanitary Report for the Year Ending 31st December, 1934* (Zomba, Nyasaland: Government Printer, April 25, 1935), Box 15, No. 20, SoMA.

66. Markku Hokkanen, "The Government Medical Service and British Missions in Colonial Malawi, c. 1891–1940: Crucial Collaboration, Hidden Conflicts," in *Beyond the State: The Colonial Medical Service in British Africa* (Manchester, UK: Manchester University Press, 2016), 53.

67. Medical officers were still overwhelmed by the scale of the work with which they had been tasked. See W. L. Gopsill, "A Few Notes on My Life in Zanzibar and Nyasaland from 1926 to 1945," n.d., MSS.Afr.s.883, BLOU, 34.

68. Gopsill, "Few Notes on My Life in Zanzibar and Nyasaland," 21.

69. Ibid., 20.

70. Gopsill, "Few Notes on My Life in Zanzibar and Nyasaland," 22.

71. Tom Burgis, *The Looting Machine: Warlords, Oligarchs, Corporations, Smugglers, and the Theft of Africa's Wealth* (London: Public Affairs, 2015); John Perkins, *Confessions of an Economic Hit Man* (New York: Plume, 2005); Léonce Ndikumana and James K. Boyce, *Africa's Odious Debts: How Foreign Loans and Capital Flight Bled a Continent* (London: Zed Books, 2011).

72. As Allan Megill explains, "historians must engage in counterfactual reasoning" in order to make any manner of causal claims, though such reasoning should not take the historian too far afield from actual events if they are to claim any authority. See Megill, *Historical Knowledge, Historical Error: A Contemporary Guide to Practice* (Chicago: University of Chicago Press, 2007), 151–56.

Chapter 3

1. "Mota Engil Earnings Release 2014" (Lisbon, Portugal: Mota Engil Group, 2015).

2. "Mota-Engil: Global Leader Transforming Malawi's Infrastructure," *European Times*, December 11, 2013.

3. Mundango Nyirenda, "Chaos in Mangochi: Two Killed as Malawi Police Clash with Villagers over Land for Mota Engil Hotel," *Nyasa Times*, February 5, 2015.

4. Aubrey Mbuju, "Disincentives to Investment," *[Malawi] Nation*, April 16, 2015.

5. Ntchindi Meki, "Peter Mutharika, Motor-Engil Hold Secret Talks," *[Malawi] Times*, June 2, 2015.

6. "Precis of Relevant Correspondence with the Colonial Office on Medical and Health Services in Nyasaland," May 3, 1939, S40/1/8/1, Document No. 204, MNA.

7. A. D. J. Bedward Williams, *Annual Medical & Sanitary Report for the Year Ending 31st December 1935* (Zomba, Nyasaland: Government Printer, April 5, 1936), Box 15, No. 19, SoMA, 6–7.

8. Harold Kittermaster, "Extract from a Despatch from the Governor's Deputy, No. 379 of the 22nd October, 1935," n.d., CO 525/161/4, 36–38, UKNA.

9. Marcus A. Greenhill, "Minute on Extract from a Despatch from the Governor's Deputy, No. 379 of the 22nd October, 1935," December 19, 1935, CO 525/161/4, UKNA, 1–2 (emphasis in original).

10. H. S. de Boer, "Proposals by Director of Medical Services, Nyasaland, for Reorganization of Medical and Health Services," June 17, 1939, CO 525/178/1, UKNA.

11. Greenhill, "Minute on Extract from a Despatch from the Governor's Deputy."

12. "Obituary: H.S. de Boer," *BMJ* 1, no. 5034 (1957): 1533–34.

13. H. S. de Boer, "Proposals by Director of Medical Services, Nyasaland, for Reorganization of Medical and Health Services," June 17, 1939, CO 525/178/1, UKNA.

14. Many officials in Nyasaland shared this view. See Harold Baxter Kittermaster, "Minute on Extract from Report on Lilongwe District 1937, MP. 18/38.C. to Director of Medical Services for Comment," March 1, 1938, S40/1/3/2, No. 40, MNA.

15. "Extract from Memorandum by DMS on Medical Policy, MP 49/35," 1938, S40/1/3/2, No. 44, MNA.

16. For more on the health consequences of labor migration, particularly for the communities left behind by migrants, see Meredith Turshen, *The Political Economy of Disease in Tanzania* (New Brunswick, NJ: Rutgers University Press, 1984), 109–31.

17. De Boer, "Proposals by Director of Medical Services, Nyasaland, for Reorganization of Medical and Health Services."

18. Ibid.

19. *Annual Medical Report on the Health and Sanitary Condition of the Nyasaland Protectorate for the Year Ending the 31st December, 1930* (Zomba, Nyasaland: Government Printer, 1931), Box 15, No. 24, SoMA; and *Annual Medical & Sanitary Report for the Year Ending 31st December 1939* (Zomba, Nyasaland: Government Printer, 1940), Box 15, No. 19, SoMA.

20. "Memo from Governor DM Kennedy to Chief Secretary, Zomba, Re: Dispatch to Be Sent to Colonial Office Concerning De Boer Report," May 8, 1939, S40/1/8/1, Document No. 204, MNA.

21. "Minute by Boyd Re: De Boer Report," August 14, 1939, CO525/178/1, UKNA.

22. "Minute by Arthur John Rushton O'Brien Re: De Boer Report," August 2, 1939, CO525/178/1, UKNA.

23. For a brief discussion of the creation of the Colonial Office's Social Services Department in 1939, see Frederick Cooper, *Decolonization and African Society: The Labor Question in French and British Africa* (New York: Cambridge University Press, 1996), 69.

24. "Minute by Gerard Clauson Re: De Boer Report," August 8, 1939, CO 525/178/1, UKNA (emphasis added).

25. *Annual Medical & Sanitary Report for the Year Ending 31st December 1939*, 25.

26. William T. C. Berry, *Before the Wind of Change* (Suffolk: Halesworth Press, 1984), 4. P. R. Stephens, "Allocation of Expenditure, 1962/63" (Blantyre, Rhodesia, and Nyasaland: Ministry of Health Regional Headquarters, June 25, 1962), 4.5.9R, Box 9121, MNA.

27. Jones, Glyn, Hugh Norman-Walker, Henry Phillips, et al., "Colloquium on Nyasaland Finance," April 23, 1980, Mss.Afr.s.1742, Box 1, File 27, BLOU, 3.

28. J. C. Chakanza, "Provisional Annotated Chronological List of Witch-Finding Movements in Malawi, 1850–1980," *Journal of Religion in Africa* 15, no. 3 (1985): 227–43.

29. John McCracken, *A History of Malawi* (Woodbridge, UK: James Currey, 2012), 210.

30. Richard Rotberg, editor's introduction to *Strike a Blow and Die: A Narrative of Race Relations in Colonial Africa*, by George Simeon Mwase (Cambridge, MA: Harvard University Press, 1967).

31. *Report of the Commission Appointed to Enquire into the Disturbances in the Copperbelt, Northern Rhodesia, Presented by the Secretary of State for The Colonies to Parliament by Command of His Majesty* (London: His Majesty's Stationery Office, October 1935); *Annual Report on the Social and Economic Progress of the People of Northern Rhodesia, 1935* (London: His Majesty's Stationery Office, 1936); and Ian Henderson, "East African Leadership: The Copperbelt Disturbances of 1935 and 1940," *Journal of Southern African Studies* 2, no. 1 (1975): 83–97.

32. Henderson, "East African Leadership."

33. Catherine Valentine, "Settler Visions of Health: Health Care Provision in the Central African Federation, 1953–63" (master's thesis, Portland State University, 2017), 43.

34. A. W. Pim and S. Milligan, "Report of the Commission to Enquire into the Financial and Economic Position of Northern Rhodesia," 290, 294–95.

35. Ibid., 291–93. Rita Hinden, *Plan for Africa: A Report Prepared for the Colonial Bureau of the Fabian Society* (London: George Allen and Unwin Ltd., 1941), 103. Compare this figure to the revenues garnered by the UK government from taxation of Copperbelt mining companies. Between 1930 and 1940 the UK government kept £2.4 million in such revenues, while Northern Rhodesia received from the United Kingdom only £136,000 in grants for development during that period. Andrew Roberts, *A History of Zambia* (London: Heinemann, 1976), 193.

36. W. Richard Jacobs, "The Politics of Protest in Trinidad: The Strikes and Disturbances of 1937," *Caribbean Studies* 17, no. 1/2 (1977): 5–54.

37. Jeremy Seekings, "'Pa's Pension': The Origins of Non-Contributory Old-Age Pensions in Late Colonial Barbados," *Journal of Imperial and Commonwealth History* 35, no. 4 (2007): 529–47.

38. Cooper, *Decolonization and African Society*, 58–65.

39. O. W. Phelps, "Rise of the Labour Movement in Jamaica," *Social and Economic Studies* 9, no. 4 (1960): 417–68.

40. K. W. J. Post, "The Politics of Protest in Jamaica, 1938: Some Problems of Analysis and Conceptualization," *Social and Economic Studies* 18, no. 4 (1969): 374–90; and D. H. Figueredo and Frank Argote-Freyre, *A Brief History of the Caribbean* (New York: Infobase Publishing, 2008), 201.

41. Stephen Constantine, *The Making of British Colonial Development Policy, 1914–1940* (Totowa, NJ: F. Cass, 1984), 204.

42. Arthur Creech Jones, Colonial Office Debate, *Hansard*, vol. 337, cc79–189, House of Commons Debate, 1938.

43. Constantine, *Making of British Colonial Development Policy*, 205.

44. "West India Royal Commission Report, Presented by the Secretary of State for the Colonies to Parliament by Command of His Majesty" (London: His Majesty's Stationery Office, June 1945), xiii.

45. Constantine, *Making of British Colonial Development Policy*, 207.

46. Ibid., 208–9.

47. Gareth Curless, "The Sudan Is 'Not Yet Ready for Trade Unions': The Railway Strikes of 1947–48," *Journal of Imperial and Commonwealth History* 41, no. 5 (2013): 804–22; John Iliffe, "A History of the Dockworkers of Dar Es Salaam," *Tanzania Notes and Records* 71 (1970): 119–48; and Frederick Cooper, *On the African Waterfront: Urban Disorder and Transformation of Work in Colonial Mombasa* (New Haven, CT: Yale University Press, 1987), 48–50.

48. Constantine, *Making of British Colonial Development Policy*, 214.

49. Ibid., 213.

50. Ibid., 218–19.

51. *Colonial Development: A Factual Survey of the Origins and History of British Aid to Developing Territories*, British Aid 5 (London: The Overseas Development Institute, 1964), 24.

52. See West Indies (Royal Commission's Report), *Hansard*, vol. 357, cc.1164–1166, House of Commons Debate, February 1940.

53. "West India Royal Commission Report, Presented by the Secretary of State for the Colonies to Parliament by Command of His Majesty."

54. "Lord Moyne Tells of Findings of Royal Commission," *Daily Gleaner*, February 21, 1940.

55. "West India Royal Commission Report, Presented by the Secretary of State for the Colonies to Parliament by Command of His Majesty," 6.

56. Constantine, *Making of British Colonial Development Policy*, 222.

57. Paul Kelemen, "Planning for Africa: The British Labour Party's Colonial Development Policy, 1920–1964," *Journal of Agrarian Change* 7, no. 1 (2007): 79–80.

58. "West India Royal Commission Report, Presented by the Secretary of State for the Colonies to Parliament by Command of His Majesty"; Pim and Milligan, "Report of the Commission to Enquire into the Financial and Economic Position of Northern Rhodesia"; and "Report of the Commission Appointed to Enquire into the Disturbances in the Copperbelt, Northern Rhodesia, Presented by the Secretary of State for the Colonies to Parliament by Command of His Majesty."

59. Cooper, *Decolonization and African Society*, 58, 64.

60. See Constantine, *Making of British Colonial Development Policy*, 189.

61. Charles Bathurst, Colonial Development and Welfare Bill Debate, *Hansard* vol. 116, cc723–48, House of Lords Debate, 1940.

62. Berry, *Before the Wind of Change*, 81; Cynthia Brantley, *Feeding Families: African Realities and British Ideas of Nutrition and Development in Early Colonial Africa* (Portsmouth, NH: Heinemann, 2002), 130, 140.

63. Berry, *Before the Wind of Change*, 57.

64. *Annual Medical & Sanitary Report for the Year Ending 31st December 1939*, 4–5.

65. *Annual Medical and Sanitary Report for the Year Ending 31st December 1940* (Zomba, Nyasaland: Government Printer, 1941), Box 15, No. 16, SoMA, 1.

66. Michael King and Elizabeth King, *The Story of Medicine and Disease in Malawi: The 150 Years Since Livingstone* (Blantyre, Malawi: Arco Books, 1992), 137.

67. "Provision of Rural Dispensaries in the Lilongwe District, by Chief Secretary, Zomba," November 18, 1942, S40/1/3/2, MNA.

68. J. O. Shircore, "Letter to Director of Medical Services, Zomba," September 28, 1942, S40/1/3/2, File 51a, MNA.

69. J. M. Ellis, "Letter to Director of Medical Services, Zomba, from Provincial Commissioner, Northern Province," June 4, 1943, S40/1/3/2, File 67a, MNA. Also see Juxon Barton, "Letter to JO Shircore from Chief Secretary, Zomba," November 15, 1943, S40/1/3/2, MNA.

70. McCracken, *History of Malawi*, 262. Also see Philip Short, *Banda* (Boston: Routledge & Kegan Paul, 1974).

71. For more on this episode, see Markku Hokkanen, *Medicine, Mobility and the Empire: Nyasaland Networks* (Manchester, UK: Manchester University Press, 2017), ch. 5.

72. Anna Crozier, "The Colonial Medical Officer and Colonial Identity: Kenya, Uganda and Tanzania before World War Two" (PhD diss., University College London, 2005), 214–17.

73. Ibid.

74. D. V. Altendorff, "Genealogy of the Speldewinde Family of Ceylon," *Journal of the Dutch Burgher Union* 33, no. 3 (1944): 76; and Crozier, "The Colonial Medical Officer and Colonial Identity," 62.

75. Anna Crozier, "Sensationalising Africa: British Medical Impressions of Sub-Saharan Africa 1890–1939," *Journal of Imperial and Commonwealth History* 35, no. 3 (2007): 393–415.

Chapter 4

1. GOtv Malawi, *Izeki ndi Jakobo: Matewera amwana*, published January 18, 2013, YouTube video, https://www.youtube.com/watch?v=CLkKVUPn6R8&t=9s

2. GOtvMalawi, *Izeki ndi Jakobo: Kusutsa galu mkukumba*, published September 8, 2014, YouTube video, https://www.youtube.com/watch?v=eHZ2of3vyNw.

3. J. Clyde Mitchell, *The Yao Village: A Study in the Social Structure of a Nyasaland Tribe* (Manchester, UK: The Manchester Press, 1956), 113.

4. "Statement of Policy on Colonial Development and Welfare Presented by the Secretary of State for the Colonies to Parliament by Command of His Majesty" (London: His Majesty's Stationery Office, February 1940), House of Commons Parliamentary Papers Online, 6.

5. Stephen Constantine, *The Making of British Colonial Development Policy, 1914–1940* (Totowa, NJ: F. Cass, 1984), 222.

6. "Report on the Colonial Empire (1939–1947), Presented by the Secretary of State for the Colonies to Parliament by Command of His Majesty" (London: His Majesty's Stationery Office, July 1947), House of Commons Parliamentary Papers Online, Appendix II.

7. Karen Fields, *Revival and Rebellion in Colonial Central Africa* (Portsmouth, NH: Heinemann, 1997), 253.

8. "Editorial Notes: The South African Protectorates," *Journal of the Royal African Society* 40, no. 16 (1941): 293–94.

9. "Report on the Colonial Empire (1939–1947), Presented by the Secretary of State for the Colonies to Parliament by Command of His Majesty," 9–10.

10. William Manchester and Paul Reid, *The Last Lion: Winston Spencer Churchill: Defender of the Realm, 1940–1965* (Boston: Little, Brown, 2012), 506; and *Colonial Development: A Factual Survey of the Origins and History of British Aid to Developing Territories*, British Aid 5 (London: The Overseas Development Institute, 1964), 26.

11. James Hubbard, *The United States and the End of British Colonial Rule in Africa, 1941–1968* (Jefferson, NC: McFarland, 2010), 11.

12. Ruth B. Russell and Jeannette E. Muther, *A History of the United Nations Charter: The Role of the United States, 1940–1945* (Washington, DC: Brookings Institution, 1958), 76.

13. Hubbard, *United States and the End of British Colonial Rule in Africa*, 11–12.

14. *Colonial Development: A Factual Survey.*

15. "Report on the Colonial Empire (1939–1947)," 11.

16. Ibid., 13.

17. Mark Minion, "The Fabian Colonial Society and Europe during the 1940s: The Search for a Socialist Foreign Policy," *European History Quarterly* 30, no. 2 (2000): 237–38.

18. Ibid. Also see Michael Cowen and Robert Shenton, "The Origin and Course of Fabian Colonialism in Africa," *Journal of Historical Sociology* 4, no. 2 (1991): 143–74.

19. Minion, "Fabian Colonial Society and Europe during the 1940s," 246.

20. "Report of Activities of Fabian Colonial Bureau for the Half Year, November 1940–April 1941," 1941, CO 1015/701, UKNA.

21. "Labour Party's Declaration of Policy for Colonial Peoples, Labour Party International Department, Advisory Committee on Imperial Questions," July 1940, Mss.Brit. Emp.s.365, Box 46, File 1, BLOU.

22. Leonard S. Woolf, "Draft Memorandum Formulating a Colonial Policy for the Labour Party after the War," Revenue, Expenditure & Public Finance, September 1941, Mss. Brit.Emp.s.365, Box 46, File 1, BLOU.

23. "Response by Norman Leys to Woolf's Draft Memorandum Formulating a Colonial Policy for the Labour Party after the War," September 1941, Mss.Brit.Emp.s.365, Box 46, File 1, BLOU.

24. T. Reid, "Comments on Woolf Draft Memorandum Formulating a Colonial Policy for the Labour Party after the War," September 1941, Mss.Brit.Emp.s.365, Box 46, File 1, BLOU.

25. Lord Malcolm Hailey, "A Colonial Charter: An Address at the Annual Meeting of the Anti-Slavery & Aborigines Protection Society," May 28, 1942, Mss.Brit.Emp.s.365, Box 46, File 4, BLOU.

26. Lord Malcolm Hailey, "A Colonial Charter: An Address at the Annual Meeting of the Anti-Slavery & Aborigines Protection Society," May 28, 1942, Mss.Brit.Emp.s.365, Box 46, File 4, BLOU.

27. Hubbard, *United States and the End of British Colonial Rule in Africa*, 10.

28. Rita Hinden, "A Colonial Charter," June 4, 1942, Mss.Brit.Emp.s.365, Box 46, File 4, BLOU.

29. Hinden, "Colonial Charter."

30. Beveridge proposed "a comprehensive national health service will ensure that for every citizen there is available whatever medical treatment he requires, in whatever form he requires, domiciliary or institutional, general, specialist or consultant." Service, he explained, was to be "provided where needed without contribution conditions in any individual case." See William Beveridge, "Social Insurance and Allied Services," Inter-Departmental Committee on Social Insurance and Allied Services (London: His Majesty's Stationery Office, 1942), 158–59.

31. Joseph M. Hodge, *Triumph of the Expert: Agrarian Doctrines of Development and the Legacies of British Colonialism* (Athens: Ohio University Press, 2007), 198.

32. Daniel Rodgers, *Atlantic Crossings: Social Politics in a Progressive Age* (Cambridge, MA: Harvard University Press, 1998), 492.

33. Mair had aided Lord Hailey in producing the *African Survey*. She was also Beveridge's stepdaughter by his marriage to Jessie Mair in 1942.

34. Lucy Philip Mair, *Welfare in the British Colonies* (New York: Royal Institute of International Affairs, 1944), 9.

35. Ibid., 10.

36. Ibid.

37. "Social Welfare in the Colonies" (London: Colonial Office, April 1945), Box 11, No. 9, SoMA, 2.

38. Ibid., 2.

39. Ibid., 2–3.

40. John Iliffe, "The Poor in the Modern History of Malawi," in *Malawi: An Alternative Pattern of Development* (Edinburgh: Centre of African Studies,1985).

41. Ibid.

42. John Iliffe, *The African Poor: A History* (New York: Cambridge University Press, 1987), 267.

43. Iliffe, "Poor in the Modern History of Malawi," 266.

44. Ibid., 4–5.

45. A. G. Hopkins, *An Economic History of West Africa* (New York: Addison Wesley Longman, 1973), 9–10.

46. Steven Feierman, *Peasant Intellectuals: Anthropology and History in Tanzania* (Madison: University of Wisconsin, 1990); Elias C. Mandala, *End of Chidyerano: A History of Food and Everyday Life in Malawi, 1860–2004* (Portsmouth, NH: Heinemann, 2005); and Michael Watts, *Silent Violence: Food, Famine, and Peasantry in Northern Nigeria* (Berkeley: University of California Press, 1983), 109. Also see Steven Feierman, "Struggles for Control: The Social Roots of Health and Healing in Modern Africa," *African Studies Review* 28, nos. 2/3 (1985): 118.

47. Mair, *Welfare in the British Colonies*, 72.

48. "Social Security in the Colonial Territories." Papers on Colonial Affairs. Colonial Office, June 1944. Mss Brit Emp s.332, Box 47, File 4. BLOU.

49. Beveridge, "Social Insurance and Allied Services."

50. Luke Messac, "Moral Hazards and Moral Economies: The Combustible Politics of Healthcare User Fees in Malawian History," *South African Historical Journal* 66, no. 2 (2014): 371–89.

51. "Obituary: ADJB Williams, OBE, MRCS, LRCP," *BMJ* 1, no. 5084 (1958): 1421.

52. Arthur D. J. B. Williams, "Post-War Development of Medical Services" (Zomba, Nyasaland: Government Printer, 1944).

53. Ibid.

54. Markku, Hokkanen, "Towards a Cultural History of Medicine(s)," in *Crossing Colonial Historiographies: Histories of Colonial and Indigenous Medicines in Transnational Perspective*, ed. Anne Digby, Waltraud Ernst, and Projit Mukharji (Newcastle, UK: Cambridge Scholars Publishing, 2010),151–54. For classic works in this vein, see Nancy Rose Hunt, *A Colonial Lexicon: Of Birth Ritual, Medicalization, and Mobility in the Congo* (Durham, NC: Duke University Press, 1999); and Anne Digby, *Diversity and Division in Medicine* (Bern: Peter Lang, 2006).

55. Nyasaland Protectorate, "Report of the Post-War Development Committee" (Zomba, Nyasaland: Government Printer, 1945).

56. "An Address by Rt. Hon A. Creech Jones, Secretary of State for the Colonies, to the Annual Meeting of the Anti-Slavery and Aborigines Protection Society" (London, UK, October 24, 1946), Mss.Brit.Emp.s.332, Box 47, File 4, BLOU.

57. This act was passed before Creech Jones began his tenure as secretary of state for the colonies.

58. *Colonial Development: A Factual Survey*, 32.

59. "Editorial: Colonial Tasks," *Times (of London)*, January 10, 1945, The Times Digital Archive.

60. "Nyasaland Protectorate Development Programme, Revised 1947" (Zomba, Nyasaland: Government Printer, 1947).

61. Constantine, *Making of British Colonial Development Policy*, 201. Also see "An Address by Rt Hon A. Creech Jones, Secretary of State for the Colonies, to the Annual Meeting of the Anti-Slavery and Aborigines Protection Society," 4.

62. "Return of Schemes Made Under the Colonial Development and Welfare Acts, by the Secretary of State for the Colonies with the Concurrence of the Treasury in the Period from 1st April, 1946 to 31st March 1947" (London: His Majesty's Stationery Office, July 1947), House of Commons Parliamentary Papers Online.

63. "Nyasaland Protectorate Development Programme, Revised 1947."

64. John Iliffe, "A History of the Dockworkers of Dar Es Salaam," *Tanzania Notes and Records* 71 (1970): 119–48.

65. Frederick Cooper, *Decolonization and African Society: The Labor Question in French and British Africa* (New York: Cambridge University Press, 1996), 226.

66. Gareth Curless, "The Sudan Is "Not Yet Ready for Trade Unions: The Railway Strikes of 1947–48," *Journal of Imperial and Commonwealth History* 41, no. 5 (2013): 804–22.

67. Cooper, *Decolonization and African Society*, 226.

68. Roy Lewis, *10 Years of Colonial Development and Welfare, 1946–1955* (London: Central Office of Information, 1956), 16.

69. Stanley Awbery, Colonial Development and Welfare Bill, *Hansard*, vol. 480, cols. 1135–251, House of Commons Debate, February 1940.

70. Steven Feierman has made a similar argument about the link between colonial health-care spending and protest. In a 1985 review article on "the social roots of health and healing in modern Africa," he explained: "In the colonial situation the ultimate arbiter was in the metropole; employers of labor were well-represented there, but the potential African beneficiaries of improved health care had little influence in the colonial mother-country. What influence they had emerged from the politics of resistance and of nationalism." See Feierman, "Struggles for Control."

71. Lewis, *10 Years of Colonial Development and Welfare*.

72. Ibid., 19.

73. Michael Cowen and Robert Shenton, "The Origin and Course of Fabian Colonialism in Africa," *Journal of Historical Sociology* 4, no. 2 (1991): 143–74. Also see Paul Kelemen, "Planning for Africa: The British Labour Party's Colonial Development Policy, 1920–1964," *Journal of Agrarian Change* 7, no. 1 (2007): 76–98.

74. "Committee on Colonial Development: Export to the Colonies of Items of Equipment Which Are in Short Supply in the United Kingdom, Memorandum by the Colonial Office," February 7, 1949, MH79/629, UKNA.

75. Henry Wilkinson, "Export to the Colonies of Items of Equipment Which Are in Short Supply in the United Kingdom, a Note by the Ministry of Health," February 14, 1949, MH79/629, UKNA.

76. "Cabinet Committee on Colonial Development" (Cabinet Office, Great George Street, SW, March 28, 1949), MH79/629, UKNA.

77. Ibid.

78. *Annual Report of the Medical Department for the Year 1950* (Zomba, Nyasaland: Government Printer, 1951), University of Malawi Library; *Annual Report of the Medical Department for the Year 1952* (Zomba, Nyasaland: Government Printer, 1953), Box 15, No. 2, SoMA, 19.

79. "Shortage of X-Ray Films," *BMJ* 1, no. 94 (1952): 94–95.

80. *Annual Report of the Medical Department for the Year Ended 31st December, 1945* (Zomba, Nyasaland: Government Printer, 1946), Box 15, No. 11, SoMA; *Annual Report of the Medical Department for the Year 1952*.

81. *Annual Reports of the Medical Department, 1948–1953*.

82. Colin Baker, *Development Governor: Sir Geoffrey Colby—A Biography* (New York: I. B. Tauris & Co. Ltd., 1994), 91.

Chapter 5

1. Jim Paul, "Medicine and Imperialism in Morocco," *Middle East Research and Information Project Reports* 60 (1977): 3–12.
2. George Monbiot, "Deny the British Empire's Crimes? No, We Ignore Them," *Guardian*, April 23, 2012; Caroline Elkins, *Imperial Reckoning: The Untold Story of Britain's Gulag in Kenya* (New York: Holt, 2005).
3. John Allen, "To Talk about British Atrocities in Kenya during the Mau Mau Era Is Nonsense," *Guardian*, May 9 2012.
4. Tom Burgis, *The Looting Machine: Warlords, Oligarchs, Corporations, Smugglers, and the Theft of Africa's Wealth* (London: PublicAffairs, 2015).
5. Paul Kagame, "Reflecting on Rwanda's Past—While Looking Ahead," *Wall Street Journal*, April 7, 2014.
6. Paul Farmer, Matthew Basilico, and Luke Messac, "After McKeown: The Changing Roles of Biomedicine, Public Health and Economic Growth in Mortality Declines," in *Therapeutic Revolutions: Pharmaceuticals and Social Change in the Twentieth Century*, ed. Jeremy Greene, Flurin Condrau, and Elizabeth Watkins (Chicago: University of Chicago Press, 2016), 186–217.
7. Agnes Binagwaho, Paul Farmer, Sabin Nsanzimana, et al., "Rwanda 20 Years on: Investing in Life," *Lancet* 384, no. 9940 (2014): 371–75; and Paul Farmer, Cameron Nutt, Claire Wagner, et al., "Reduced Premature Mortality in Rwanda: Lessons from Success," *BMJ* 346 (2013): f65.
8. "Abuja+12: Shaping the Future of Health in Africa" (UNAIDS, July 2013).
9. H.S. de Boer to Honorable Chief Secretary, Ref. Cen. Regy. MP No. 1273/21, June 21, 1941, S40/1/3/2, no. 124, MNA.
10. Native Authority Mbwana to Senior Medical Officer, Medical Department, Lilongwe, June 10, 1941, S40/1/3/2, no. 127, MNA.
11. Austin C. Mkandawire, *Living My Destiny: A Medical and Historical Narrative* (Limbe, Malawi: Popular Publications, 1998), 47.
12. De Boer to Honorable Chief Secretary, Ref. Cen. Regy. MP No. 1273/21.
13. John Goodall, *Goodbye to Empire: A Doctor Remembers* (Edinburgh: Pentland Press, 1987), 79.
14. R. M. Morris, *Annual Report on the Public Health of the Federation of Rhodesia and Nyasaland for the Year 1956* (Salisbury, Rhodesia: Government Printer, 1957), BL, 15.
15. A. Hurst, H. M. Maier, and R. Dwork, "A Critical Study of Pneumoperitoneum and Phrenic Nerve Crush in Pulmonary Tuberculosis," *Diseases of the Chest* 13, no. 4 (1947): 345–59; R. Y. Keers, "Pneumoperitoneum: Its Place in Treatment," *British Journal of Tuberculosis and Diseases of the Chest* 42, no. 3 (1948): 58–66; and James L. Livingstone, "Observations on the Treatment of Pulmonary Tuberculosis at the Present Time," *BMJ* 1, no. 4908 (1955): 243–50.
16. John B. Christopherson, "The UMCA and Medical Work at Magila," *Central Africa* 39 (1921): 86–91.
17. John Lwanda, *Politics, Culture and Medicine in Malawi: Historical Continuities and Ruptures with Special Reference to HIV/AIDS* (Zomba, Malawi: Michigan

State University Press, 2005), 76, 95. Also see Markku Hokkanen, "Towards a Cultural History of Medicine(s) in Colonial Central Africa," in *Crossing Colonial Historiographies: Histories of Colonial and Indigenous Medicines in Transnational Perspective*, ed. Anne Digby, Waltraud Ernst, and Projit Mukharji (Newcastle, UK: Cambridge Scholars Publishing, 2010), 157–58.

18. Gopsill, "A Few Notes on My Life in Zanzibar and Nyasaland," Mss.Afr.s.883, BLOU, 11.

19. Caroline Bledsoe and Monica Goubaud, "The Reinterpretation of Western Pharmaceuticals among the Mende of Sierra Leone," *Social Science & Medicine* 21, no. 3 (1985): 275–82.

20. S. de Villiers, "Tuberculosis in Anthropological Perspective," *South African Journal of Ethnology* 14, no. 3 (1991): 69. Also see J. I. Mata, "Integrating the Client's Perspective in Planning a Tuberculosis Education and Treatment Program in Honduras," *Medical Anthropology* 9, no. 1 (1985): 62. For a thorough critique of culturalist perspectives on health-seeking behavior, see Paul Farmer, "Social Scientists and the New Tuberculosis," *Social Science & Medicine* 44, no. 3 (1997): 347–58.

21. For a brief and (somewhat dated) review of this literature, see Sjaak van der Geest, Anita Hardon, and Susan Reynolds Whyte, "Planning for Essential Drugs: Are We Missing the Cultural Dimension?," *Health Policy and Planning* 5, no. 2 (1990): 182–85. A more recent bibliography of this literature is provided in Susan Reynolds Whyte, Sjaak van der Geest, and Anita Hardon, *Social Lives of Medicines* (New York: Cambridge University Press, 2002).

22. For a West African study of care-seeking behavior that uses colonial disease returns, see S. Kojo Addae, *The Evolution of Modern Medicine in a Developing Country: Ghana, 1880–1960* (Rickmansworth, UK: Durham Academic Press, 1997).

23. See John M. Janzen, *The Quest for Therapy in Lower Zaire* (Berkeley: University of California Press, 1978), 221. Also see S. C. McCombie, "Treatment Seeking for Malaria: A Review of Recent Research," *Social Science and Medicine* 43, no. 6 (1996): 933–45.

24. Anne Digby, *Diversity and Division in Medicine: Health Care in South Africa from the 1800s* (Bern, Switzerland: Peter Lang, 2006), 384–98.

25. Judith Walzer Leavitt, *Brought to Bed: Child-Bearing in America, 1750–1950* (New York: Oxford University Press, 1986), 56–57.

26. Walsh McDermott, "Medicine: The Public's Good and One's Own," *World Health Forum* 1 (1980): 128; and Farmer, Basilico, and Messac, "After McKeown."

27. Gerhard Anders, *In the Shadow of Good Governance: An Ethnography of Civil Service Reform in Africa* (Boston: Brill, 2010).

28. P. S. Bell, *Report of the Medical Department for the Year 1947*, Nyasaland Protectorate, 1948, 1, Box 15, No. 9, SoMA, 5.

29. David J. D. Stevenson, "The Health Services of Malawi" (MD thesis, University of Glasgow, 1964), 38.

30. *Malawi Population Census, 1966, Final Report, Department of Census and Statistics* (Zomba, Malawi: Government Printer, 1967), i.

31. William J. House and George Zimalirana, "Rapid Population Growth and Poverty Generation in Malawi," *Journal of Modern African Studies* 30, no. 1 (1992): 141–61.

32. Harry Gear, "Some Problems of the Medical Services of the Federation of Rhodesia and Nyasaland," *BMJ* 2, no. 5197 (1960): 528.

33. Maurice King, *Development Plan for Health Services, 1970–1985* (Zomba, Malawi: Ministry of Health and Community Development, 1970), UMMC.

34. *Annual Report on the Public Health of the Federation of Rhodesia and Nyasaland for the Year 1962* (Salisbury, Rhodesia: Government Printer, 1963), CSD 607, BL.

35. H. S. Gear, "Some Problems of the Medical Services of the Federation of Rhodesia and Nyasaland," *BMJ* 2, no. 5197 (1960): 525–31.

36. John McCracken, *A History of Malawi: 1859–1966* (Woodbridge, UK: James Currey, 2012), 265.

37. Randall M. Packard, *White Plague, Black Labor: Tuberculosis and the Political Economy of Health and Disease in South Africa* (Berkeley, University of California Press, 1989), 81.

38. Miles Larmer, "Permanent Precarity: Capital and Labour in the Central African Copperbelt," *Labor History* 5, no.2 (2017): 170–84. Also see J. L. Parpart, *Labour and Capital in the African Copperbelt* (Philadelphia: Temple University Press, 1983), 136–41; and Ian Phimister, "Proletarians in Paradise: The Historiography and Historical Sociology of White Miners on the Copperbelt," in *Living the End of Empire: Politics and Society in Late Colonial Zambia*, ed. Jan-Bart Gewald, M. Hinfelaar, and G. Macola (Leiden: Brill, 2011), 129–46.

39. McCracken, *History of Malawi*, 258.

40. For illuminating studies of the historical links forged by migration between Malawi, Zimbabwe, and nearby colonies and nations, see Markku Hokkanen, *Medicine, Mobility and the Empire: Nyasaland Networks, 1859–1960* (Manchester, UK: Manchester University Press, 2017), chapter 1; and Zoë Groves, "Urban Migrants and Religious Networks: Malawians in Colonial Salisbury, 1920–1970," *Journal of Southern African Studies* 38, no. 3 (2012): 491–511. Also see Zoë Groves, "Transnational Networks and Regional Solidarity: The Case of the Central African Federation, 1953–1963," *African Studies* 72, no. 2 (2013): 155–75.

41. *Rural Radio Listenership Survey for 1968: Special Report for Malawi Broadcasting Corporation, Department of Census and Statistics* (Zomba, Malawi: Government Printer, 1968), Table 6.

42. McCracken, *History of Malawi*, 322–24.

43. Maurice King, *Development Plan for Health Services*, 2.

44. The value of bicycle imports rose from £26,000 in 1945 to £310,000 in 1953. John McCracken, "Bicycles in Colonial Malawi: A Short History," *Society of Malawi Journal* 64, no. 1 (2011): 1–12.

45. Even at the district hospital in the small lakeshore town of Nkhata Bay, 61 percent of outpatients came from less than two miles away. E. R. de Winter, *Health Services of a District Hospital in Malawi* (Assen, Netherlands: Van Gorcum and Co., 1972), 106.

46. Arthur Hazlewood and Patrick D. Henderson, "Nyasaland: The Economics of Federation," *Bulletin of the Oxford University Institute of Statistics* 22, no. 1 (1960): 1–91; and Daniel Thomson Jack, *Report on an Economic Survey of Nyasaland, 1958–1959* (Salisbury: Federation of Rhodesia and Nyasaland, 1959).

47. James Le Fanu, *The Rise and Fall of Modern Medicine* (New York: Basic Books, 2002); and Luke Messac, "Moral Hazards and Moral Economies: The Combustible Politics of Healthcare User Fees in Malawian History." *South African Historical Journal* 66, no. 2 (2014): 371–89.

48. William T. C. Berry, *Before the Wind of Change* (Suffolk, UK: Halesworth Press, 1984), 14–15. "M&B" stood for May & Baker, the British firm where the drug was discovered.

49. Gopsill recalled an epidemic of cerebrospinal meningitis in Mlanje that killed "thousands." Once the new drugs arrived, such outbreaks became less common and less devastating, as "one was able to protect contacts and carriers were in large degree eradicated." Gopsill, "A Few Notes on My Life in Zanzibar and Nyasaland," 34–35.

50. *Annual Medical and Sanitary Report for the Year Ending 31st December 1941* (Zomba, Nyasaland: Government Printer, 1942), Box 15 No. 15, SoMA, 8

51. Edmund Charles Smith Richards, "CDWAC No 527: Nyasaland. Venereal Disease: Purchase of Drugs for Treatment. Application for Free Grant of £42,000," January 23, 1945, CO 525/199/5, UKNA.

52. *Annual Report of the Medical Department for the Year Ended 31st December 1944* (Zomba, Nyasaland: Government Printer, 1945), Box 15 No. 12, SoMA.

53. G. Currie, "A Clinical Trial of Etisul in Lepromatous Leprosy," *Transactions of the Royal Society of Tropical Medicine and Hygiene* 57 (May 1963): 196–205.

54. John Iliffe, "The Poor in the Modern History of Malawi," in *Malawi: An Alternative Pattern of Development* (Edinburgh: Centre of African Studies,1985), 257.

55. Colin Baker, *Expatriate Experience of Life and Work in Nyasaland*, vol. 3 (Cardiff: Mpemba Books, 2013), 286.

56. Baker, *Expatriate Experience*, 40, 44. Also see Electra Dory, *Leper Country: A Candid, at Times Shocking, Account of a Medical Missionary's Life among Primitive People in Africa* (London: Frederick Muller Ltd, 1963).

57. Megan Vaughan, *Curing Their Ills: Colonial Power and African Illness* (Redwood City, CA: Stanford University Press, 1991), 84.

58. Berry, *Before the Wind of Change*, 17.

59. Ibid., 18.

60. Berry, *Before the Wind of Change*, 9. For more on the history of injections and their popularity, as well as a discussion on injections as placebos in late colonial Nyasaland, see Hokkanen, "Towards a Cultural History of Medicine(s)," 154–55.

61. H. de Boer, "Annual Medical & Sanitary Report for the Year Ending 31st December 1938" (Zomba, Nyasaland: Government Printer, 1939), Box 15 No. 18, SoMA, 27.

62. Megan Vaughan, "Health and Hegemony: Representation of Disease and the Creation of the Colonial Subject in Nyasaland," in *Contesting Colonial Hegemony: State and Society in African and India*, ed. Dagmar Engels and Shula Marks (London: British Academic Press, 1994), 191.

63. H. S. Gear, "Some Problems of the Medical Services of the Federation of Rhodesia and Nyasaland," *BMJ* 2, no. 5197 (1960): 525; and D. M. Blair, *Annual Report on the Public Health of the Federation of Rhodesia and Nyasaland for the Year 1958* (Salisbury, Rhodesia: Government Printer, April 30, 1959), BL.

64. Morris, *Annual Report on the Public Health of the Federation of Rhodesia and Nyasaland for the Year 1956*, 15.

65. Ibid.

66. David A. Walton, Paul Farmer, Wesler Lambert, et al., "Integrated HIV Prevention and Care Strengthens Primary Health Care: Lessons from Rural Haiti," *Journal of Public Health Policy*, 25, no. 2 (2004): 137–58.

67. McCracken, *History of Malawi*.

68. L. H. Gann, "Lord Malvern (Sir Godfrey Huggins): A Reappraisal," *Journal of Modern African Studies* 23, no. 4 (1985): 723–28. Also see Alex May, *The Commonwealth and International Affairs: The Roundtable Centennial Selection* (London: Routledge, 2010), 107.

69. Joan E. Wicken, "African Contrasts," Alice Horsman Travelling Fellow, 1956–1957 (paper submitted to Somerville College, Oxford, January 1958), MSS.Afr.s.1726, BLOU, 23–24, 47.

70. McCracken, *History of Malawi*.

71. *Federation and Nyasaland: The Facts* (Salisbury: Federation of Rhodesia and Nyasaland, 1962).

72. McCracken, *History of Malawi*, 275–76.

73. Ibid. Also see *Report of the Advisory Commission on the Review of the Constitution of Rhodesia and Nyasaland*, Appendix VII: Possible Constitutional Changes, 24–28.

74. Viscount Charles Bathurst Bledisloe, *Rhodesia-Nyasaland Royal Commission's Report* (London: H.M. Stationery Office, 1939).

75. Catherine Valentine, "Settler Visions of Health: Health Care Provision in the Central African Federation, 1953–63" (master's thesis, Portland State University, 2017), 70–74; Hastings Kamuzu Banda and Harry Nkumbula, *Federation in Central Africa* (Harlesden: Leveridge, 1949); and Philip Short, *Banda* (Boston: Routledge and Kegan Paul, 1974), 57–58.

76. See D. S. Pearson and W. L. Taylor, *Break-Up: Some Economic Consequences for the Rhodesias and Nyasaland* (Salisbury, Southern Rhodesia: The Phoenix Group, 1963). Also see Arthur Hazlewood and Patrick D. Henderson, *Nyasaland: The Economics of Federation* (Oxford: Basil Blackwell, 1960).

77. Valentine, "Settler Visions of Health," 59.

78. "Mr. Chirwa Exaggerates about African Neglect," *Nyasaland Times*, July 20, 1954.

79. Banda and Nkumbula, *Federation in Central Africa*.

80. McCracken, *History of Malawi*, 330.

81. John McCracken, "Coercion and Control in Nyasaland: Aspects of the History of a Colonial Police Force," *Journal of African History* 27, no. 1 (1986): 138.

82. Landeg White, *Magomero: Portrait of an African Village* (London: Cambridge University Press, 1989), 217. *Capitão* is a Portuguese word meaning "master" or "captain."

83. McCracken, *History of Malawi*, 313.

84. McCracken, "Coercion and Control in Nyasaland."

85. Pierre Bourdieu, *Acts of Resistance: Against the Tyranny of the Market*, trans. Richard Nice (New York: The New Press, 1998).

86. John W. D. Goodall, "Naming Ceremony of Queen Elizabeth Central Hospital, Blantyre," *Central African Journal of Medicine* 3, no. 8 (1957): 333–35.

87. Gear, "Some Problems of the Medical Services of the Federation of Rhodesia and Nyasaland," 525.

88. Hazlewood and Henderson, "Nyasaland"; and Daniel Thomson Jack, *Report on an Economic Survey of Nyasaland, 1958–1959* (Salisbury: Federation of Rhodesia and Nyasaland, 1959).

89. Gear, "Some Problems of the Medical Services."

90. McCracken, *History of Malawi*, 261.

91. G. F. Pollard, "Letter to the Editor from District Commissioner, Blantyre District," *Times (of Nyasaland)*, August 27, 1954, MNA; and David Frost, "The Economic Outlook for Nyasaland," *Race & Class* 4, no. 2 (1963): 61.

92. William J. Barber, "Federation and the Distribution of Economic Benefits," in *New Deal in Central Africa*, ed. Colin Leys and Cranford Pratt (New York: Praeger, 1960), 81–97.

93. Valentine, "Settler Visions of Health," 105.

94. Short, *Banda*.

95. Phillip Murphy, "A Police State? The Nyasaland Emergency and Colonial Intelligence," in *Malawi in Crisis: the 1959/60 Nyasaland State of Emergency and its Legacy*, ed. Kings M. Phiri, John McCracken, and Wapumuluka O. Mulwafu, 137–64 (Zomba, Malawi: Kachere Series, 2012).

96. Short, *Banda*.

97. *A Conspectus Including the Development Plan for 1965–69* (Blantyre, Malawi: Ministry of Health, June 14, 1965), MNA.

98. Valentine, "Settler Visions of Health," 88–91.

99. McCracken, *History of Malawi*, 261.

100. "Nkata Bay Hospital," *Nyasaland Times*, January 1, 1960, MNA, 1.

101. H. S. Gear, "Medicine and the New Africa: The Passing of Colonialism South of the Sahara," *Lancet* 276, no. 7158 (1960): 1023.

102. "Twice as Much for Health," *Nyasaland Times*, May 24, 1960. Also see Michael Gelfand, *Proud Record: An Account of the Health Services Provided for Africans in the Federation of Rhodesia and Nyasaland* (Salisbury: Federal Information Department, 1960).

103. John Iliffe, *Africans: The History of a Continent* (New York: Cambridge University Press, 2007), 253.

104. Federation of Rhodesia and Nyasaland, Office of the High Commissioner, "The First Steps in Central Africa: Let Facts Have a Hearing," *Evening Standard*, November 23, 1960, 20. BL Newspaper Collection.

105. Ibid. Also see Andrew Cohen, " 'Voice and Vision'—The Federation of Rhodesia and Nyasaland's Public Relations Campaign in Britain: 1960–63," *Historia* 54, no. 2 (2009): 113–32.

106. Valentine, "Settler Visions of Health," 100

107. Roy Welensky, "National Health Development," November 25, 1961, Mss.Welensky Papers, BLOU, 7–8.

108. Ibid.

109. McCracken, *History of Malawi*, 384.

110. *Federation and Nyasaland: The Facts.*

111. Ibid.

112. "Sick Had to Leave," *Nyasaland Times*, July 8, 1960, 1.

113. "Government Doing Everything Possible," *Nyasaland Times*, July 8, 1960.

114. "Death by Smallpox Is Stalking Nyasaland," *Nyasaland Times*, October 11, 1960, MNA.

115. "Have Your Child and Yourself Vaccinated," *Nyasaland Times*, November 25, 1960, MNA.

116. "Infant with Smallpox, Central Province, Nyasaland," *Nyasaland Times*, December 6, 1960, MNA.

117. D. M. Blair, *Annual Report on the Public Health of the Federation of Rhodesia and Nyasaland for the Year 1960* (Salisbury, Southern Rhodesia: Government Printer, May 27, 1961), 9, BL.

118. J. Mowat Sword, "Smallpox in Central Province, Nyasaland," *BMJ* 2, no. 5245 (1961): 165–66.

119. *Federation and Nyasaland: The Facts.*

120. Ibid.

121. Kanyama Chiume, "Smallpox: The Truth," *Tsopano*, January 1961, 7.

122. McCracken, *History of Malawi*; and Short, *Banda*.

123. Alister C. Munthali, "Determinants of Vaccination Coverage in Malawi: Evidence from the Demographic and Health Surveys," *Malawi Medical Journal* 19, no. 2 (2007): 79–82.

124. H. G. Bevan-Pritchard, "Letter on 'Evasion of Smallpox Vaccines,'" 1930, M2/5/16, MNA, in John Lwanda, *Politics, Culture and Medicine in Malawi: Historical Continuities and Ruptures with Special Reference to HIV/AIDS* (Zomba, Malawi: Michigan State University Press, 2005). Also see Vaughan, "Health and Hegemony," 185–87.

125. R. M. Morris, *Annual Report on the Public Health of the Federation of Rhodesia and Nyasaland for the Year 1956* (Salisbury, Rhodesia: Government Printer, 1957), 15, BL.

126. Chiume, "Smallpox: The Truth." Also see Blair, *Annual Report on the Public Health of the Federation of Rhodesia and Nyasaland for the Year 1960*, 9, 13.

127. *Annual Report on the Public Health of the Federation of Rhodesia and Nyasaland for the Year 1955* (Salisbury, Rhodesia: Government Printer, 1956), 7; and Sword, "Smallpox in Central Province, Nyasaland." Morris, *Annual Report on the Public Health of the Federation of Rhodesia and Nyasaland for the Year 1956*, 6.

128. *Annual Report on the Public Health of the Federation of Rhodesia and Nyasaland for the Year 1955*, 7.

129. Morris, *Annual Report on the Public Health of the Federation of Rhodesia and Nyasaland for the Year 1956*. Also see Stevenson, "Health Services of Malawi," 72.

130. Morris, *Annual Report on the Public Health of the Federation of Rhodesia and Nyasaland for the Year 1956*, 6.

131. "No Smallpox Epidemic in Nyasaland, Says Dr. Banda," *Rhodesia Herald*, Monday, November 28, 1960, 1, BL Newspaper Collection.

132. Short, *Banda*.

133. Stevenson, "Health Services of Malawi," 72.

134. "Medical Events: Big Drop in Nyasaland Smallpox Cases," *Central African Journal of Medicine*, March 1963, 120.

135. Frank Fenner, Donald Henderson, Isao Arita, et al., *Smallpox and Its Eradication* (Geneva: World Health Organization, 1989), 975–81.

136. DMS to Medical Officer in Charge, Zomba African Hospital, March 20, 1954, File 6186, 7.6.11R, Box 13375, MNA.

137. J. A. D. Bradfield, Provincial Medical Officer, to Medical Superintendent, Zomba, Re: Requisition for Medical Supplies, October 22, 1962, File No. 3405 (Zomba Hospital Drugs and Medical Equipment), Document No. 250, MNA.

138. Medical Officer in Charge, African Hospital, Lilongwe, to the Director of Medical Services, Zomba, Re: Streptomycin Supplies, March 5, 1954, Medical Department, Medical Requisitions, No. 27, Ref. No. MS&S, SG3/27/165, MNA; E. H. Murcott, Director of Medical Services to the Medical Officer in Charge, Karonga, March 8, 1954, Medical Department, Medical Requisitions, No. 25, M.1/15/875, MNA; and E. H. Murcott, Director of Medical Services to the Medical Officer in Charge, African Hospital, Zomba, March 20, 1954, Medical Department, Medical Requisitions, No. 32, MNA.

139. Medical Officer in Charge, Mzimba to Director of Medical Services, Zomba, April 29, 1954, Medical Department, Medical Requisitions, No. 49, Ref. No. 19/54/69, MNA.

140. J. W. D. Goodall (Medical Specialist, Zomba African Hospital) to E. H. Murcott (Director of Medical Services), June 8, 1956, File No. 3405 (Zomba Hospital Drugs and Medical Equipment), MNA; and E. H. Murcott (Director of Medical Services, Nyasaland) to Secretary to the Federal Ministry of Health, Southern Rhodesia, June 12, 1956, File No. 3405 (Zomba Hospital Drugs and Medical Equipment), MNA.

141. Wallace Fox, "Realistic Chemotherapeutic Policies for Tuberculosis in Developing Countries," *BMJ* 1, no. 5376 (1964): 135–42. Also see Stevenson, " Health Services of Malawi," 87; and *Annual Report on the Work of the Nyasaland/Malawi Ministry of Health for the Year 1964* (Zomba, Malawi: Government Printer, 1965), UMMC.

142. Goodall, *Goodbye to Empire*, 92.

143. H. R. Durrant (for Director of Medical Services) to Medical Officer, Karonga (through Provincial Medical Officer, Northern Province), November 1, 1961, File 2205 (Karonga Hospital Medical Requisitions), MNA.

144. Medical Officer, Karonga Hospital to Director of Medical Services (through Provincial Medical Officer, Northern Province, Mzuzu), December 18, 1961, File 2205 (Karonga Hospital Medical Requisitions), MNA.

145. Colin Baker, "The Government Medical Service in Malawi: An Administrative History, 1891–1974," *Medical History* 20, no. 3 (1976): 296–311.

146. Paul Farmer, "An Anthropology of Structural Violence," *Current Anthropology* 45, no. 3 (2004): 305–25. See also Luke Messac and Krishna Prabhu, "Redefining the

Possible: The Global AIDS Response," in *Reimagining Global Health: An Introduction*, ed. Paul Farmer, Arthur Kleinman, Jim Yong Kim, et al. (Berkeley: University of California Press, 2013), 111–32.

147. Wicken, "African Contrasts," 67.

148. E. H. Murcott to Senior Hospital Assistant in Charge, Fort Manning (through Provincial Medical Officer, Central Province, Lilongwe), April 13, 1954, File No. 3405 (Zomba Hospital Drugs and Medical Equipment), Document Number 44, MNA.

149. E. H. Murcott, Director of Medical Services, Zomba, to All Officers in Charge of Stations and Provincial Medical Officers, n.d., Ref. No. M. 1/13/1114, No. 36, MNA.

150. McCracken, *History of Malawi*, 380–81.

151. Ibid., 384–89.

152. Andrew Roberts, *A History of Zambia* (London: Oxford University Press, 1976), 225.

153. Baker, "Government Medical Service in Malawi." Also see Michael King and Elizabeth King, *The Story of Medicine and Disease in Malawi: The 150 Years Since Livingstone* (Blantyre, Malawi: Arco Books, 1992), 155.

154. Sally Hubbard, "Nursing in Zomba, 1963–64," in *Expatriate Experience of Life and Work in Nyasaland*, vol. 3, ed. Colin Baker (Cardiff: Mpemba Books, 2014), 303–11.

155. Glyn Jones, Hugh Norman-Walker, Henry Phillips, et al, "Colloquium on Nyasaland Finance," April 23, 1980, Mss.Afr.s.1742, Box 1, File 27, BLOU, 56.

156. McCracken, *History of Malawi*, 423; H. Phillips, *From Obscurity to Bright Dawn: How Nyasaland Became Malawi, an Insider's Account* (London: I. B. Tauris, 1998), 177.

157. Goodall, *Goodbye to Empire*; *Annual Report on the Public Health of the Federation of Rhodesia and Nyasaland for the Year 1962* (Salisbury, Rhodesia: Government Printer, 1963), CSD 607, BL; *Annual Report on the Work of the Nyasaland/Malawi Ministry of Health for the Year 1964*.

Chapter 6

1. Mpambira Kambewa, "The Malawian Extended Family, Promoting 'Dependency Syndrome'?," *Pabwalo*, March 22, 2015, http://www.pabwalo.com/debate/the-malawian-extended-family-promoting-dependency-syndrome/ (accessed July 1, 2015).

2. Megan Vaughan, *Curing Their Ills: Colonial Power and African Illness* (Redwood City, CA: Stanford University Press, 1991).

3. Markku Hokkanen, *Medicine, Mobility and the Empire: Nyasaland Networks, 1859–1960* (Manchester, UK: Manchester University Press, 2017).

4. John McCracken, *A History of Malawi: 1859–1966* (Woodbridge, UK: James Currey, 2012).

5. Colin Baker, "The Government Medical Service in Malawi: An Administrative History, 1891–1974," *Medical History* 20, no. 3 (1976): 296–311.

6. John Lwanda, *Politics, Culture and Medicine in Malawi: Historical Continuities and Ruptures with Special Reference to HIV/AIDS* (Zomba, Malawi: Michigan State

University Press, 2005) and *Colour, Class and Culture: A Preliminary Communication into the Creation of Doctors in Malawi* (Glasgow: Dudu Nsomba, 2008).

7. For one example of a seminal ethnography, see Claire L. Wendland, *A Heart for the Work: Journeys through an African Medical School* (Chicago: University of Chicago Press, 2010).

8. Eric de Winter, *Health Services of a District Hospital in Malawi* (Assen, Netherlands: Van Gorcum and Co., 1972), 85.

9. Lwanda, *Colour, Class and Culture*, 10.

10. Austin C. Mkandawire, *Living My Destiny: A Medical and Historical Narrative* (Limbe, Malawi: Popular Publications, 1998), 114–15.

11. Kathryn Morton, *Aid and Dependence: British Aid to Malawi* (London: Routledge, 2011), 45. Also see Harvey J. Sindima, *Malawi's First Republic: An Economic and Political Analysis* (Lanham, MD: University Press of America, 2002), 127.

12. In a letter to the Colonial Office in 1939, Banda wrote of his "project of acquiring a British medical qualification to return to Nyasaland in the service of my people." H. K. Banda to N. V. Boyd, 29 June 1939, CO525/177/17, File No. 10, UKNA.

13. Jack Mapanje, in John Lwanda, "Hastings Kamuzu Banda," *British Medical Journal* 316, no. 7134 (1998), 868.

14. Colin Baker, "The Government Medical Service in Malawi: An Administrative History, 1891–1974," *Medical History* 20, no. 3 (1976): 308.

15. Luke Messac, "Moral Hazards and Moral Economies: The Combustible Politics of Healthcare User Fees in Malawian History," *South African Historical Journal* 66, no. 2 (2014): 371–89.

16. James Ferguson, *Give a Man a Fish: Reflections on the New Politics of Distribution* (Durham, NC: Duke University Press, 2015).

17. See Steven Feierman, "Colonizers, Scholars and the Creation of Invisible Histories," in *Beyond the Cultural Turn: New Directions in the Study of Society and Culture*, ed. Lynn Hunt and Victoria Bonnell (Berkeley: University of California Press, 1999), 182-215.

18. Jürgen Habermas, *The Structural Transformation of the Public Sphere: An Inquiry into a Category of Bourgeois Society*, trans. Thomas Burger (Cambridge, MA: MIT Press, 1991), 232.

19. Hector L. Duff, *Nyasaland under the Foreign Office* (London: George Bell, 1906), 361. Also see P. G. Chinguwo, *In the Parliament of Malawi, Official Report of the Proceedings, First Session-Second Meeting*, 1964.

20. Messac, "Moral Hazards and Moral Economies," 377; and Patrick Malloy, "'Holding [Tanganyika] by the Sindano: Networks of Medicine in Colonial Tanganyika" (PhD diss., University of California Los Angeles, 2003), 231–32.

21. "'Something for Nothing Days' Over," *Nyasaland Times*, November 25, 1960, MNA.

22. Harry S. Gear, "Some Problems of the Medical Services of the Federation of Rhodesia and Nyasaland," *BMJ* 2, no. 5197 (1960), 530.

23. J. R. T. Wood, *The Welensky Papers: A History of the Federation of Rhodesia and Nyasaland* (Durban, South Africa: Graha Publications, 1983), 1107–8.

24. Ibid., 1140–41.

25. Glyn Jones, Hugh Norman-Walker, Henry Phillips, et al., "Colloquium on Nyasaland Finance," April 23, 1980, Mss.Afr.s.1742, Box 1, File 27, BLOU, 64–65.

26. Security Liaison Officer, Salisbury, to Special Branch, Nyasaland Police, Zomba, re: "Dr. Banda's Previous History," November 13, 1960, KV 2/4075, UKNA.

27. A. F. Hewlett, Security Liaison Officer, Ghana, to SLO Central Africa, December 6, 1960, File No. 498a, KV2/4075, UKNA.

28. See, e.g., Philip Short, *Banda* (Boston: Routledge and Kegan Paul, 1974).

29. "Medical Events: Territorial Government Takes over Hospitals in Nyasaland," *Central African Journal of Medicine* (April 1963): 159.

30. Sally Hubbard, "Nursing in Zomba, 1963–64," in *Expatriate Experience of Life and Work in Nyasaland, vol. 3*, ed. Colin Baker (Cardiff, UK: Mpemba Books, 2014), 308.

31. Megan Vaughan, "Maternal Mortality in Malawi: History and Moral Responsibility," in *Death, Belief and Politics in Central African History*, ed. Walima T. Kalusa and Megan Vaughan (Lusaka, Zambia: The Lembani Trust, 2013), 303.

32. Megan Vaughan, *The Story of an African Famine: Gender and Famine in Twentieth-Century Malawi* (New York: Cambridge University Press, 1987).

33. As Eric de Winter, a Dutch physician who had worked in Nkhata Bay in the late 1960s, pointed out, "It is often considered acceptable in developing countries not to let all pregnant women deliver in a hospital, but only to select high-risk patients." *Health Services of a District Hospital in Malawi*, 122.

34. Robert Park, "General Notice No. 3: Ministry of Health: Out-Patient and Maternity Fees," *Malawi Government Gazette*, 1, no. 1 (1964), 1. .

35. Stevenson, "Health Services of Malawi".

36. Kanyama Chiume, *Kwacha: An Autobiography* (Nairobi: East African Publishing House, 1975), 211.

37. For such histories of the Cabinet Crisis, see Andrew C. Ross, *Colonialism to Cabinet Crisis: A Political History of Malawi* (Zomba, Malawi: Kachere, 2009); and Colin Baker, *Revolt of the Ministers: The Malawi Cabinet Crisis, 1964–65* (New York: I. B. Tauris, 2001).

38. Messac, "Moral Hazards and Moral Economies," 384.

39. *In the Parliament of Malawi: Official Report of the Proceedings* (Zomba: Government Printer, September 9, 1964), 98, MNA. Also see Henry B. M. Chipembere, *Hero of the Nation: Chipembere of Malawi; An Autobiography* (Blantyre: Christian Literature Association of Malawi, 2001).

40. "Chipembere Addresses Rally at Fort Johnston," *Times (of Malawi)*, September 15, 1964.

41. Baker, *Revolt of the Ministers*, 212–15.

42. Harry Franklin, "Malawi: Dr Banda Faces the Rebels," *Spectator*, April 1, 1965.

43. Chipembere died in the United States in 1975 at age forty-five from complications of diabetes. Earl H. Phillips, "HBM Chipembere, 1930–1975, Malawi Patriot," *Ufahamu: A Journal of African Studies* 7, no. 1 (1976): 5–18.

44. "Premier Addresses Rally at Palombe: Dr. Banda: 'Man of Honour': Repeats Charges against Some of the Ministers," *Times (of Malawi)*, September 15, 1964.

45. "Outpatient Attendances, 1963–64," in *A Conspectus Including the Development Plan for 1965–1969* (Blantyre, Malawi: Ministry of Health, 1965), MNA.

46. "Tour of the Fort Johnston Area Commencing on Sunday, 25th June, 1967 at Monkey Bay," File 195, Folder 6835, MNA. Also see *Annual Report on the Work of the*

Nyasaland/Malawi Ministry of Health for the Year 1964 (Zomba: Government Printer, 1965), 5, UMMC.

47. "Banda Gift for Poor African Patients," *Times (of Malawi)*, September 18, 1964.
48. "Dr. Banda at Queen Elizabeth Hospital," *Times*, September 25, 1964, 1, 5.
49. Hastings Kamuzu Banda, "Prime Minister's Speech to the Nation, Transcript, Ministry of Information, Blantyre," February 18, 1965, HK Banda Speech Collection, MNA.
50. Baker, *Revolt of the Ministers*, 319.
51. Paul Brietzke, "The Chilobwe Murders Trial," *African Studies Review* 17, no. 2 (1974): 361–79.
52. De Winter, *Health Services of a District Hospital in Malawi*.
53. Catherine Valentine, "Settler Visions of Health: Health Care Provision in the Central African Federation, 1953–63" (master's thesis, Portland State University, 2017), 161. Also see Marcia Burdette, *Zambia: Between Two Worlds* (London: Routledge, 1988), 68; and P. J. Freund, "Health Care in a Declining Economy: The Case of Zambia," *Social Science and Medicine* 23, no. 9 (1986): 875–88.
54. Stevenson, "Health Services of Malawi," 176; World Bank, "Table 21: Government Development Expenditure," Economic Memorandum on Tanzania: Prepared for the May 1977 Meeting of the East Africa Consultative Group—Tanzania," Report No. 1567-TA, April 12, 1977.
55. Maurice King, *Development Plan for Health Services in Malawi, 1970–1985*. Zomba: Ministry of Health, 1970.
56. *Building the Nation: Malawi, 1964–1974: Issued to Commemorate the Tenth Anniversary of Malawi's Independence* (Blantyre, Malawi: Department of Information, 1974), 30.
57. W. P. Junde, "Letter from Secretary for Health and Community Development to the District Commissioner, Fort Johnston, Re: Nankumba Health Unit-Construction of Staff Housing," July 15, 1970, 22-20-8F, Box 53423, No. 43, MNA.
58. C. G. Kumwembe, "V.I.P. Debtors Accounts Referred to Ministry Headquarters as at 31st March, 1973, from Auditor-General to Secretary for Health," October 22, 1973, 9-12-3F, Box 34105, Folder C2/90, MNA.
59. SFO to US, Re: Mr JZU Tembo, March 19, 1971, 9-12-3F, Box 34105, Folder C2/90, Folio 145, MNA. Also see Accountant General, Zomba, to Secretary for Health, Blantyre, Re: Hospital Accounts: Invoicing and Collection of Accounts Outstanding, November 12, 1973, 9-12-3F, Box 34105, Folder C2/90, Folio 302, MNA.
60. King, *Development Plan for Health Services in Malawi*; and *Annual Report of the Ministry of Health for the Year 1965* (Zomba, Malawi: Government Printer, 1968).
61. King, *Development Plan for Health Services in Malawi*.
62. De Winter, *Health Services of a District Hospital in Malawi*, 121.
63. Ibid., 124.
64. John Bryant, *Health and the Developing World* (Ithaca, NY: Cornell University Press, 1969), 59–60.
65. Memorandum from G. E. Okurume, Re: Annual Meeting Departmental Discussions Held on September 29, 1969, October 17, 1969, Item No. 1860299, WBGA.
66. John Adelman, Back-to-Office Report, Mission to Malawi. Submitted to Mr. Abdel G. El Emary, July 31, 1969, Item No. 1860299, WBGA, 15.

67. Malawi President Hastings Kamuzu Banda to World Bank Group President Robert McNamara, delivered by Aleke Banda on July 14, 1969, September 12, 1969, 2, Item No. 1860299, WBGA.

68. World Bank Group President Robert McNamara to Malawi President Hastings Kamuzu Banda, October 20, 1969, WBGA File No. 1860299, WBGA.

69. Matthew Connelly, *Fatal Misconception: The Struggle to Control World Population* (Cambridge, MA: Belknap Press, 2010), 206.

70. Ibid., 233.

71. Devesh Kapur, John Lewis, and Richard Webb, *The World Bank: Its First Half Century* (Washington, DC: Brookings, 1997), 249–50.

72. "Recent Economic Developments: Malawi" (International Bank for Reconstruction and Development, International Development Association, Eastern Africa Department, August 27, 1971), 5, WBGA website.

73. "Recent Economic Developments: Malawi" (International Bank for Reconstruction and Development, International Development Association, Eastern Africa Department, August 27, 1971), 5, WBGA website.

74. Short, *Banda*, 279–80.

75. H. R. Durrant, Officer in Charge to Medical Superintendent, Zomba Hospital, re "Medical Supplies," February 2, 1965, 2-1-1F, Box 12484, Folder 3405, MNA.

76. Kathryn Morton, *Aid and Dependence: British Aid to Malawi* (London: Routledge, 2011), 117–18.

77. Short, *Banda*, 280.

78. Hastings Kamuzu Banda and Cullen Young, Preface to *Our African Way of Life*, ed. Hastings Kamuzu Banda and Cullen Young (London: Lutterworth Press, 1946), 24.

79. See Suzanne Miers and Igor Kopytoff, *Slavery in Africa: Historical and Anthropological Perspectives* (Madison: University of Wisconsin Press, 1979). Also see Jan Vansina, *Paths in the Rainforest: Toward a History of Political Tradition in Equatorial Africa*. Madison: University of Wisconsin Press, 1990.

80. "Kamuzu Speaks to His Amazon Army, by Our Staff Reporter," *Malawi News: The Voice of the Congress Party*, January 21, 1961.

81. "Speech Made by His Excellency the President, Ngwazi Dr. Kamuzu Banda at Neno, on Sunday, December 8, 1968," in *The President Speaks* (Blantyre, Malawi: Department of Information), 3, H. K. Banda Speech Collection, MNA.

82. Wiseman C. Chirwa, "Dancing towards Dictatorship: Political Songs and Popular Culture in Malawi," *Nordic Journal of African Studies* 10, no. 1 (2001): 1–27.

83. "Speech by His Excellency the Life President, Ngwazi Dr. H. Kamuzu Banda at the Official Opening of Dedza District Hospital," December 4, 1975, 12, HK Banda Speech Collection, MNA. For more on these singers, see Chirwa, "Dancing towards Dictatorship," 1–27; and Lisa Gilman, *The Dance of Politics: Gender, Performance, and Democratization in Malawi* (Philadelphia: Temple University Press, 2009).

84. Jonathan Kydd and Robert Christiansen, "Structural Change in Malawi since Independence: Consequences of a Development Strategy Based on Large-Scale Agriculture," *World Development* 10, no. 5 (1982): 355–75.

85. "Address by His Excellency the Life President, Ngwazi Dr. H. Kamuzu Banda after Inspecting and Approving the Site for the Kamuzu College of Nursing, Lilongwe,

8 December 1975," in *His Excellency the Life President's Speeches: Central Region Tour, December 2–15, 1975*, 18–25, H. K. Banda Speech Collection, MNA; and Louis Joseph Chimango, Minister of Health, to Life President Hastings Kamuzu Banda, "Annual Report on Gift of K160,000 to Four Hospitals," 1979, 9-12-1F, MNA.

86. Wendland, *Heart for the Work*, 57–58; also see Wakisa Mulwafu and Adamson Muula, *The First Medical School in Malawi: Including a Short Biography of its Architect, Professor John Chiphangwi* (Lilongwe, Malawi: Sunrise Publications, 2001), 114–15.

87. B. W. Malunga, "Obituary: Professor J.D. Chiphangwi," *Malawi Medical Journal* 14, no. 2 (2002): 4.

88. Paul M. Meo, "World Bank/IFC Office Memorandum to Mr. IMD Little, Adviser, Development Economics Department," April 20, 1976, Item No. 1417224, WBGA, 1-2.

89. Joey Power, *Building Kwacha: Political Culture and Nationalism in Malawi* (Rochester, NY: University of Rochester Press, 2010), 206. Also see Sindima, *Malawi's First Republic*, 204.

90. Reuben Makayiko Chirambo, "'Mzimu Wa Soldier': Contemporary Popular Music and Politics in Malawi," in *A Democracy of Chameleons: Politics and Culture in the New Malawi*, ed. Harri Englund (Stockholm, Sweden: Elanders Gotab, 2002), 103–22.

91. "His Excellency the Life President's Speeches: Opening of the Education Conference, Soche Hill College" (Zomba, Malawi: Ministry of Information and Broadcasting, April 14, 1972), 4, H.K. Banda Speech Collection, MNA.

92. Jane Harrigan, "Malawi," in *Aid and Power: The World Bank and Policy-Based Lending*, vol. 2, *Case Studies*, ed. Paul Mosley, Jane Harrigan, and John Toye (London: Routledge, 1991), 204–8.

93. Jones, Norman-Walker, Phillips, et al., "Colloquium on Nyasaland Finance," 74–75.

94. Simon Thomas, "Economic Developments in Malawi Since Independence," *Journal of Southern African Studies* 2, no. 1 (1975): 50.

95. "Speech by His Excellency the Life President, Ngwazi Dr. H. Kamuzu Banda at the Official Opening of Dedza District Hospital, December 4, 1975," 17; Jones, Norman-Walker, Phillips, et al., "Colloquium on Nyasaland Finance," 76.

96. "Address by His Excellency the Life President, Ngwazi Dr. H. Kamuzu Banda after Inspecting and Approving the Site for the Kamuzu College of Nursing, Lilongwe, 8 December 1975," in *His Excellency the Life President's Speeches: Central Region Tour, December 2–15, 1975*, 23, H. K. Banda Speech Collection, MNA.

97. For a description of a similar political dynamic in postcolonial Lesotho, see John Aerni-Flessner, "Development, Politics and the Centralization of State Power in Lesotho, 1960–75," *Journal of African History* 55, no. 3 (2014): 401–21.

98. "Speech Made by His Excellency the President, Ngwazi Dr. Kamuzu Banda at Neno, on Sunday, December 8, 1968," in *The President Speaks* (Blantyre, Malaawi: Department of Information, 1968), 2, H. K. Banda Speech Collection, MNA.

99. Sindima, *Malawi's First Republic*, 69.

100. Colin Baker, "The Development of the Civil Service in Malawi from 1891 to 1972" (PhD diss, University of London, 1981), 332.

101. Henry Mowschenson, "Dr. H. Kamuzu Banda: President of the Republic of Malawi," *Central African Journal of Medicine* 12, no. 8 (1966): 152–53. Also see Valentine, "Settler Visions of Health," 157.

102. See Harri Englund, "Extreme Poverty and Existential Obligations: Beyond Morality in the Anthropology of Africa?," *Social Analysis: The International Journal of Social and Cultural Practice* 52, no. 3 (2008): 36.

103. "Speech by His Excellency the Life President, Ngwazi Dr. H. Kamuzu Banda at the Official Opening of Dedza District Hospital, December 4, 1975."

104. Short, *Banda*, 239–40.

105. *Annual Report on the Work of the Nyasaland/Malawi Ministry of Health for the Year 1964*, 3. Also see Henry Mowschenson, "Dr. H Kamuzu Banda: President of the Republic of Malawi," *Central African Journal of Medicine* 12, no 8 (1966): 152–53.

106. Baker, "The Development of the Civil Service in Malawi," 330.

107. Joel Peters, *Israel and Africa: The Problematic Friendship* (New York: I. B. Tauris, 1992), 37–38. The others were Swaziland, Lesotho, and Mauritius.

108. *What Is Communism? Speech by Ngwazi Dr. Kamuzu Banda, Prime Minister of Malawi, to Zomba Debating Society* (Ministry of Information, April 1964), 19–20, H. K. Banda Speech Collection, MNA.

109. *A Conspectus Including the Development Plan for 1965–69*. Also see Short, *Banda*, 239–40. Also see Lemson Chitsamba, "Malawi and the Politics of Foreign Aid" (PhD diss, London School of Economics, 1990), 104.

110. "Staff Appraisal Report, Republic of Malawi Health Project" (World Bank, Population, Health and Nutrition Department, March 24, 1983), 12, WBGA website.

111. "Malawi Growth and Structural Change: A Basic Economic Report" (World Bank, East Africa Regional Office, February 8, 1982), 183, WBGA website.

112. W. Arthur Lewis, *Development Planning: The Essentials of Economic Policy* (New York: Harper & Row, 1966), 161–63; and Walt Rostow, *The Stages of Economic Growth: A Non-Communist Manifesto* (Cambridge, UK: Cambridge University Press, 1960). For more on the influence of modernization theorists on Malawian leaders, see John McCracken, "In the Shadow of Mau Mau: Detainees and Detention Camps during Nyasaland's State of Emergency," in *Malawi in Crisis: the 1959/60 Nyasaland State of Emergency and its Legacy*, ed. Kings M. Phiri, John McCracken, and Wapulumuka Mulwafu (Zomba, Malawi: Kachere, 2012), 165–91.

113. J. R. Peberdy to Kasuko Hashimoto, EA1DB, Re: "First Draft Issues Paper for Malawi Basic Economic Report," July 26, 1978, Item No. 1417224, WBGA; and Peter Hansen to A. A. Upindi, June 23, 1978, Item No. 1417224, WBGA website.

114. Max Gluckman, *The Ideas in Barotseland Jurisprudence* (New Haven, CT: Yale University Press, 1965), 173.

115. Meyer Fortes, *The Web of Kinship among the Tallensi* (London: Oxford University Press, 1949), 293. Also see Englund, "Extreme Poverty and Existential Obligations," 33–50.

116. Lwanda, *Colour, Class and Culture*, 32.

117. W. J. Chikakuda, "The Expanded Programme on Immunization in Malawi," *Malawi Epidemiological Quarterly* 2 (1983): 3–12.
118. "Malawi Growth and Structural Change," 180.

Chapter 7

1. United Nations Food & Agriculture Organization, "Malawi: GIEWS Country Briefs" (January 14, 2016).
2. Jane Harrigan, "Malawi," in *Aid and Power: The World Bank and Policy-Based Lending*, vol. 2, *Case Studies*, ed. Paul Mosley, Jane Harrigan, and John Toye (London: Routledge, 1991), 201–69.
3. Harrigan, "Malawi."
4. Wycliffe Chilowa, "Structural Adjustment Program in Malawi: Perspectives on Public and Private Sectors," in *Africa's Experience with Structural Adjustment: Proceedings of the Harare Seminar, May 23–24, 1994*, ed. Kapil Kapoor (Washington, DC: The World Bank, 1995), 100.
5. Elias Banda and Gill Walt, "The Private Health Sector in Malawi: Opening Pandora's Box?," *Journal of International Development* 7 (1995): 405.
6. Chinyamata Chipeta, "Malawi," in *The Impact of Structural Adjustment on the Population of Africa: The Implications for Education, Health and Employment*, ed. Aderanti Adepoju (London: James Currey, 1993), 112.
7. Banda and Walt, "Private Health Sector in Malawi," 405.
8. Munthali, "Determinants of Vaccination Coverage in Malawi: Evidence from the Demographic and Health Surveys," *Malawi Medical Journal* 19, no. 2 (June 2007): 79–82.
9. Matthew Basilico, Jonathan Weigel, Anjali Motgi, et al., "Health for All? Competing Theories and Geopolitics," in *Reimagining Global Health: An Introduction*, ed. Paul Farmer, Jim Yong Kim, Arthur Kleinman, et al. (Berkeley: University of California Press, 2013), 74–110.
10. Harrigan, "Malawi," 217–23.
11. Chipeta, "Malawi," 116.
12. Harrigan, "Malawi," 245.
13. Ibid., 246; and Chilowa, "Structural Adjustment Program in Malawi," 103.
14. Gilbert M. Burnham, George Pariyo, Edward Galiwango, et al., "Discontinuation of Cost Sharing in Uganda," *Bulletin of the World Health Organization* 82, no. 3 (2004), 187–95; Aurelia Lepine, Mylene Lagarde, and Alexis Le Nestour, "Free Primary Care in Zambia: An Impact Evaluation Using a Pooled Synthetic Control Method," Health, Econometrics and Data Group Working Papers, University of York, September 2015, 5; and Hansjörg Dilger, "Targeting the Empowered Individual: Transnational Policymaking, the Global Economy of Aid, and the Limitations of Biopower in Tanzania," in *Medicine, Mobility, and Power in Global Africa: Transnational Health and Healing*, ed. Hansjörg Dilger, Abdoulaye Kane, and Stacey Langwick (Bloomington: Indiana University Press, 2012), 65.

15. Barbara McPake, Nouria Brikci, Giorgiao Cometto, et al., "Removing User Fees: Learning from International Experience to Support the Process," *Health Policy and Planning* 26, suppl. 1 (2011), ii104–17.

16. Paul Mosley, "Development Economics and the Underdevelopment of Sub-Saharan Africa," *Journal of International Development* 7, no. 5 (1995): 685–706.

17. Ezekiel Kalipeni, "Structural Adjustment and the Health Care Crisis in Malawi," *Proteus* 21, no. 1 (2004): 23.

18. John Iliffe, *The African AIDS Epidemic: A History* (Athens: Ohio University Press, 2005), 44.

19. Malcolm Molyneux, "A Medical Career in Malawi—Personal Reflections," *Malawi Medical Journal* 28, no. 3 (2016): 82–83.

20. Bizwick Mwale, "HIV/AIDS in Malawi," *Malawi Medical Journal* 14, no. 2 (2002): 2–3.

21. Claire L. Wendland, *A Heart for the Work: Journeys through an African Medical School* (Chicago: University of Chicago Press, 2010), 48.

22. Iliffe, *African AIDS Epidemic*, 44.

23. Ibid., 113.

24. G. C. Matchaya, "Trends in Life Expectancy and the Macroeconomy in Malawi," *Malawi Medical Journal* 19, no. 4 (2007): 154–58.

25. D. J. Wakin, "AIDS Wildfire Ravages Southern Africa," *News Gazette* (Urbana-Champaign, IL), October 25, 1998, B–4, cited in Kalipeni, "Structural Adjustment and the Health Care Crisis in Malawi," 26.

26. Kalipeni, "Structural Adjustment and the Health Care Crisis in Malawi."

27. Michael King, "AIDS: Are We Really Serious?," *Malawi Medical Journal* 15, no. 2 (2003), 79.

28. Vicky Levy, "Reply to 'AIDS: Are We Really Serious?,'" *Malawi Medical Journal* 15, no. 2 (2003), 79.

29. Catherine Valentine, "Settler Visions of Health: Health Care Provision in the Central African Federation, 1953–63" (master's thesis, Portland State University, 2017), 158.

30. Wendland, *Heart for the Work*, 64.

31. Bizwick Mwale, "HIV/AIDS in Malawi." *Malawi Medical Journal* 14, no. 2 (2002): 2–3.

32. UNAIDS Country Profile: Malawi. Also see Andreas Jahn, Sian Floyd, and Amelia C. Crampin, "Population-Level Effect of HIV on Adult Mortality and Early Evidence of Reversal after Introduction of Antiretroviral Therapy in Malawi," *Lancet* 371, no. 9624 (2008): 1603–11.

33. Katharina Kober and Wilm Van Damme, "Scaling up Access to Antiretroviral Treatment in Southern Africa: Who Will Do the Job?," *Lancet* 364, no. 9428 (2004): 103–7.

34. Kober and Van Damme, "Scaling up Access to Antiretroviral Treatment in Southern Africa."

35. Malawi Ministry of Health, *Treatment of AIDS: Guidelines for the Use of Antiretroviral Therapy in Malawi* (Lilongwe, April 2008), iii.

36. J. Chiona, F. Mikhori, M. A. Chimole, et al., "Living Our Faith: Pastoral Letter of the Catholic Bishops of Malawi," March 8, 1992, 5.

37. Joey Power, *Building Kwacha: Political Culture and Nationalism in Malawi* (Rochester, NY: University of Rochester Press, 2010), 1.

38. Wendland, *Heart for the Work*, 51.

39. Bakili Muluzi, *Mau Anga: The Voice of a Democrat: Past, Present & Future* (Pretoria, South Africa: Skotaville Media, 2002), 17.

40. Bakili Muluzi, "The State Opening of Parliament, Thursday, 30th June, 1999, The New State House, Lilongwe," in Muluzi, *Mau Anga*, 183.

41. Anne Conroy, "Malawi and the Poverty Trap—A First Person Account," in *Poverty, AIDS and Hunger: Breaking the Poverty Trap in Malawi*, ed. Anne Conroy, Malcolm Blackie, Alan Whiteside, et al. (New York: Palgrave Macmillan, 2006), 120–21.

42. Roshni Menon, "Famine in Malawi: Causes and Consequences," Human Development Report Office Occasional Paper (United Nations Development Programme, 2007).

43. Interview with Patrick Mwale, Ward Councilor, Matope, February 2015.

44. Bridget Msolomba, Lakdini Pathirana, B. Purcell, et al., "Vaccines or Latrines? Debating Spending on Health," *Malawi Medical Journal* 15, no. 1 (2003): 18–19.

45. Tarak Meguid and Elled Mwenyekonde, *The Department of Obstetrics & Gynaecology at Kamuzu Central Hospital and Bottom Hospital, Lilongwe, Malawi: A Situational Analysis*, January 2005, 13.

46. Meguid and Mwenyekonde, *Situational Analysis*, 16.

47. Ibid., 33.

48. Nirmala Ravishankar, Paul Gubbins, Rebecca Cooley, et al., "Financing of Global Health: Tracking Development Assistance for Health from 1990 to 2007," *Lancet* 373, no. 9681 (2009): 2113–24.

49. See, for instance, Mandisa Mbali, *South African AIDS Activism and Global Health Politics* (London: Palgrave Macmillan, 2013); and Raymond Smith and Patricia Siplon, *Drugs into Bodies: Global AIDS Treatment Activism* (New York: Praeger, 2006).

50. Jesse Helms, *Here's Where I Stand: A Memoir* (New York: Random House, 2005), 145.

51. Joshua Busby, "Bono Made Jesse Helms Cry: Jubilee 2000, Debt Relief, and Moral Action in International Politics," *International Studies Quarterly* 51, no. 2 (2007): 247–75.

52. Greg Behrman, *The Invisible People: How the U.S. Has Slept Through the Global AIDS Pandemic, the Greatest Humanitarian Catastrophe of Our Time* (New York: Free Press, 2004), 246.

53. Franklin Graham, interview for *Frontline: Age of AIDS*, PBS, January 31, 2005.

54. George W. Bush, interview with Matt Frei, *BBC World News America*, February 14, 2008.

55. Paul Farmer, interview in *Bending the Arc* (documentary, directed by Pedro Kos and Kief Davidson, 2017).

56. George W. Bush, "President Bush Announces a Five-Year, $30 Billion HIV/AIDS Plan" (speech presented at White House, May 30, 2007).

57. Luke Messac and Krishna Prabhu, "Redefining the Possible: The Global AIDS Response," in *Reimagining Global Health: An Introduction*, ed. Paul Farmer, Jim Yong Kim, Arthur Kleinman, et al. (Berkeley: University of California Press, 2013), 111–32.

58. Ramesh Govindaraj, *World Bank Project Information Document, Appraisal Stage*, Health Sector Support Project, Report No. AB862, November 2004, 2; and *Health Equity and Financial Protection Report—Malawi*, Report No. 71255 (Washington, DC: World Bank, 2012).

59. "World Development Indicators: Health Expenditure, Total (% of GDP)" (World Bank).

60. Messac and Prabhu, "Redefining the Possible."

61. Edwin Libamba, Simon Makombe, Anthony Harries, et al., "Malawi's Contribution to '3 by 5': Achievements and Challenges," *Bulletin of the World Health Organization* 85, no. 2 (2007): 156–60.

62. UNITAID, "Audited Financial Report for the Year Ended 31 December 2014," 35.

63. *Malawi Antiretroviral Treatment Quarterly Report* (HIV Unit, Ministry of Health, March 2011).

64. Sian Floyd, Anna Molesworth, and Albert Dube, "Population-Level Reduction in Adult Mortality after Extension of Anti-Retroviral Therapy Provision into Rural Areas in Northern Malawi," *PLoS One* 5, no. 10 (2010): 9.

65. David McCoy, Barbara McPake, and Victor Mwapasa, "The Double Burden of Human Resource and HIV Crises: A Case Study of Malawi," *Human Resources for Health* 6, no. 16 (2008): 6–16.

66. For US international health spending between 2006 and 2015, see "The U.S. Government and Global Health" (Kaiser Family Foundation, April 23, 2015). For an overview of multilateral and bilateral spending levels between 1990 and 2014, see *Financing Global Health 2014: Shifts in Funding as the MDG Era Closes* (Seattle, WA: Institute for Health Metrics and Evaluation, 2015), 18.

67. Gates, Bill. "Rich Countries' Aid Generosity: 2010 Annual Letter from Bill Gates." January 2010, https://www.gatesfoundation.org/who-we-are/resources-and-media/annual-letters-list/annual-letter-2010.

68. *Financing Global Health 2017* (Seattle: Institute for Health Metrics and Evaluation, 2018).

69. International Treatment Preparedness Coalition, *Rationing Funds, Risking Lives: World Backtracks on HIV Treatment*, April 2010, 6.

70. Ryan Lizza, "The Obama Memos: The Making of a Post-Post-Partisan Presidency," *New Yorker*, January 30, 2012.

71. John Donnelly, "Emanuel on TB: 'The Challenge Is Enormous,'" *Science Speaks: Global ID News*, October 28, 2010.

72. The most important illicit financial flow, according to most analyses, involves the mis-attribution of profits earned in Africa to low-tax nations in Europe. See "Report of the High Level Panel on Illicit Financial Flows from Africa" (United Nations Economic Commission for Africa, 2011). Also see Martha Khonje, "Corporate Tax Deals Are Robbing Poor Countries of Teachers and Nurses," *Guardian*, July 2, 2015.

73. Luke Messac, "Malawi's Health Care Subject of Intense Worry for Country's Poor," *Pulitzer Center on Crisis Reporting*, August 2, 2013.

74. Interview with Dorothy Ngoma, July 8, 2011, Lilongwe, Malawi.

75. "Editorial: Revealed: How the Malawian Cabinet Nearly Committed Treason," *London Evening Post*, May 10, 2012.
76. "Malawi's 'Cashgate' Scandal: The $32m Heist," *Economist*, February 27, 2014.
77. Aidspan, "Accountability for Global Fund Grants in Malawi," November 2016, 8. http://www.aidspan.org/publication/accountability-global-fund-grants-malawi.
78. "Medical Drug Shortages Hit Malawi Public Hospitals as DHOs Exhaust Budgets," *Nyasa Times*, February 5, 2017.
79. See Alister Munthali, Hasheem Mannan, Malcolm MacLachlan, et al., "Non-Use of Formal Health Services in Malawi: Perceptions from Non-Users," *Malawi Medical Journal* 26, no. 4 (2014): 129.
80. World Health Organization, *Malawi: WHO Statistical Profile, Updated January 2015*. https://www.who.int/gho/countries/mwi.pdf?ua=1

Conclusion: Breaking the Spell of Scarcity

1. William Easterly, *The White Man's Burden: Why the West's Efforts to Aid the Rest Have Done So Much Ill and So Little Good* (New York: Penguin Books, 2006), 255.
2. Andrew Creese, Katherine Floyd, Anita Alban, et al., "Cost-Effectiveness of HIV/AIDS Interventions in Africa: A Systematic Review of the Evidence," *Lancet* 359, no. 9318 (2002): 1635–42.
3. Colleen Denny and Ezekiel Emanuel, "US Health Aid Beyond PEPFAR: The Mother and Child Campaign," *Journal of the American Medical Association* 300, no. 17 (2008): 2048–51.
4. Paul Farmer, *AIDS and Accusation: Haiti and the Geography of Blame* (Berkeley: University of California Press, 1992), 256–57.
5. Ted Schrecker, "Interrogating Scarcity: How to Think About 'Resource-Scarce Settings,'" *Health Policy and Planning* 28 (2013): 400–409. Also see Peter Ubel, "'Rationing' Health Care: Not All Definitions Are Created Equal," *Archives of Internal Medicine* 158 (1998): 211.
6. Economic historians have begun to include such forced labor in calculations of the burden of taxation placed on the colonized and have found that "labor taxes constituted in most places the largest component of early colonial budgets." See Marlous van Waijenburg, "Financing the African Colonial State: The Revenue Imperative and Forced Labor," *Journal of Economic History* 78, no. 1 (2018): 40.
7. In 2016, Malawi's government spent $32.30 per person on health care (including foreign aid), while the US government spent $8,077.93. See "Domestic General Government Heatlh Expenditure per Capita, PPP (Current International $)," World Health Organization Global Health Expenditure database.
8. Mike Davis, "Planet of Slums" (speech presented at Rhodes College, Memphis, TN, November 5, 2015).

Bibliography

Archival Records Consulted

Bodleian Library, Oxford University (BLOU)
Mss.Afr.s.332; Papers of Arthur Creech Jones (1904–1965)
Mss.Afr.s.883; Papers of Walter Gopsill (1926–1945)
Mss.Afr.s.1726; Papers of Joan Wicken (1956–1958)
Mss.Afr.s.1742; "Colloquium on Nyasaland Finance," in Papers of Glyn Jones (1980)
Mss.Brit.Emp.s.365; Papers of the Fabian Colonial Bureau (1929–1967)
Mss.Welensky; Papers of the Rt. Hon. Sir Roy Welensky, KCMG (1936–1990)

British Library, London (BL)
Newspaper Collection
Evening Standard
Rhodesia Herald

Malawi National Archives (MNA)

Director of Medical Services
2-1-1F, 12456, 6548/1; Drugs, Advertisements, Medical Supplies (1957–1968)
2-1-1F, 12484, 2013.I; Fort Johnston Hospital Branch IV Advances
2-1-1F, 12484, 6968VI; Annual Report, Ministry of Health (1963)
2-1-1F, 12484, 3405; Zomba General Hospital, Drugs & Equipment (1953–1965)
2-5-8F, 788, M1/13V; Requisitions for Medical Stores
2-5-8F, 788, M1/59; Medical Stores & Equipment, Fort Johnston Hospital (1948–1955)
2-14-2F, 12571, 6970; Annual Confidential Reports
2-27-1F, 12567, 1225; Central Hospital, Hospital Fees
2-28-1F, 12569, 6245; Dangerous Drugs Legislation
2-28-1, 12569, 6292; Government Gazette, Regulation of Doctors
2-28-1F, 12570, 7671; Controller of Stores, General
2-28-3F, 10628, ANI; C. L. Kadzamira (1959–1961)
2-29-11R, 10641; Federal Information Sheets (1961–1962)
3-15-1F, 12481, 4501B; Medical Stores Monthly Returns
4-5-8R, 9113, P1.3; Old Age Pensions and Hardship Cases (1955–1959)
4-5-9R, 9121, 6443C; Analysis of Hospital Expenditure (1962–1963)
4-5-9R, 9121, 6571; Care of the Aged Infirm (1956–1961)
4-5-11R, 9131, 6956: Tour on Inspections and Reports by Secretary, Medical HQ
4-1-10R, 8535, 5956; Medical Stores Accounts

7-6-10R, 13371, 8304I; Tenders for Hospital Provisions
7-6-10R, 13371, 8329; Monthly Health Reports, Fort Johnston
7-6-10F, 13374, 2205; Karonga Hospital Drugs and Medical Equipment (1961)
7-6-11R, 13375, 8299; Hospital Provisions (1968)
7-6-11R, 13375, 6186II; Tuberculosis and Treatment, General (1954)
7-6-11R, 13376, 6835; Monkey Bay Dispensary
7-6-11R, 13377, 6905; Transport of Patients Policy
7-6-11R, 13377, MP4205, Laboratory Drugs and Medical Equipment
7-6-11R, 13377, 2019I; Fort Johnston Hospital
7-6-11F, 13379, 6561; Pharmacy & Poisons, Regulation Issues and Licenses
7-6-11F, 13380, 6291III; Development Plans

Malawi Ministry of Development Planning

7-7-9R, 13381, DEV/1A; Development Plans
7-7-9R, 13381, 6504II; WHO Publication and Statistics
7-7-9R, 13383, Dev/1B; Development Plan
7-7-9R, 13383, 1225IV; Central Hospital, Hospital Fees
7-7-9F, 13385, D/D/L/1; Dangerous Drugs License No. 5
14-2-8R, 20610; Papers of Henry Ord (1968–1969)
12-7-4F, 42592, DEV/74/5; New Karonga Hospital and Health Subcentres
12-7-4F, 42596, DEV/41/20; Economic Planning Division Circulars (1975–1984)
12-7-4F, 42597, DEV/74/30/Vol. II; Improvements to Hospitals (1977–1984)
12-7-5R, 42600, DEV/74/10; Replacement of Rural Health Centres, CIDA (1978–1983)
12-7-6R, 42603, DEV/74/4/31/41: Peripheral Health Units, Blantyre/Lilongwe and Mzuzu (1975–1982)
12-6-6F, 42604, DEV/74/50, Nutrition and Rehabilitation Unit, Domasi (1977–1982)
20-12-3F, 52002; Kamuzu Central Hospital (1978)
22-20-8F, 53423, DEV/74/2; Nankumba Health Unit
22-20-9F, 53427, DEV/74/8; Nkhata Bay District Hospital (1968–1972)

Malawi Office of the President

9-12-1AF, 34096, C4/11/V; Complaints, General Correspondence (1975–1980)
9-12-1AF, 34096; Memoranda to His Excellency the Life President (1979–1980)
9-12-1F, 34098; Memoranda to His Excellency the Life President (1978)
9-12-3F, 34103; Development Proposals of the Ministry of Health, 1976/1977 to 1978–1979 (1976)
9-12-3F, 34103; Development Programme, 1970–1972/1973 (1970)
9-12-3F, 34103, C4/11/II; Complaints (1970–1974)
9-12-3F, 34104, C1/24A; World Bank Economic Mission (1972–1974)
9-12-3F, 34104, C1/15; Ministry of Health Development Programme (1960–1974)
9-12-3F, 34104, C1/14; Papers on Possible Health Development (1966–1973)
9-12-3F, 34105, C2/90; Hospital/Medical Fees
9-12-4F, 34106, C7/3; Disturbances in Malawi (1964–1972)
9-12-4F, 34107, C/1/26/II: Economic Indicators (1970–1971)

Society of Malawi Archives, Blantyre
Medical Department Annual Reports

United Kingdom National Archives (UKNA)

ACT 1/717; Government Actuary's Department, Advice on Social Insurance for the Colonies (1943–1947)

CA 25/26/6; Rioting in Nyasaland: interdepartmental Central Africa Committee (1959)

CAOG 12/98; Purchase of foreign commonwealth goods: drugs (1947–1965)

CO 323/665; Crown Agents (1915)

CO 525/1 to CO 525/221; Nyasaland Original Correspondence (1904–1952)

CO 626/41: Colonial Office: Nyasaland (Malawi): Sessional Papers (1963)

CO 859/66/5; Social Services Department and Successors, Nyasaland, Memorandum on Medical Policy (1943)

CO 970: Colonial Office: Colonial Development Advisory Committee (1929–1940)

CO 1015/227: Functions of the Federal Public Service: Health Services (1952)

CO 1015/701; Discussions with the Fabian Colonial Bureau on Matters Affecting Central Africa (1940–1953)

CO 1015/1547; Commission of Enquiry into Unrest in Nyasaland Held by Lord Devlin (1959)

DO 183/403; Dissolution of the Central African Federation: Health (1963)

DO 224/17; Malawi: Internal Political Situation (1964)

DO 224/23; Malawi: Internal Political Situation (1965–1966)

FCO 29/202; US Aid to Malawi (1967–1968)

FCO 29/214; Policy and Review of Financial Aid to Malawi (1968)

FCO 29/217; Malawi: Budget and Financial Assistance (1968)

FCO 29/219; Development Aid for Malawi (1968)

FCO 141/14152; Nyasaland: Opposition to the Malawi Congress Party (1963–1964)

FCO 141/14202; Nyasaland: Records of Discussions between the Governor and Dr. Hastings Banda (1963–1964)

FCO 141/14212; Nyasaland: Monthly Colonial Intelligence Summaries from the Colonial Office (1963–1964)

FCO 141/14218; Nyasaland: Malawi Congress Party (1963–1964)

FCO 141/14234; Nyasaland: Political Reports to the Foreign Office; Nyasaland Intelligence Committee Reports (1963–1964)

Hansard (Mentions of Nyasaland, Colonial Office, and Colonial Development and Welfare Bill in House of Commons and House of Lords Debates) (1900–2014)

INF 10/186; Nyasaland; Photographs Compiled by the Central Office of Information (1955–1964)

INF 10/194; British Empire Collection of Photographs (1949–1962)

KV 2/4071; Security Service: Personal Files, Hastings Walter Kamuzu Banda (1958)

KV 2/4077; Security Service: Pernal Files, Hastings Walter Kamuzu Banda (1962–1963)

MH 55/2; Sir Basil Blackett, "A Layman's Plea for a Positive Health Policy" (1932–1933)

MH 79/629; Ministry of Health Committee on Colonial Development (1949)

T 1/11348; Treasury Board Paper and In-letters (1911)

T 1/11954; Nyasaland War Expenditure (1916)

T 1/12467; Financial Arrangements for the Construction of a Railway from Beira to the Zambesi (1920)

T 161/156/1; Countries. Africa: Nyasaland: Estimates (1922–1923)
T 161/1384; Colonial Development Advisory Committee: Nyasaland (1932–1935)

University of Edinburgh Library Archives (UoELA)
George Shepperson Papers
University of Malawi Malawiana Collection (UMMC)

Development Plans for Health Services
Medical Department Reports

World Bank Group Archives (WBGA)
Documents and Reports Online

Africa Department
Current Economic Position and Prospects of Malawi, 1967, AF-68A.

Agriculture Projects Department
Appraisal of Karonga Rural Development Project, Malawi, 1971, PA-106a.

Eastern Africa Department
The Current Economic Position and Prospects of Malawi, 1969, AE-5a.
Recent Economic Developments, Malawi, 1971, AE-17a.

Eastern Africa Regional Office
Malawi Basic Needs, 1981, 3461-MAI.
Malawi: The Development of Human Capital, 1981, 3462-MAI.
Malawi Growth and Structural Change: A Basic Economic Report, 1982, 3082a-MAI.
Recent Economic Developments and Prospects of Malawi, 1973, 67a-MAI.
Recent Economic Development and Prospects of Malawi, 1975, 560a-MAI.

Population, Health, and Nutrition Department
Staff Appraisal Report: Republic of Malawi Health Project, 1983, 4342-MAI.

President's Office
Report and Recommendation of the President of the IBRD to the Executive Directors on a
   Proposed Loan to the Republic of Malawi for a Karonga Rural Development Project—
   Phase II, 1976, P-1806.

World Bank Archival Holdings
Malawi-General-1964–1968: 1860267; 1060279; 1860282; 10860294
Malawi- General-1969/1971 Correspondence, Volume 1: 1860268
Malawi-General-1964/1978 Correspondence: 1047167
Malawi-General-Consultative Group-Correspondence 01-1966-1967: 1860303
Malawi-General-Economic Mission-1967-Correspondence-Volume 1; 1860281
Malawi-General-Mission-Mr. Shoaib-Malawi-Correspondence-1967: 1870266
Malawi-General Negotiations-1963–1965: 1860297
Malawi-General Negotiations-Correspondence-Volume 2-1966–1968; 1860298

Malawi-General Negotiations-1969/1971 Correspondence-Volume 2; 1860299; 1860300

Malawi-Lending, Economy and Program [LEAP]-General-1975/1980 Correspondence-Volume 1; 1417224

Malawi-Lending, Economy and Program [LEAP]-1975/1980 Correspondence-Volume 2; 30241524

Malawi-Lending, Economy and Program [LEAP]0General-1975/1980 Correspondence-Volume 3; 30241525

Malawi-Lending, Economy and Program [LEAP]-General-1981/1983 Correspondence-Volume 1; 1158183

Malawi-Lending, Economy and Program [LEAP]-General-1981/1983 General-Correspondence-Volume 2; 30241509

Malawi-Lending, Economy and Program[LEAP]-General-1975/1980 Correspondence-Volume 4; 30241526

Oral History Interviews

Mwale, Patrick. Interview conducted by Luke Messac in Matope, Malawi. February 2015.

Ngoma, Dorothy. Interview conducted by Luke Messac in Lilongwe, Malawi. July 8, 2011.

Periodicals

Central African Journal of Medicine
IRIN News
Malawi News
Nyasa Times
Nyasaland Times (later *The Times [of Malawi]*)
Tsopano
The Economist
The Guardian
The Hindu
The London Evening Post
The Scotsman
The Times [of London]

Government Reports

Bell, R. D. *Report of the Commission Appointed to Enquire into the Financial Position and Further Development of Nyasaland.* London, 1938.

Beveridge, William. *Social Insurance and Allied Services.* London, 1942.

Chinguwo, P. G. *In the Parliament of Malawi, Official Report of the Proceedings, First Session-Second Meeting,* 1964.

Federation of Rhodesia and Nyasaland. *Annual Report on the Public Health.* Salisbury, 1956–1959, 1961, 1963.

Federation of Rhodesia and Nyasaland. *Federation and Nyasaland: The Facts.* Salisbury, 1962.

Gelfand, Michael. *Proud Record: An Account of the Health Services Provided for Africans in the Federation of Rhodesia and Nyasaland*. Salisbury: Federal Information Department, 1960.

Jack, Daniel T. *Report on an Economic Survey of Nyasaland, 1958–1959*. Ministry of Economic Affairs, Federation of Rhodesia and Nyasaland, 1959.

King, M. *Development Plan for Health Services in Malawi, 1970–1985*. Zomba, 1970.

Lord Moyne. *West India Royal Commission Report*. London, 1945.

Malawi. *Annual Report on the Work of the Nyasaland/Malawi Ministry of Health*. Zomba, 1965.

Malawi. *Annual Report of the Ministry of Health for the Year 1965*. Zomba, 1968.

Malawi. *Antiretroviral Treatment Quarterly Report*. Lilongwe, 2011.

Malawi. *Building the Nation: Malawi, 1964–1974*. Blantyre,1974.

Malawi. *A Conspectus Including the Development Plan for 1965–69*. Blantyre, 1965.

Malawi. *Developing Malawi: Office of the President and Cabinet, Economic Planning Division*. Zomba, 1971.

Malawi. *Economic Report*. Zomba, 1970, 1975, 1977.

Malawi. *Government Gazette*. Zomba, 1964.

Malawi. *His Excellency the Life President's Speeches: Central Region Tour, 2–15 December 1975*. Lilongwe, 1976.

Malawi. *His Excellency the Life President's Speeches: Opening of the Education Conference, Soche Hill College, 17 April 1972*. Zomba, 1972.

Malawi. *His Excellency the President's Speeches: State Opening of Parliament, 2 July 1971*. Zomba, 1971.

Malawi. *In the Parliament of Malawi, Official Report of the Proceedings*. Zomba, 1964.

Malawi. *Population Census, 1966, Final Report*. Zomba, 1967.

Malawi. *The President Speaks*. Blantyre, 1969.

Malawi. *Treatment of AIDS: Guidelines for the Use of Antiretroviral Therapy in Malawi*. Lilongwe, 2008.

Malawi Congress Party. *Manifesto for the General Election*. Limbe, 1961.

Northern Rhodesia. *Annual Report on the Social and Economic Progress of the People*. London, 1936.

Nyasaland Protectorate. *Annual Medical and Sanitary Reports*. Zomba, 1935–1936, 1939, 1940, 1942.

Nyasaland Protectorate. *Annual Medical Reports on the Health and Sanitary Condition*. Zomba, 1919, 1926, 1928–1929, 1931–1932.

Nyasaland Protectorate. *Annual Report of the Medical Department*. Zomba, 1945–1946, 1948, 1951, 1953.

Nyasaland Protectorate. *Development Programme, Revised*. Zomba, 1947

Nyasaland Protectorate. *Proclamations, Rules and Notices*. Zomba, 1915.

Nyasaland Protectorate. *Report of the Post-War Development Committee*. Zomba, 1945.

Nyasaland Protectorate. *What Is Communism? Speech by Ngwazi Dr. Kamuzu Banda, Prime Minister of Malawi, to Zomba Debating Society*. Zomba, 1964.

Pearson, D. S., and W. L. Taylor. *Break-up: Some Economic Consequences for the Rhodesias and Nyasaland*. Salisbury, 1963.

Pim, Alan W., and S. Milligan. *Report of the Commission to Enquire into the Financial and Economic Position of Northern Rhodesia*. London, 1938.

Shircore, John O. *Report on the Nyasaland Medical Service with Special Reference to a Grant Under the Colonial Development Fund*. Zomba, 1930.

Stephens, P. R. *Allocation of Expenditure, 1962/63*. Blantyre, 1962.

United Kingdom. *Report of the Advisory Commission on the Review of the Constitution of Rhodesia and Nyasaland*. London, 1960.

United Kingdom Colonial Office. *Colonial Office List*. 1913–1950.

United Kingdom Colonial Office. *Report of the Commission Appointed to Enquire into the Disturbances in the Copperbelt, Northern Rhodesia*. London, 1935.

United Kingdom Colonial Office. *Report on the Colonial Empire, 1939–1947*. London, 1947.

United Kingdom Colonial Office. *Return of Schemes Made Under the Colonial Development and Welfare Acts*. London, 1947.

United Kingdom Colonial Office. *Social Welfare in the Colonies*. London, 1945.

United Kingdom Colonial Office. *Statement of Policy on Colonial Development and Welfare*. London, 1940.

United Kingdom Treasury Department. *Memorandum Explaining the Financial Resolution of the Colonial Development Act*. London, 1929.

Viscount Bledisloe. *Rhodesia-Nyasaland Royal Commission's Report*. London, 1939.

Williams, A. D. J. B. "Post-War Development of Medical Services." Zomba, 1944.

Nongovernmental Reports

Chiona, J., F. Mikhori, M. A. Chimole, et al. "Living Our Faith: Pastoral Letter of the Catholic Bishops of Malawi." March 8, 1992.

Aidspan, "Accountability for Global Fund Grants in Malawi," November 2016. http://www.aidspan.org/publication/accountability-global-fund-grants-malawi

Fabian Colonial Bureau. *Labour in the Colonies*. London, Fabian Colonial Bureau, 1942

Institute for Health Metrics and Evaluation. *Financing Global Health 2014: Shifts in Funding as the MDG Era Closes*. Seattle, WA: IHME, 2015.

International Monetary Fund. *2015 Article IV Consultation—Press Release; Staff Report; and Statement by the Executive Director for Malawi*. Washington, DC: IMF, 2015.

International Treatment Preparedness Coalition. *Rationing Funds, Risking Lives: World Backtracks on HIV Treatment*. April 2010.

Kaiser Family Foundation. *The Global HIV/AIDS Epidemic: Global Health Policy Fact Sheet*. Washington, DC: Kaiser Family Foundation, 2015.

Kaiser Family Foundation. *The U.S. Government and Global Health*. Washington, DC: Kaiser Family Foundation, 2015.

"Maternal Mortality Ratio (Modeled Estimate, per 100,000 Live Births)." World Bank Data. https://data.worldbank.org/indicator/SH.STA.MMRT?locations=MW

Meguid, Tarak, and Elled Mwenyekonde. *The Department of Obstetrics & Gynaecology at Kamuzu Central Hospital and Bottom Hospital, Lilongwe, Malawi: A Situational Analysis*. January 2005.

Oxfam. *Missing Medicines in Malawi: Campaigning against 'Stock-Outs' of Essential Drugs*. London: Oxford University Press, 2011.

UNAIDS. *Abuja+12: Shaping the Future of Health in Africa*. Geneva: UNAIDS, 2013.

UNAIDS. *The Gap Report: Beginning the End of the AIDS Epidemic*. Geneva: UNAIDS, 2014.

UNAIDS Country Profile: Malawi. http://www.unaids.org/en/regionscountries/countries/malawi.

United Nations Economic Commission for Africa. *Report of the High Level Panel on Illicit Financial Flows from Africa*. New York: United Nations Economic Commission for Africa, 2011.

UNFAO. "Malawi: GIEWS Country Briefs." http://www.fao.org/giews/countrybrief/country.jsp?code=MWI.

UNITAID. *Audited Financial Report* Vernier: UNITAID, 2015.

World Bank. *The Changing Wealth of Nations: Measuring Sustainable Development for the New Millennium.* Washington, DC: The World Bank, 2011.

World Bank. *Economic Memorandum on Tanzania: Prepared for the May 1977 Meeting of the East Africa Consultative Group—Tanzania.* Report No. 1567-TA, April 12, 1977.

World Bank. "World Development Indicators: Health Expenditure, Total (% of GDP)." World Bank. http://datatopics.worldbank.org/health/

World Health Organization. *Malawi: WHO Statistical Profile, Updated January 2015.* http://www.who.int/gho/countries/mwi.pdf?ua=1.

Published Sources

Addae, S. Kojo. *The Evolution of Modern Medicine in a Developing Country: Ghana 1880–1960.* Rickmansworth, UK: Durham Academic Press, 1997.

Aerni-Flessner, John. "Development, Politics and the Centralization of State Power in Lesotho, 1960–1975." *Journal of African History* 55, no. 3 (2014): 401–21.

Altendorff, D. V. "Genealogy of the Speldewinde Family of Ceylon." *Journal of the Dutch Burgher Union* 33, no. 3 (1944): 76.

Anders, Gerhard. *In the Shadow of Good Governance: An Ethnography of Civil Service Reform in Africa.* Boston: Brill, 2010.

Aronowitz, Robert. *Risky Medicine: Our Quest to Cure Fear and Uncertainty.* Chicago: University of Chicago Press, 2015.

Baily, Francis. *Twenty-Nine Years' Hard Labour.* London: Hutchinson and Co., 1934.

Baker, Colin. *Development Governor: Sir Geoffrey Colby—A Biography.* London: I.B. Tauris, 1994.

Baker, Colin. "The Development of the Civil Service in Malawi from 1891 to 1972." PhD diss., University of London, 1981.

Baker, Colin. *Expatriate Experience of Life and Work in Nyasaland,* Volume 3. Cardiff, UK: Mpemba Books, 2013.

Baker, Colin. "The Government Medical Service in Malawi: An Administrative History, 1891–1974." *Medical History* 20, no. 3 (1976): 296–311.

Baker, Colin. *Revolt of the Ministers: The Malawi Cabinet Crisis, 1964–1965.* New York: I. B. Tauris, 2001.

Baker, Colin. "Tax Collection in Malawi: An Administrative History, 1891–1972." *International Journal of African Historical Studies* 8, no. 1 (1975): 40–62.

Baldwin, Peter. *The Politics of Social Solidarity: Class Bases of the European Welfare State, 1875–1975.* Cambridge, UK: Cambridge University Press, 1990.

Banda, Elias, and Gill Walt. "The Private Health Sector in Malawi: Opening Pandora's Box?" *Journal of International Development* 7 (1995): 403–21.

Banda, Hastings Kamuzu, and Harry Nkumbula. *Federation in Central Africa.* Harlesden: Leveridge, 1949.

Bandawe, Lewis Mataka. *Memoirs of a Malawian: The Life and Reminiscences of Lewis Mataka Bandawe.* Blantyre, Malawi: Claim, 1971.

Barber, William J. "Federation and the Distribution of Economic Benefits." In *New Deal in Central Africa*, edited by Colin Leys and Cranford Pratt, 81–97. New York: Frederick A. Praeger, 1960.

Basilico, Matthew, Jonathan Weigel, Anjali Motgi, et al. "Health for All? Competing Theories and Geopolitics." In *Reimagining Global Health: An Introduction*, edited by Paul Farmer, Jim Yong Kim, Arthur Kleinman, et al., 74–110. Berkeley: University of California Press, 2013.

Beck, Ann. *A History of the British Medical Administration of East Africa, 1900–1950.* Cambridge, MA: Harvard University Press, 1970.

Beck, Ann. *Medicine, Tradition, and Development in Kenya and Tanzania, 1920–1970.* Waltham, MA: African Studies Association, 1981.

Behrman, Greg. *The Invisible People: How the U.S. Has Slept Through the Global AIDS Pandemic, the Greatest Humanitarian Catastrophe of Our Time.* New York: Free Press, 2004.

Berger, Peter, and Thomas Luckmann. *The Social Construction of Reality: A Treatise in the Sociology of Knowledge.* New York: Penguin, 1966.

Berry, William T. C. *Before the Wind of Change.* Suffolk, UK: Halesworth Press, 1984.

Binagwaho, Agnes, Paul E. Farmer, Sabin Nsanzimana, et al. "Rwanda 20 Years on: Investing in Life." *Lancet* 384, no. 9940 (2014): 371–75.

Birungi, H. "Injections and Self-Help: Risk and Trust in Ugandan Health Care." *Social Science and Medicine* 47, no. 10 (1998): 1455–67.

Bledsoe, Caroline, and Monica Goubaud. "The Reinterpretation of Western Pharmaceuicals among the Mende of Sierra Leone." *Social Science and Medicine* 21, no. 3 (1985): 275–82.

Bloch, Marc. *The Historian's Craft: Reflections on the Nature and Uses of History and the Techniques and Methods of the Men Who Write It.* Translated by Peter Putnam. New York: Vintage, 1953.

Boeder, Robert. *Alfred Sharpe of Nyasaland, Builder of Empire.* Blantyre: Society of Malawi, 1981.

Bourdieu, Pierre. *Acts of Resistance: Against the Tyranny of the Market.* Translated by Richard Nice. New York: The New Press, 1998.

Brantley, Cynthia. *Feeding Families: African Realities and British Ideas of Nutrition and Development in Early Colonial Africa.* Portsmouth, NH: Heinemann, 2002.

Brett, Edward. *Colonialism and Underdevelopment in East Africa : The Politics of Economic Change, 1919–1939.* London: Heinemann, 1973.

Brietzke, Paul. "The Chilobwe Murders Trial." *African Studies Review* 17, no. 2 (1974): 361–79.

Brown, Barbara. "Facing the 'Black Peril': The Politics of Population Control in South Africa." *Journal of Southern African Studies* 13, no. 2 (1987): 256–73.

Bruchhausen, Walter. "Medical Pluralism as a Historical Phenomenon: A Regional and Multi-Level Approach to Health Care in German, British and Independent East Africa." In *Crossing Colonial Historiographies*, edited by Anne Digby, Waltraud Ernst, and Projit B. Mukharji, 99–113. Newcastle, UK: Cambridge Scholars Press, 2010.

Bryant, John. *Health and the Developing World.* Ithaca, NY: Cornell University Press, 1969.

Burdette, Marcia. *Zambia: Between Two Worlds.* London: Routledge, 1988.

Burgis, Tom. *The Looting Machine: Warlords, Oligarchs, Corporations, Smugglers, and the Theft of Africa's Wealth.* London: PublicAffairs, 2015.

Burnham, Gilbert M., George Pariyo, Edward Galiwango, et al. "Discontinuation of Cost Sharing in Uganda." *Bulletin of the World Health Organization* 82, no. 3 (2004): 187–95.

Busby, Joshua. "Bono Made Jesse Helms Cry: Jubilee 2000, Debt Relief, and Moral Action in International Politics." *International Studies Quarterly* 51, no. 2 (2007): 247–75.

Bush, George W. Interview with Matt Frei. *BBC World News America*, February 14, 2008.

Bush, George W. "President Bush Announces a Five-Year, $30 Billion HIV/AIDS Plan." Speech presented at the White House, May 30, 2007.

Cain, P. J., and A. G. Hopkins. *British Imperialism, 1688–2000.* 2nd ed. London: Longman, 2001.

Chakanza, J. C. "Provisional Annotated Chronological List of Witch-Finding Movements in Malawi, 1850–1980." *Journal of Religion in Africa* 15, no. 3 (1985): 227–43.

Chikakuda, W.J. "The Expanded Programme on Immunization in Malawi." *Malawi Epidemiological Quarterly* 2 (1983): 3–12.

Chilowa, Wycliffe. "Structural Adjustment Program in Malawi: Perspectives on Public and Private Sectors." In *Africa's Experience with Structural Adjustment: Proceedings of the Harare Seminar, May 23–24, 1994,* edited by Kapil Kapoor, 97–122. Washington, DC: The World Bank, 1995.

Chipembere, Henry B. M. *Hero of the Nation: Chipembere of Malawi; An Autobiography.* Blantyre: Christian Literature Association of Malawi, 2001.

Chipeta, Chinyamata. "Malawi." In *The Impact of Structural Adjustment on the Population of Africa: The Implications for Education, Health and Employment,* edited by Aderanti Adepoju, 105–18. London: James Currey, 1993.

Chirambo, Reuben. "'Mzimu Wa Soldier': Contemporary Popular Music and Politics in Malawi." In *A Democracy of Chameleons: Politics and Culture in the New Malawi,* edited by Harri Englund, 103–22. Stockholm, Sweden: Elanders Gotab, 2002.

Chirwa, Wiseman. "Dancing Towards Dictatorship: Political Songs and Popular Culture in Malawi." *Nordic Journal of African Studies* 10, no. 1 (2001): 1–27.

Chitsamba, L. S. "Malawi and the Politics of Foreign Aid." PhD diss., London School of Economics, 1990.

Chiume, Kanyama. *Kwacha: An Autobiography.* Nairobi, Kenya: East African Publishing House, 1975.

Christopherson, John B. "The UMCA and Medical Work at Magila." *Central Africa* 39 (1921): 86–91.

Cohen, Andrew. "'Voice and Vision'—The Federation of Rhodesia and Nyasaland's Public Relations Campaign in Britain: 1960–63." *Historia* 54, no. 2 (2009): 113–32.

Colbourn, Tim, Sonia Lewycka, Bejoy Nambiar, Iqbal Anwar, Ann Phoya, and Chisale Mhango. "Maternal Mortality in Malawi, 1977–2012." *BMJ Open* 3, no. 12 (2013): e004150.

Colby, Geoffrey. "Recent Developments in Nyasaland." *African Affairs* 55, no. 221 (1956): 273–82.

Colonial Development: A Factual Survey of the Origins and History of British Aid to Developing Territories. London: The Overseas Development Institute Ltd., 1964.

Connelly, Matthew. *Fatal Misconception: The Struggle to Control World Population.* Cambridge, MA: Harvard University Press, 2010.

Conroy, Anne. "Malawi and the Poverty Trap—A First Person Account." In *Poverty, AIDS and Hunger: Breaking the Poverty Trap in Malawi,* edited by Anne Conroy, Malcolm Blackie, Alan Whiteside et al., 118–37. New York: Palgrave Macmillan, 2006.

Constantine, Stephen. *The Making of British Colonial Development Policy, 1914–1940.* Totowa, NJ: F. Cass, 1984.

Cooper, Frederick. *Decolonization and African Society: The Labor Question in French and British Africa.* New York: Cambridge University Press, 1996.

Cooper, Frederick. *On the African Waterfront: Urban Disorder and Transformation of Work in Colonial Mombasa.* New Haven, CT: Yale University Press, 1987.

Coudenhove, Hans. *My African Neighbors: Man, Bird, and Beast in Nyasaland.* Boston: Little, Brown, and Company, 1925.

Cowen, Michael, and Robert Shenton. "The Origin and Course of Fabian Colonialism in Africa." *Journal of Historical Sociology* 4, no. 2 (1991): 143–74.

Creese, Andrew, Katherine Floyd, Anita Alban, et al. "Cost-Effectiveness of HIV/AIDS Interventions in Africa: A Systematic Review of the Evidence." *Lancet* 359, no. 9318 (2002): 1635–42.

Crosby, Cynthia Ann. "A History of the Nyasaland Railway, 1895–1935: A Study in Colonial Economic Development." PhD diss., Syracuse University, 1974.

Crozier, Anna. "The Colonial Medical Officer and Colonial Identity: Kenya, Uganda and Tanzania before World War Two." PhD diss., University College London, 2005.

Crozier, Anna. "Sensationalising Africa: British Medical Impressions of Sub-Saharan Africa 1890–1939." *Journal of Imperial and Commonwealth History* 35, no. 3 (2007): 393–415.

Curless, Gareth. "The Sudan Is 'Not Yet Ready for Trade Unions': The Railway Strikes of 1947–48." *Journal of Imperial and Commonwealth History* 41, no. 5 (2013): 804–22.

Currie, G. "A Clinical Trial of Etisul in Lepromatous Leprosy." *Transactions of the Royal Society of Tropical Medicine and Hygiene* 57 (1963): 196–205.

Curtin, Philip. "Medical Knowledge and Urban Planning in Tropical Africa." *American Historical Review* 90, no. 3 (1985): 594–613.

Davis, Lance, and Robert Huttenback. *Mammon and the Pursuit of Empire: The Political Economy of British Imperialism, 1860–1912.* Cambridge, UK: Cambridge University Press, 1986.

Davis, Mike. "Planet of Slums." Speech presented at Rhodes College, Memphis, TN, November 5, 2015.

de Villiers, S. "Tuberculosis in Anthropological Perspective." *South African Journal of Ethnology* 14, no. 3 (1991): 69–72.

de Winter, Eric. *Health Services of a District Hospital in Malawi.* Assen, Netherlands: Van Gorcum and Co., 1972.

Denman, Paul, and Paul McDonald. "Unemployment Statistics from 1881 to the Present Day." *Labour Market Trends* 104, no. 1 (1996): 5–18.

Denny, Colleen, and Ezekiel Emanuel. "US Health Aid Beyond PEPFAR: The Mother and Child Campaign." *Journal of the American Medical Association* 300, no. 17 (2008): 2048–51.

Digby, Anne. *Diversity and Division in Medicine: Health Care in South Africa from the 1800s.* Bern, Switzerland: Peter Lang, 2006.

Dilger, Hansjörg. "Targeting the Empowered Individual: Transnational Policymaking, the Global Economy of Aid, and the Limitations of Biopower in Tanzania." In *Medicine, Mobility, and Power in Global Africa: Transnational Health and Healing,* edited by Hansjörg Dilger, Abdoulaye Kane, and Stacey Langwick, 60–91. Bloomington: Indiana University Press, 2012.

Donnelly, John. "Emanuel on TB: 'The Challenge Is Enormous.'" *Science Speaks: Global ID News*, October 28, 2010.

Dory, Electra. *Leper Country: A Candid, at Times Shocking, Account of a Medical Missionary's Life among Primitive People in Africa*. London: Frederick Muller Ltd., 1963.

Doyle, Shane *Before HIV: Sexuality, Fertility and Mortality in East Africa, 1900–1980*. Oxford: Oxford University Press, 2013.

Drummond, Ian M. "More on British Colonial Aid Policy in the Nineteen-Thirties." *Canadian Journal of History* 6, no. 2 (1971): 189–95.

Duff, Hector L. *Nyasaland under the Foreign Office*. London: George Bell, 1906.

Easterly, William. "Human Rights are the Wrong Basis for Health Care." *Financial Times*, October 12, 2009.

Easterly, William. *The White Man's Burden: Why the West's Efforts to Aid the Rest Have Done So Much Ill and So Little Good*. New York: Penguin Books, 2006.

Eckart, Wolfgang U. "The Colony as Laboratory: German Sleeping Sickness Campaigns in German East Africa and in Togo, 1900–1914." *History and Philosophy of the Life Sciences* 24, no. 1 (2002): 69–89.

Elkins, Caroline. *Imperial Reckoning: The Untold Story of Britain's Gulag in Kenya*. New York: Holt, 2005.

Englund, Harri. "Extreme Poverty and Existential Obligations: Beyond Morality in the Anthropology of Africa?" *Social Analysis: The International Journal of Social and Cultural Practice* 52, no. 3 (2008): 33–50.

Fabian, Johannes. *Time and the Other: How Anthropology Makes Its Object*. New York: Columbia University Press, 1983.

Farley, John. *Bilharzia: A History of Imperial Tropical Medicine*. New York: Cambridge University Press, 1991.

Farmer, Paul. *AIDS and Accusation: Haiti and the Geography of Blame*. Berkeley: University of California Press, 1992.

Farmer, Paul. "An Anthropology of Structural Violence." *Current Anthropology* 45, no. 3 (2004): 305–25.

Farmer, Paul. "Global AIDS: New Challenges for Health and Human Rights." *Perspectives in Biology and Medicine* 48, no. 1 (2005): 10–16.

Farmer, Paul. Interview in *Bending the Arc*. Documentary. Directed by Pedro Kos and Kief Davidson, 2017.

Farmer, Paul. "Social Scientists and the New Tuberculosis." *Social Science and Medicine* 44, no. 3 (1997): 347–58.

Farmer, Paul. "Who Lives and Who Dies." *London Review of Books*, February 5, 2015.

Farmer, Paul, Matthew Basilico, and Luke Messac. "After McKeown: The Changing Roles of Biomedicine, Public Health and Economic Growth in Mortality Declines." In *Therapeutic Revolutions: Pharmaceuticals and Social Change in the Twentieth Century*, edited by Jeremy Greene, Flurin Condrau, and Elizabeth Watkins, 186–217. Chicago: University of Chicago Press, 2016.

Farmer, Paul, Cameron Nutt, Claire Wagner, et al. "Reduced Premature Mortality in Rwanda: Lessons from Success." *BMJ* 346, no. 18 (2013): f65.

Feierman, Steven. "Change in African Therapeutic Systems." *Social Science and Medicine* 13B (1979): 277–84.

Feierman, Steven. "Colonizers, Scholars and the Creation of Invisible Histories." In *Beyond the Cultural Turn: New Directions in the Study of Society and Culture*, edited by Lynn Hnt and Victoria Bonnelly, 182–215. Berkeley: University of California Press, 1999.

Feierman, Steven. *Peasant Intellectuals: Anthropology and History in Tanzania.* Madison: University of Wisconsin Press, 1990.

Feierman, Steven. "Struggles for Control: The Social Roots of Health and Healing in Modern Africa." *African Studies Review* 28, nos. 2/3 (1985): 73–147.

Fenner, Frank, Donald A. Henderson, Isao Arita, et al. *Smallpox and Its Eradication.* Geneva: World Health Organization,1989.

Ferguson, James. *Give a Man a Fish: Reflections on the New Politics of Distribution.* Durham, NC: Duke University Press, 2015.

Fields, Karen E. *Revival and Rebellion in Colonial Central Africa.* Portsmouth, NH: Heinemann, 1997.

Figueredo, D. H., and Frank Argote-Freyre. *A Brief History of the Caribbean.* New York: Infobase Publishing, 2008.

Floyd, Sian, Anna Molesworth, and Albert Dube. "Population-Level Reduction in Adult Mortality after Extension of Anti-Retroviral Therapy Provision into Rural Areas in Northern Malawi." *PLoS One* 5, no. 10 (2010): e13499.

Fortes, Meyer. *The Web of Kinship among the Tallensi.* London: Oxford University Press, 1949.

Fox, Wallace. "Realistic Chemotherapeutic Policies for Tuberculosis in Developing Countries." *BMJ* 1, no. 5376 (1964): 135–42.

Frankema, Ewout. "Colonial Taxation and Government Spending in British Africa, 1880–1940: Maximizing Revenue or Minimizing Effort?" *Explorations in Economic History* 48, no. 1 (2011): 136–49.

Freund, P. J. "Health Care in a Declining Economy: The Case of Zambia." *Social Science and Medicine* 23, no. 9 (1986): 875–88.

Frost, David. "The Economic Outlook for Nyasaland." *Race and Class* 4, no. 2 (1963): 59–72.

Frykberg, Eric. "Popliteal Vascular Injuries." *Surgical Clinics of North America* 82, no. 1 (2002): 67–89.

Gallagher, John. *The Decline, Revival and Fall of the British Empire: The Ford Lectures and Other Essays.* Edited by Anil Seal. London: Cambridge University Press, 1982.

Gann, Lewis H. "Lord Malvern (Sir Godfrey Huggins): A Reappraisal." *Journal of Modern African Studies* 23, no. 4 (1985): 723–28.

Gardner, Leigh. *Taxing Colonial Africa: The Political Economy of British Imperialism.* New York: Oxford University Press, 2012.

Gates, Bill. "Rich Countries' Aid Generosity: 2010 Annual Letter from Bill Gates." January 2010, http://www.gatesfoundation.org/annual-letter/2010/Pages/rich-countries-foreign-aid.aspx.

Gear, Harry S. "Medicine and the New Africa: The Passing of Colonialism South of the Sahara." *Lancet* 276, no. 7158 (1960): 1020–23.

Gear, Harry S. "Some Problems of the Medical Services of the Federation of Rhodesia and Nyasaland." *BMJ* 2, no. 5197 (1960): 525–31.

Gelfand, Michael. *Lakeside Pioneers: Socio-Medical Study of Nyasaland, 1875-1920.* Oxford: Basil Blackwell, 1964.

Gelfand, Michael. *A Service to the Sick: A History of the Health Services for Africans in Southern Rhodesia, 1890-1953.* Gwelo, Southern Rhodesia: Mambo Press, 1976.

Gewald, Jan-Bart. *Forged in the Great War: People, Transport and Labour: The Establishment of Colonial Rule in Zambia, 1890-1920.* Leiden: African Studies Centre, 2015.

Gilman, Lisa. *The Dance of Politics: Gender, Performance, and Democratization in Malawi.* Philadelphia: Temple University Press, 2009.

Gluckman, Max. *The Ideas in Barotseland Jurisprudence.* New Haven, CT: Yale University Press, 1965.

Good, Charles M. *The Steamer Parish: The Rise and Fall of Missionary Medicine on an African Frontier.* Chicago: University of Chicago Press, 2004.

Goodall, John. *Goodbye to Empire: A Doctor Remembers.* Edinburgh: Pentland Press, 1987.

Goodall, John. "Naming Ceremony of Queen Elizabeth Hospital, Blantyre." *Central African Journal of Medicine* 3, no. 8 (1957): 333–35.

GOtvMalawi, *Izeki ndi Jakobo Kusutsa galu mkukumba.* published September 8, 2014, YouTube video, https://www.youtube.com/watch?v=eHZ2of3vyNw.

GOtv Malawi, *Izeki ndi Jakobo: Matewera amwana,* published January 18, 2013, YouTube video, https://www.youtube.com/watch?v=CLkKVUPn6R8&t=9s

Graham, Franklin. Interview for *Frontline: Age of AIDS.* PBS, January 31, 2005. http://www.pbs.org/wgbh/pages/frontline/aids/interviews/graham.html.

Greene, Jeremy. "Colonial Medicine and Its Legacies." In *Reimagining Global Health: An Introduction,* edited by Paul Farmer, Jim Yong Kim, Arthur Kleinman, et al., 33–73. Berkeley: University of California Press, 2013.

Groves, Zoë. "Transnational Networks and Regional Solidarity: The Case of the Central African Federation, 1953–1963," *African Studies* 72, no. 2 (2013): 155–75.

Groves, Zoë. "Urban Migrants and Religious Networks: Malawians in Colonial Salisbury, 1920–1970," *Journal of Southern African Studies* 38, no. 3 (2012): 491–511.

Guthe, T. "Clinical, Serological and Epidemiological Features of Fambosia Tropica (Yaws) and Its Control in Rural Communities." *Acta Derm-Venereol* 49 (1969): 343–68.

Habermas, Jürgen. *The Structural Transformation of the Public Sphere: An Inquiry into a Category of Bourgeois Society.* Translated by Thomas Burger. Cambridge, MA: MIT Press, 1991.

Hailey, Malcolm. *An African Survey: A Study of Problems Arising in Africa South of the Sahara.* London: Oxford University Press, 1938.

Han, Song, and Casey B. Mulligan. "Inflation and the Size of Government." *Federal Reserve Bank of St. Louis Review* 90, no. 3 (2008): 245–68.

Harrigan, Jane. "Malawi." In *Aid and Power: The World Bank and Policy-Based Lending,* Volume 2, *Case Studies,* edited by Paul Mosley, Jane Harrigan, and John Toye, 201–69. London: Routledge, 1991.

Havinden, Michael, and David Meredith. *Colonialism and Development: Britain and Its Tropical Colonies, 1850–1960.* London: Routledge, 1996.

Hazlewood, Arthur, and Patrick D. Henderson. "Nyasaland: The Economics of Federation." *Bulletin of the Oxford University Institute of Statistics* 22, no. 1 (1960): 1–91.

Headrick, D. R. "Sleeping Sickness Epidemics and Colonial Responses in East and Central Africa, 1900–1940." *PLoS Neglected Tropical Diseases* 8, no. 4 (2014): e2772.

Helms, Jesse. *Here's Where I Stand: A Memoir.* New York: Random House, 2005.

Henderson, Ian. "East African Leadership: The Copperbelt Disturbances of 1935 and 1940." *Journal of Southern African Studies* 2, no. 1 (1975): 83–97.

Hinden, Rita. *Plan for Africa: A Report Prepared for the Colonial Bureau of the Fabian Society.* London: George Allen and Unwin Ltd., 1941.

Hodge, Joseph M. *Triumph of the Expert: Agrarian Doctrines of Development and the Legacies of British Colonialism.* Athens: Ohio University Press, 2007.

Hokkanen, Markku. "The Government Medical Service and British Missions in Colonial Malawi, c. 1891–1940: Crucial Collaboration, Hidden Conflicts." In *Beyond the State: The Colonial Medical Service in British Africa*, 39–63. Manchester, UK: Manchester University Press, 2016.

Hokkanen, Markku. *Medicine, Mobility and the Empire: Nyasaland Networks, 1859–1960*. Manchester, UK: Manchester University Press, 2017.

Hokkanen, Markku. *Medicine and Scottish Missionaries in the Northern Malawi Region 1875–1930: Quests for Health in a Colonial Society*. Lewiston, NY: Edwin Mellen Press, 2007.

Hokkanen, Markku. "Towards a Cultural History of Medicine(s) in Colonial Central Africa." In *Crossing Colonial Historiographies: Histories of Colonial and Indigenous Medicines in Transnational Perspective*, edited by Anne Digby, Waltraud Ernst, and Projit Mukharji, 143–64. Newcastle, UK: Cambridge Scholars Publishing, 2010.

Hopkins, A. G. *An Economic History of West Africa*. New York: Addison Wesley Longman, 1973.

House, William, and George Zimalirana. "Rapid Population Growth and Poverty Generation in Malawi." *Journal of Modern African Studies* 30, no. 1 (1992): 141–61.

Hubbard, James P. *The United States and the End of British Colonial Rule in Africa, 1941–1968*. Jefferson, NC: McFarland and Co., 2010.

Hubbard, Sally. "Nursing in Zomba, 1963–64." In *Expatriate Experience of Life and Work in Nyasaland*, Volume 3, edited by Colin Baker, 303–11. Cardiff, UK: Mpemba Books, 2014.

Huillery, Elise. "The Black Man's Burden—The Cost of Colonization of French West Africa." *Journal of Economic History* 74, no. 1 (2013): 1–38.

Hunt, Nancy Rose. *A Colonial Lexicon: Of Birth Ritual, Medicalization, and Mobility in the Congo*. Durham, NC: Duke University Press, 1999.

Hurst, Allan, H. M. Maier, and R. Dwork. "A Critical Study of Pneumoperitoneum and Phrenic Nerve Crush in Pulmonary Tuberculosis." *Diseases of the Chest* 13, no. 4 (1947): 345–59.

Iliffe, John. *The African AIDS Epidemic: A History*. Athens: Ohio University Press, 2005.

Iliffe, John. *The African Poor: A History*. New York: Cambridge University Press, 1987.

Iliffe, John. *Africans: The History of a Continent*. New York: Cambridge University Press, 2007.

Iliffe, John. *East African Doctors: A History of the Modern Profession*. New York: Cambridge University Press, 1998.

Iliffe, John. "A History of the Dockworkers of Dar Es Salaam." *Tanzania Notes and Records* 71 (1970): 119–48.

Iliffe, John. "The Poor in the Modern History of Malawi." In *Malawi: An Alternative Pattern of Development*. Edinburgh: Centre of African Studies, 1985, 243–93.

International Monetary Fund. *World Economic Outlook Database—April 2017*.

Jack, James William. *Daybreak in Livingstonia: The Story of the Livingstonia-Mission, British Central Africa*. London: Forgotten Books, 2012.

Jacobs, W. Richard. "The Politics of Protest in Trinidad: The Strikes and Disturbances of 1937." *Caribbean Studies* 17, nos. 1/2 (1977): 5–54.

Jahn, Andreas, Sian Floyd, and Amelia C. Crampin. "Population-Level Effect of HIV on Adult Mortality and Early Evidence of Reversal after Introduction of Antiretroviral Therapy in Malawi." *Lancet* 371, no. 9624 (2008): 1603–11.

Janzen, John M. *The Quest for Therapy in Lower Zaire*. Berkeley: University of California Press, 1978.

Jennings, Michael. "'Healing of Bodies, Salvation of Souls': Missionary Medicine in Colonial Tanganyika, 1870s–1939." *Journal of Religion in Africa* 38, no. 1 (2008): 27–56.

Jerven, Morton. *Poor Numbers: Why We Are Misled by African Development Statistics and What to Do About It*. Ithaca, NY: Cornell University Press, 2013.

Jones, Griffith Bevan. *Britain and Nyasaland*. London: Allen and Unwin, 1964.

Kagame, Paul. "Reflecting on Rwanda's Past—While Looking Ahead." *Wall Street Journal*, April 7, 2014.

Kalipeni, Ezekiel. "Structural Adjustment and the Health Care Crisis in Malawi." *Proteus* 21, no. 1 (2004): 23–30.

Kapur, Devesh, John P. Lewis, and Richard C. Webb. *The World Bank: Its First Half Century*. Washington, DC: Brookings Institution Press, 1997.

Keers, R. Y. "Pneumoperitoneum: Its Place in Treatment." *British Journal of Tuberculosis and Diseases of the Chest* 42, no. 3 (1948): 58–66.

Kelemen, Paul. "Planning for Africa: The British Labour Party's Colonial Development Policy, 1920–1964." *Journal of Agrarian Change* 7, no. 1 (2007): 76–98.

Kesner, Richard M. *Economic Control and Colonial Development: Crown Colony Financial Management in the Age of Joseph Chamberlain*. Westport, CT: Greenwood Press, 1981.

Khonje, Martha. "Corporate Tax Deals Are Robbing Poor Countries of Teachers and Nurses." *Guardian*, July 2, 2015.

King, Michael. "AIDS: Are We Really Serious?" *Malawi Medical Journal* 15, no. 2 (2003): 79.

King, Michael, and Elizabeth King. *The Story of Medicine and Disease in Malawi: The 150 Years Since Livingstone*. Blantyre, Malawi: Arco Books, 1992.

Klinker, Phillip A., and Rogers M. Smith. *The Unsteady March: The Rise and Decline of Racial Equality in America*. Chicago: University of Chicago Press, 1999.

Kober, Katharina, and Wilm van Damme. "Scaling up Access to Antiretroviral Treatment in Southern Africa: Who Will Do the Job?" *Lancet* 364, no. 9428 (2004): 103–7.

Kydd, Jonathan, and Robert Christiansen. "Structural Change in Malawi since Independence: Consequences of a Development Strategy Based on Large-Scale Agriculture." *World Development* 10, no. 5 (1982): 355–75.

Landau, Paul S. "Explaining Surgical Evangelism in Colonial Southern Africa: Teeth, Pain and Faith." *Journal of African History* 37, no. 2 (1996): 261–81.

Langwick, Stacey A. "Articulate(d) Bodies: Traditional Medicine in a Tanzanian Hospital." *American Ethnologist* 35, no. 3 (2008): 428–39.

Larmer, Miles. "Permanent Precarity: Capital and Labour in the Central African Copperbelt." *Labor History* 5, no.2 (2017): 170–84.

Le Fanu, James. *The Rise and Fall of Modern Medicine*. New York: Basic Books, 2002.

Leavitt, Judith Walzer. *Brought to Bed: Child-Bearing in America, 1750–1950*. New York: Oxford University Press, 1986.

Lepine, Aurelia, Mylene Lagarde, and Alexis Le Nestour. "Free Primary Care in Zambia: An Impact Evaluation Using a Pooled Synthetic Control Method." Health, Econometrics and Data Group Working Papers, University of York, September 2015.

Levy, Vicky. "Reply to 'AIDS: Are We Really Serious?'" *Malawi Medical Journal* 15, no. 2 (2003): 79.

Lewis, Roy. *10 Years of Colonial Development and Welfare, 1946–1955*. London: Central Office of Information, 1956.

Lewis, W. Arthur. *Development Planning: The Essentials of Economic Policy.* New York: Harper and Row, 1966.

Libamba, Edwin, Simon D. Makombe, Anthony D. Harries, et al. "Malawi's Contribution to '3 by 5': Achievements and Challenges." *Bulletin of the World Health Organization* 85, no. 2 (2007): 156–60.

Livingston, Julie. *Improvising Medicine: An African Oncology Ward in an Emerging Cancer Epidemic.* Durham, NC: Duke University Press, 2012.

Livingston, Julie, Keith Wailoo, and Barbara M. Cooper. "Vaccination as Governance: HPV Skepticism in the United States and Africa, and the North-South Divide." In *Three Shots at Prevention: The HPV Vaccine and the Politics of Medicine's Simple Solutions*, edited by Keith Wailoo, Julie Livingston, Steven Epstein, et al., 231–53. Baltimore, MD: Johns Hopkins University Press, 2010.

Livingstone, David. *David Livingstone's Shire Journal 1861–1864.* Edited by G. W. Clendennen. Aberdeen, UK: Scottish Cultural Press, 1993.

Livingstone, David. *Missionary Travels and Researches in South Africa.* London: John Murray, 1857.

Livingstone, James L. "Observations on the Treatment of Pulmonary Tuberculosis at the Present Time." *BMJ* 1, no. 4908 (1955): 243–50.

Livingstone, W. P. *Laws of Livingstonia: A Narrative of Missionary Adventure and Achievement.* Toronto: University of Toronto Libraries, 2011 (1921).

Lizza, Ryan. "The Obama Memos: The Making of a Post-Post-Partisan Presidency." *New Yorker*, January 30, 2012.

Lugard, Lord F. J. D. *The Dual Mandate in British Tropical Africa.* New York: Routledge, 2013.

Lwanda, John. *Colour, Class and Culture: A Preliminary Communication into the Creation of Doctors in Malawi.* Glasgow, UK: Dudu Nsomba, 2008.

Lwanda, John. "Hastings Kamuzu Banda." *British Medical Journal* 316, no. 7134 (1998): 868.

Lwanda, John. *Politics, Culture and Medicine in Malawi: Historical Continuities and Ruptures with Special Reference to HIV/AIDS.* Zomba, Malawi: Michigan State University Press, 2005.

Lyall Grant, R. W., A .M. D. Turnbull, J. C. Casson, et al. "Report of the Commission Appointed by His Excellency the Governor to Inquire into Various Matters and Questions Concerned with the Native Rising within the Nyasaland Protectorate, 14 January 1916." In *Voices from the Chilembwe Rising*, edited by John McCracken, 586–96. Oxford: Oxford University Press, 2015.

Lyons, Maryinez. *The Colonial Disease: A Social History of Sleeping Sickness in Northern Zaire, 1900–1940.* New York: Cambridge University Press, 1992.

Magrath, I., and J. Litvak. "Cancer in Developing Countries: Opportunity and Challenge." *Journal of the National Cancer Institute* 85, no. 11 (1993): 863.

Maier, D. "Nineteenth Century Asante Medical Practices." *Comparative Studies in Society and History* 21, no. 1 (1979): 63–81.

Mair, Lucy P. *Welfare in the British Colonies.* New York: Royal Institute of International Affairs, 1944.

Malik, Kenan. "The Great British Empire Debate." *New York Review of Books*, January 26, 2018.

Malloy, Patrick. "'Holding [Tanganyika] by the Sindano': Networks of Medicine in Colonial Tanganyika." PhD diss., University of California Los Angeles, 2003.

Malmsten, Neal R. "British Government Policy toward Colonial Development, 1919–1939." *Journal of Modern History* 49, no. 2 (1977): D1249–87.

Malunga, B. W. "Obituary: Professor J. D. Chiphangwi." *Malawi Medical Journal* 14, no. 2 (2002): 4.

Manchester, William, and Paul Reid. *The Last Lion: Winston Spencer Churchill: Defender of the Realm, 1940–1965.* Boston: Little, Brown, 2012.

Mandala, Elias C. *The End of Chidyerano: A History of Food and Everyday Life in Malawi, 1860–2004.* Portsmouth, NH: Heinemann, 2005.

Mandala, Elias C. "Feeding and Fleecing the Native: How the Nyasaland Transport System Distorted a New Food Market, 1890s–1920s." *Journal of Southern African Studies* 32, no. 3 (2006): 505–24.

Marks, Shula. "What Is Colonial about Colonial Medicine? And What Has Happened to Imperialism and Health?" *Society for the Social History of Medicine* 10, no. 2 (1997): 205–19.

Marseille, Elliott, Paul B. Hofmann, and James G. Kahn. "HIV Prevention before HAART in Sub-Saharan Africa." *Lancet* 359, no. 9320 (2002): 1851–56.

Marshall, T. H. *Citizenship and Social Class: And Other Essays.* Cambridge, UK: Cambridge University Press, 1950.

Masebo, Oswald. "Society, State and Infant Welfare: Negotiating Medical Interventions in Colonial Tanzania, 1920–1950." PhD diss., University of Minnesota, 2010.

Mata, J. I. "Integrating the Client's Perspective in Planning a Tuberculosis Education and Treatment Program in Honduras." *Medical Anthropology* 9, no. 1 (1985): 57–64.

Matchaya, G. C. "Trends in Life Expectancy and the Macroeconomy in Malawi." *Malawi Medical Journal* 19, no. 4 (2007): 154–58.

May, Alex. *The Commonwealth and International Affairs: The Roundtable Centennial Selection.* London: Routledge, 2010.

Mbali, Mandisa. *South African AIDS Activism and Global Health Politics.* London: Palgrave Macmillan, 2013.

McCombie, S. C. "Treatment Seeking for Malaria: A Review of Recent Research." *Social Science and Medicine* 43, no. 6 (1996): 933–45.

McCoy, David, Barbara McPake, and Victor Mwapasa. "The Double Burden of Human Resource and HIV Crises: A Case Study of Malawi." *Human Resources for Health* 6, no. 16 (2008): 6–16.

McCracken, John. "Bicycles in Colonial Malawi: A Short History." *Society of Malawi Journal* 64, no. 1 (2011): 1–12.

McCracken, John. "Coercion and Control in Nyasaland: Aspects of the History of a Colonial Police Force." *Journal of African History* 27, no. 1 (1986): 127–47.

McCracken, John. *A History of Malawi: 1859–1966.* Woodbridge, UK: James Currey, 2012.

McCracken, John. "In the Shadow of Mau Mau: Detainees and Detention Camps during Nyasaland's State of Emergency." In *Malawi in Crisis: The 1959/60 Nyasaland State of Emergency and its Legacy,* edited by Kings M. Phiri, John McCracken, and Wapulumuka O. Mulwafu, 165–91. Zomba, Malawi: Kachere, 2012.

McCulloch, Mary. *A Time to Remember: The Story of the Diocese of Nyasaland.* London: Charles Birchall and Sons, 1959.

McDermott, Walsh. "Medicine: The Public's Good and One's Own." *World Health Forum* 1 (1980): 128.

McPake, Barbara, Nouria Brikci, Giorgiao Cometto, et al. "Removing User Fees: Learning from International Experience to Support the Process." *Health Policy and Planning* 26, no. 1 (2011): S104–17.

Megill, Allan. *Historical Knowledge, Historical Error: A Contemporary Guide to Practice.* Chicago: University of Chicago Press, 2007.

Mehta, Lyla, ed. *The Limits to Scarcity: Contesting the Politics of Allocation.* London: Earthscan, 2010.

Menon, Roshi. *Famine in Malawi: Causes and Consequences.* New York: United Nations Development Programme, 2007.

Messac, Luke. "Malawi's Health Care Subject of Intense Worry for Country's Poor." *Pulitzer Center on Crisis Reporting,* August 2, 2013.

Messac, Luke. "Moral Hazards and Moral Economies: The Combustible Politics of Healthcare User Fees in Malawian History." *South African Historical Journal* 66, no. 2 (2014): 371–89.

Messac, Luke, and Krishna Prabhu. "Redefining the Possible: The Global AIDS Response." In *Reimagining Global Health: An Introduction,* edited by Paul Farmer, Jim Yong Kim, Arthur Kleinman, et al., 111–32. Berkeley: University of California Press, 2013.

Miers, Suzanne, and Igor Kopytoff. *Slavery in Africa: Historical and Anthropological Perspectives.* Madison: University of Wisconsin Press, 1979.

Milner, Viscount. *Questions of the Hour.* London: Hodder and Stoughton Ltd., 1923.

Minion, Mark. "The Fabian Colonial Society and Europe during the 1940s: The Search for a Socialist Foreign Policy." *European History Quarterly* 30, no. 2 (2000): 237–70.

Mitchell, Clyde. *The Yao Village: A Study in the Social Structure of a Nyasaland Tribe.* Manchester, UK: The Manchester Press, 1956.

Mkandawire, Austin C. *Living My Destiny: A Medical and Historical Narrative.* Limbe, Malawi: Popular Publications, 1998.

Molyneux, Malcolm. "A Medical Career in Malawi—Personal Reflections." *Malawi Medical Journal* 28, no. 3 (2016): 82–83.

Monbiot, George. "Deny the British Empires' Crimes? No, We Ignore Them." *Guardian,* April 23, 2012.

Morgan, David J. *The Official History of Colonial Development: The Origins of British Aid Policy, 1924–1945.* London: Humanities Press,1980.

Morgan, David J. *The Origins of British Aid Policy, 1924–1945.* London: Brill, 1980.

Morton, Kathryn. *Aid and Dependence: British Aid to Malawi.* London: Routledge, 2011.

Mosley, Paul. "Development Economics and the Underdevelopment of Sub-Saharan Africa." *Journal of International Development* 7, no. 5 (1995): 685–706.

Mossop, R. T. *History of Western Medicine in Zimbabwe.* Lewiston, NY: Edwin Mellen Press,1997.

Mota Engil Group. "Mota Engil Earnings Release 2014." Lisbon, Portugal: Mota Engil Group, 2015.

Mowschenson, Henry. "Dr. H Kamuzu Banda: President of the Republic of Malawi." *Central African Journal of Medicine* 12, no 8 (1966): 152–53.

Msolomba, Bridget, Lakdini Pathirana, B. Purcell, et al. "Vaccines or Latrines? Debating Spending on Health." *Malawi Medical Journal* 15, no.1 (2003): 18–19.

Mullenix, Philip, Scott Steele, and Charles Andersen. "Limb Salvage and Outcomes among Patients with Traumatic Popliteal Vascular Injury: An Analysis of the National Trauma Data Bank." *Journal of Vascular Surgery* 44, no. 1 (2006): 94–99.

Muluzi, Bakili. *Mau Anga: The Voice of a Democrat: Past, Present and Future.* Pretoria, South Africa: Skotaville Media, 2002.

Mulwafu, Wakisa, and Adamson Muula. *The First Medical School in Malawi: Including a Short Biography of Its architect, Professor John Chiphangwi.* Lilongwe, Malawi: Sunrise Publications, 2001.

Munthali, Alister C. "Determinants of Vaccination Coverage in Malawi: Evidence from the Demographic and Health Surveys." *Malawi Medical Journal* 19, no. 2 (2007): 79–82.

Munthali, Alister, Hasheem Mannan, Malcolm MacLachlan, et al. "Non-Use of Formal Health Services in Malawi: Perceptions from Non-Users." *Malawi Medical Journal* 26, no. 4 (2014): 126–32.

Murphy, Phillip. "A Police State? The Nyasaland Emergency and Colonial Intelligence." In *Malawi in Crisis: The 1959/60 Nyasaland State of Emergency and its Legacy*, edited by Kings M. Phiri, John McCracken, and Wapumuluka O. Mulwafu, 137–64. Zomba, Malawi: Kachere, 2012.

Mwale, Bizwick. "HIV/AIDS in Malawi." *Malawi Medical Journal* 14, no. 2 (2002): 2–3.

Mwase, George Simeon. *Strike a Blow and Die: A Narrative of Race Relations in Colonial Africa*. Cambridge, MA: Harvard University Press, 1967.

Ndikumana, L., and J. K. Boyce. *Africa's Odious Debts: How Foreign Loans and Capital Flight Bled a Continent*. London: Zed Books, 2011.

Ngoma, T. A. "World Health Organization Cancer Priorities in Developing Countries." *Annals of Oncology* 17, no. 8 (2006): S9–14.

Nthenda, L. J. L. "H.M. Treasury and the Nyasaland Administration, 1919–40." PhD diss., Oxford University, 1972.

O'Neil, Mary, Zina Jarah, and Leonard Nkosi. *Evaluation of Malawi's Emergency Human Resources Programme*. Cambridge, MA: Management Sciences for Health, 2010.

Packard, Randall M. *A History of Global Health: Interventions into the Lives of Other Peoples*. Baltimore, MD: Johns Hopkins University Press, 2016.

Packard, Randall M. "The Invention of the 'Tropical Worker': Medical Research and the Quest for Central African Labor on the South African Gold Mines, 1903–36." *Journal of African History* 34, no. 2 (1993): 271–92.

Packard, Randall M. *The Making of a Tropical Disease: A Short History of Malaria*. Baltimore, MD: Johns Hopkins University Press, 2011.

Packard, Randall M. *White Plague, Black Labor: Tuberculosis and the Political Economy of Health and Disease in South Africa*. Berkeley, University of California Press, 1989.

Page, Melvin E. *The Chiwaya War: Malawians in the First World War*. Boulder, CO: Westview Press, 2000.

Paice, Edward. *Tip and Run: The Untold Tragedy of the Great War in Africa*. London: Weidenfeld and Nicolson, 2007.

Parpart, J. L. *Labour and Capital in the African Copperbelt*. Philadelphia: Temple University Press, 1983.

Paul, Jim. "Medicine and Imperialism in Morocco." *Middle East Research and Information Project Reports* 60 (1977): 3–12.

Pearson, D. S., and W. L. Taylor. *Break-Up: Some Economic Consequences for the Rhodesias and Nyasaland*. Salisbury, Southern Rhodesia: The Phoenix Group, 1963.

Perkins, John. *Confessions of an Economic Hit Man*. New York: Plume, 2005.

Peters, Joel. *Israel and Africa: The Problematic Friendship*. London: I. B. Tauris, 1992.

Petryna, Adriana, and Arthur Kleinman, "The Pharmaceutical Nexus." In *Global Pharmaceuticals: Ethics, Markets, Practices*, edited by Adriana Petryna, Arthur Lakoff, and Arthur Kleinman, 1–32. Durham, NC: Duke University Press, 2006.

Phelps, Orme W. "Rise of the Labour Movement in Jamaica." *Social and Economic Studies* 9, no. 4 (1960): 417–68.

Phillips, Earl H. "HBM Chipembere, 1930–1975, Malawi Patriot." *Ufahamu: A Journal of African Studies* 7, no. 1 (1976): 5–18.

Phillips, Henry. *From Obscurity to Bright Dawn: How Nyasaland Became Malawi, an Insider's Account.* London: I. B. Tauris, 1998.

Phimister, Ian. "Proletarians in Paradise: The Historiography and Historical Sociology of White Miners on the Copperbelt." In *Living the End of Empire: Politics and Society in Late Colonial Zambia*, edited by J. B. Gewald, M. Hinfelaar, and G. Macola, 129–46. Leiden: Brill, 2011.

Phiri, D. D. *Dunduzu K. Chisiza: Malawi Congress Party Secretary-General, Parliamentary-Secretary, Brilliant Thinker, Pamphleteer and Essayist.* Blantyre, Malawi: Longman Ltd.,1974.

Phiri, D. D. *History of Malawi.* Blantyre: Christian Literature Association of Malawi, 2004.

Pirie, Gordon. "The Decivilizing Rails: Railways and Underdevelopment in Southern Africa." *Journal of Economic and Social Geography* 73, no. 4 (1982): 221–28.

Post, K. W. J. "The Politics of Protest in Jamaica, 1938: Some Problems of Analysis and Conceptualization." *Social and Economic Studies* 18, no. 4 (1969): 374–90.

Power, Joey. *Building Kwacha: Political Culture and Nationalism in Malawi.* Rochester, NY: University of Rochester Press, 2010.

Ranger, Terence O. "Godly Medicine: The Ambiguities of Medical Mission in Southeastern Tanzania, 1900–1945." In *The Social Basis of Health and Healing in Africa*, edited by Steven Feierman and John Janzen, 256–84. Berkeley: University of California Press, 1992.

Ravishankar, Nirmala, Paul Gubbins, Rebecca Cooley, et al. "Financing of Global Health: Tracking Development Assistance for Health from 1990 to 2007." *Lancet* 373, no. 9681 (June 2009): 2113–24.

Reader, John. *Africa: A Biography of the Continent.* New York: Vintage Press, 1999.

Rennick, Agnes. "Church and Medicine: The Role of Medical Missionaries in Malawi, 1875–1914." PhD diss., University of Stirling, 2003.

Roberts, Andrew. *A History of Zambia.* London: Oxford University Press, 1976.

Rockel, Stephen. "'A Nation of Porters': The Nyamwezi and the Labour Market in Nineteenth-Century Tanzania." *Journal of African History* 41, no. 2 (2000): 173–95.

Rodgers, Daniel. *Atlantic Crossings: Social Politics in a Progressive Age.* Cambridge, MA: Harvard University Press, 1998.

Rodney, Walter. *How Europe Underdeveloped Africa.* London: Bogle-L'Ouverture Publications, 1972.

Rorty, Richard. "Human Rights, Rationality, and Sentimentality." In *Truth and Progress: Philosophical Papers*, Volume 3, edited by Richard Rorty, 167–85. Cambridge, MA: Harvard University Press, 1998.

Ross, Andrew C. *Colonialism to Cabinet Crisis: A Political History of Malawi.* Zomba, Malawi: Kachere, 2009.

Rostow, Walt. *The Stages of Economic Growth: A Non-Communist Manifesto.* Cambridge, UK: Cambridge University Press, 1960.

Rotberg, Richard. Introduction to *Strike a Blow and Die: A Narrative of Race Relations in Colonial Africa*, by George Simeon Mwase. Cambridge, MA: Harvard University Press, 1967.

Rotberg, Richard. *The Rise of Nationalism in Central Africa: The Making of Malawi and Zambia, 1873–1964.* Cambridge, MA: Harvard University Press, 1965.

Russell, Ruth, and Jeannette Muther. *A History of the United Nations Charter: The Role of the United States, 1940–1945.* Washington, DC: Brookings Institution, 1958.

Schram, Ralph. *A History of the Nigerian Health Services.* Ibadan, Nigeria: Ibadan University Press, 1971.

Schrecker, Ted. "Interrogating Scarcity: How to Think About 'Resource-Scarce Settings.'" *Health Policy and Planning* 28 (2013): 400–409.

Scott, James C. *Two Cheers for Anarchism: Six Easy Pieces on Autonomy, Dignity, and Meaningful Work and Play.* Princeton, NJ: Princeton University Press, 2012.

Seekings, Jeremy. "'Pa's Pension': The Origins of Non-Contributory Old-Age Pensions in Late Colonial Barbados." *Journal of Imperial and Commonwealth History* 35, no. 4 (2007): 529–47.

Sen, Amartya. *Development as Freedom.* New York: Anchor, 2000.

Sen, Amartya. *Poverty and Famines: An Essay on Entitlement and Deprivation.* New York: Oxford University Press, 1983.

Shepperson, George, and Thomas Price. *Independent African: John Chilembwe and the Origins, Setting and Significance of the Nyasaland Native Rising of 1915.* Edinburgh: Edinburgh University Press, 1969.

Shircore, John Owen. "Yaws and Syphilis in Tropical Africa: Mass Treatment with Bismuth-Arsenic Compounds." *Lancet* 208, no. 5366 (1926): 43–44.

Short, Philip. *Banda.* Boston: Routledge and Kegan Paul, 1974.

Sindima, Harvey J. *Malawi's First Republic: An Economic and Political Analysis.* Lanham, MD: University Press of America, 2002.

Smith, Raymond, and Patricia Patricia Siplon. *Drugs into Bodies: Global AIDS Treatment Activism.* New York: Praeger, 2006.

Stevenson, David. "The Health Services of Malawi." MD thesis, University of Glasgow, 1964.

Strebhardt, Klaus, and Axel Ullrich. "Paul Ehrlich's Magic Bullet Concept: 100 Years of Progress." *Nature Reviews Cancer* 8 (2008): 473–80.

Swanson, Maynard W. "The Sanitation Syndrome: Bubonic Plague and Urban Native Policy in the Cape Colony, 1900–1909." *Journal of African History* 18, no. 3 (1977): 387–410.

Sword, J. Mowat. "Smallpox in Central Province, Nyasaland." *BMJ* 2, no. 5245 (1961): 165–66.

Tanzi, Vito, and Ludger Schuknecht. *Public Spending in the 20th Century: A Global Perspective.* Cambridge, UK: Cambridge University Press, 2000.

Tengatenga, James. *The UMCA in Malawi: A History of the Anglican Church 1861–2010.* Zomba, Malawi: Kachere, 2010.

Tharoor, Shashi. *Inglorious Empire: What the British Did to India.* London: Hurst Publishers, 2017.

Thomas, Simon. "Economic Developments in Malawi Since Independence." *Journal of Southern African Studies* 2, no. 1 (1975): 30–51.

Tilley, Helen. *Africa as a Living Laboratory: Empire, Development, and the Problem of Scientific Knowledge, 1870–1950.* Chicago: University of Chicago Press, 2011.

Titmuss, Richard. *Problems of Social Policy.* London: His Majesty's Stationary Office, 1950.

Turshen, Meredith. *The Political Economy of Disease in Tanzania.* New Brunswick, NJ: Rutgers University Press, 1984.

Ubel, Peter. "'Rationing' Health Care: Not All Definitions Are Created Equal." *Archives of Internal Medicine* 158 (1998): 209–14.

Vail, Leroy. "The Making of an Imperial Slum: Nyasaland and Its Railways, 1895–1935." *Journal of African History* 16, no. 1 (1975): 89–112.

Valentine, Catherine. "Settler Visions of Health: Health Care Provision in the Central African Federation, 1953–63." Master's thesis, Portland State University, 2017.

van der Geest, Sjaak, Anita Hardon, and Susan Reynolds Whyte. "Planning for Essential Drugs: Are We Missing the Cultural Dimension?" *Health Policy and Planning* 5, no. 2 (1990): 182–85.

van Etten, G. "Toward Research on Health Development in Tanzania." *Social Science and Medicine* 6, no. 3 (1972): 335–52.

van Waijenburg, Marlous. "Financing the African Colonial State: The Revenue Imperative and Forced Labor." *Journal of Economic History* 78, no. 1 (2018): 40–80.

Vansina, Jan. *Paths in the Rainforest: Toward a History of Political Tradition in Equatorial Africa*. Madison: University of Wisconsin Press, 1990.

Vaughan, Megan. *Curing Their Ills: Colonial Power and African Illness*. Redwood City, CA: Stanford University Press, 1991.

Vaughan, Megan. "Health and Hegemony: Representation of Disease and the Creation of the Colonial Subject in Nyasaland." In *Contesting Colonial Hegemony: State and Society in African and India*, edited by Dagmar Engels and Shula Marks, 173–201. London: British Academic Press, 1994.

Vaughan, Megan. "Maternal Mortality in Malawi: History and Moral Responsibility." In *Death, Belief and Politics in Central African History*, edited by Walima T. Kalusa and Megan Vaughan, 293–326. Lusaka, Zambia: Lembani Trust, 2013.

Vaughan, Megan. *The Story of an African Famine: Gender and Famine in Twentieth-Century Malawi*. New York: Cambridge University Press, 1987.

von Albertini, Rudolf. *Decolonization: The Administration and Future of the Colonies, 1919–1960*. New York: Holmes & Meier Publications, 1982.

Wakin, D. J. "AIDS Wildfire Ravages Southern Africa." *News Gazette* (Urbana-Champaign, IL), October 25, 1998, B-4.

Walton, David A., Paul E. Farmer, Wesler Lambert, et al. "Integrated HIV Prevention and Care Strengthens Primary Health Care: Lessons from Rural Haiti." *Journal of Public Health Policy* 25, no. 2 (2004): 137–58.

Watts, Michael. *Silent Violence: Food, Famine, and Peasantry in Northern Nigeria*. Berkeley: University of California Press, 1983.

Wendland, Claire L. *A Heart for the Work: Journeys through an African Medical School*. Chicago: University of Chicago Press, 2010.

White, Landeg. *Bridging the Zambesi: A Colonial Folly*. London: Macmillan, 1993.

White, Landeg. *Magomero: Portrait of an African Village*. London: Cambridge University Press, 1989.

Whyte, Susan Reynolds, Sjaak van der Geest, and Anita Hardon. *Social Lives of Medicines*. New York: Cambridge University Press, 2002.

Williamson, Philip. "Percy, Eustace Sutherland Campbell, Baron Percy of Newcastle (1887–1958), Politician and Educationist." In *Oxford Dictionary of National Biography* New York: Oxford University Press, 2004. https://www.oxforddnb.com/view/10.1093/ref:odnb/9780198614128.001.0001/odnb-9780198614128-e-35473

Williamson, Philip. "'Safety First': Baldwin, the Conservative Party, and the 1929 General Election." *Historical Journal* 25, no. 2 (1982): 385–409.

Williamson, Philip. *Stanley Baldwin: Conservative Leadership and National Values*. Cambridge, UK: Cambridge University Press, 1999.

Wood, J. R. T. *The Welensky Papers: A History of the Federation of Rhodesia and Nyasaland*. Durban, South Africa: Graham Publications, 1983.

Worboys, Michael. "Colonial Medicine." In *Companion to Medicine in the Twentieth Century*, edited by Roger Cooter and John V. Pickston, 67–80. London: Routledge, 2002.

Worboys, Michael. "Manson, Ross and Colonial Medical Policy: Tropical Medicine in London and Liverpool, 1899–1914." In *Disease, Medicine and Empire: Perspectives on Western Medicine and the Experience of European Expansion*, edited by Milton Lewis and Roy Macleod, 21–38. London: Routledge, 1988.

Wormell, Jeremy. "Blackett, Sir Basil Phillott (1882–1935), Civil Servant." In *Oxford Dictionary of National Biography*. New York: Oxford University Press, 2004.

Young, Cullen, and Hastings Kamuzu Banda. *Our African Way of Life*. London: Lutterworth Press, 1946.

Index

Figures are indicated by *f* following the page number

For the benefit of digital users, indexed terms that span two pages (e.g., 52–53) may, on occasion, appear on only one of those pages.